CANCER AND ELDERS OF COLOR:
OPPORTUNITIES FOR REDUCING HEALTH DISPARITIES

Cancer and Elders of Color: Opportunities for Reducing Health Disparities

Evidence Review and Recommendations for
Research and Policy

JOHN A. CAPITMAN
SARITA BHALOTRA
MATHILDA RUWE

ASHGATE

Published by
Ashgate Publishing Limited
Gower House
Croft Road
Aldershot
Hampshire GU11 3HR
England

Ashgate Publishing Company
Suite 420
101 Cherry Street
Burlington, VT 05401-4405
USA

Ashgate website: http://www.ashgate.com

British Library Cataloguing in Publication Data
Capitman, John A.
    Cancer and elders of color : opportunities for reducing
    health disparities
    1.Cancer - Age factors - United States 2.Cancer - Social
    aspects - United States 3.Cancer - United States -
    Prevention 4.Cancer - Treatment - United States
    5.Minorities - Medical care - United States
    I.Title II.Bhalotra, Sarita III.Ruwe, Mathilda
    362.1'98976994

Library of Congress Cataloging-in-Publication Data
Capitman, John A.
    Cancer and elders of color : opportunities for reducing health disparities
    : evidence review and recommendations for research and policy / by John A. Capitman ;
    co-authors, Sarita Bhalotra and Mathilda Ruwe.
        p. cm.
    Includes index.
    ISBN 0-7546-4212-7
    1. Cancer--Age factors. 2. Cancer--Social aspects. 3. Minorities--Medical care--
    United States. I. Title

    RC262.C298 2004
    362.196'994--dc22

                                                        2004020408

ISBN 0 7546 4212 7

Printed and bound in Great Britain by TJ International Ltd, Padstow, Cornwall

Contents

List of Tables

List of Figures

Acknowledgements

On a warm August day in 2001, we noticed an announcement about an opportunity to perform a study to determine what was known about racial and ethnic disparities in cancer prevention and treatment among elders in the United States. Our messages inquiring about the interest of the others in applying for this opportunity crossed in e-mails. The resulting collaboration amongst the three authors and many other colleagues gave rise to a study that was both intellectually and ideologically challenging. As we explored the potential approaches to performing this study, we realized that we needed to go beyond the traditional strategies of literature searches and syntheses.

We needed to reconcile the potential moral dilemma associated with abhorrence for healthcare inequities and inadequate healthcare access for elders in this rich nation with the push by policy elites and many in the public for overall reduction in national health expenditures. We have kept these competing agenda in mind and have sought to understand both the healthcare cost and human cost consequences of racial/ethnic cancer disparities and the broader opportunities for cost-effective healthcare system enhancements associated with potential solutions.

From our previous experiences, we recognized that much of the most innovative work on eliminating cancer disparities was occurring in community health providers and neighborhood organizations outside the purview of traditional research institutions. The evaluative research needed to bring the potential for replicating these innovations to national audiences was unlikely to reach the academic press in a timely manner. Our solution has been a 'both-and' approach. We conducted a thorough, rigorous and scholarly search of the literature and we used a snowball sampling approach to identify promising interventions that were then examined in detailed case studies. This two-pronged approach turned out to be worthwhile. We found much that was critical in understanding disparities from publications. And we also learned from our case studies and interviews about the complex, multi-factorial etiology of disparities and the culturally respectful, community participatory approaches evolving at the local level.

Much has been written about racial and ethnic disparities in health, even more has been written about cancer prevention and treatment, and far more has been written about the elderly and chronic illnesses. These literatures are complex and rich in technological and organizational wisdom, yet existing reports have not offered ways to integrate rapid improvements in cancer prevention and treatment with increasing awareness of the professional, organizational, and community contributions to eliminating racial/ethnic and related social class health inequity. We are pleased to present in this book, a framework for the analysis and synthesis of what is known about racial and ethnic disparities in cancer prevention and treatment among elders in the United States. Our findings point both to specific changes that Medicare may wish to explore in planned demonstrations and a new understanding of cancer control that draws on emerging culturally-tailored chronic disease management models.

We gratefully acknowledge the contributions of many to this book. Our project personnel at the Centers for Medicare and Medicaid Services (CMS) were remarkable in their support; without the leadership of Catherine Gordon, then Director of the Division of Prevention and Health Promotion at CMS, and her colleagues Diane Merriman, Chris Gibbons, John Hebb and Bertha Williams, this work would not have been possible. We were very fortunate to have as consultants to the project, a fine team of accomplished clinicians and researchers that included Drs. Sheila Chapman, Michelle David, Karen Freund, Marianne Prout, Nicole Prudent, Paul Schroy, (all at Boston University Medical Center) Michelle Holmes (Harvard University), and Thomas LaVeist (Johns Hopkins school of Medicine). Ms. Tracy Schneider at Boston University ably managed the coordination of work between Brandeis and BU.

A technical advisory group consisting of Elise Berryhill, PhD (Muscogee - Creek - Nation Behavioral Health Services), Marcella Blinka, MD (Johns Hopkins University), Harold Freeman, MD (NIH-NCI Center to Reduce Health Disparities) Richard Gram (Grace Hill Health Centers, St. Louis), Agnes Hinton (University of Mississippi), Marsha Lillie-Blanton, PhD (The Henry J. Kaiser Family Foundation), Selma Morris, RN (American Medical Team for Africa), Ana Navarro, PhD (University of California at San Diego), Alan R. Nelson, MD (American College of Physicians, American Society of Internal Medicine), Karen Rezai, PhD (Pacific Community Health Organizations, Susan Shinagawa, PhD (Intercultural Cancer Council) and John S. Yao, MD (Office of Public Health) provided valuable insights in their review of the final version of the report. Chris Gibbons, MD was an impressive chair of the national advisors group. He combined his considerable enthusiasm and seemingly encyclopedic knowledge of racial/ethnic cancer control issues with gracious attention to ensuring that all viewpoints of the causes and solutions to racial/ethnic disparities in Medicare utilization were considered.

Our home base for this work was the Schneider Institute for Health Policy, the Heller School for Social Policy and Management, Brandeis University. Vanessa Calderon-Rosado, PhD served as an able Project Manager, keeping the various tasks and members operating in an efficient and seamless manner. We are deeply indebted to our project team that included Aaron Beaston-Blaakman, Eric Cahow, Roberta Constantine, Almas Dossa, DiJon Fasoli, Deborah Gurewich, Brad Krevor, Walter Leutz, Melissa Morley, Susan Moscou, Laurie Nsiah-Jefferson, Leslie Oblak, Susan Pfefferle, Jeffrey Prottas, Mark Sciegaj, and Jose Suaya.

The twenty-six case study sites we visited provided us some of the most interesting and significant findings in our report, and we are grateful for the time and energy they spared for us. We hope that long-term benefit of your generous sharing about model project experiences will be the national replication of the racially aware, culturally responsive, and community directed cancer control and disparity elimination strategies you have developed. None of this work would have been possible without the dedicated assistance of Sylvia Pendleton, project librarian, who developed a coherent strategy for managing volumes of bibliographic data and herding a balky group of researchers into consistent patterns in searching, extracting, and summarizing the published literature. Without Ellen Alper who got the manuscript camera-ready, this publication would not have come into being. Alper approached this seemingly endless task with unflagging attention, turning our sometime murky text into clear communications. Lois McNally and Linda Purrini provided the administrative support that kept the project organized and moving forward.

Needless to say, we owe an immense debt of gratitude to our families, whose patience and moral support kept us going. To all who helped and contributed, we extend our deepest and heartfelt gratitude; this work is a product of your generosity, skills and knowledge. On the other hand, errors or omissions are our responsibility, and ours alone.

JAC
SMB
MBR

Chapter 1

Racial/Ethnic Cancer Disparities: A Medicare Policy Challenge

The Medicare, Medicaid, and SCHIP Benefits Improvement and Protection Act (BIPA) of 2000, Section 122, 'Cancer Prevention and Treatment Demonstrations for Ethnic and Racial Minorities' required that the Centers for Medicare and Medicaid Services (CMS) conduct demonstrations that explore how Medicare might reduce racial and ethnic (R/E) group disparities in cancer prevention, treatment, and outcomes. Nine demonstrations were called for including eight projects that address African Americans, Latinos, Asian Americans, and American Indian/Alaska Native beneficiary populations living in both urban and rural communities, and a project in Guam. The Schneider Institute for Health Policy at Brandeis University in collaboration with Boston University Center of Excellence in Women's Health (BUCEWH) and other consultants were contracted to conduct a comprehensive review of evidence that could guide the design of these demonstrations (Capitman, Bhalotra, Calderon-Rosado, et al., 2003). The project sought to identify concepts and models that have a high probability of reducing risk factors, increasing use of Medicare-covered services, and improving health and related outcomes for Medicare beneficiaries who are members of traditionally underserved R/E groups. To achieve these goals, the project team considered information derived from (1) systematic reviews of epidemiological and intervention research on race/ethnicity and cancer disparities in elders, and (2) case studies of emerging models and innovative programs targeting cancer control in traditionally under-served communities. Expert consultants and a national advisory panel reviewed drafts of the evidence report, and their suggestions and recommendations have been incorporated. Proposed interventions to reduce or eliminate R/E cancer disparities for Medicare beneficiaries were also explored with organizations representative of potential demonstration hosts.

In the following chapters, we present a conceptual framework method used for systematic reviews and case studies, findings on barriers to equitable care and potential solutions to R/E disparities in cancer prevention and treatment. In the final chapter, we develop recommendations for demonstration design and cost-effectiveness assessment, while also noting gaps in current knowledge that may be explored in other contexts. The recommended interventions have relevance to other initiatives to address R/E and correlated socio-economic disparities in health and healthcare. This chapter provides a context for the study and overview of our method and approach.

Cancer, Medicare, and Race/Ethnicity

In 2004, it is estimated that there will be 1,368,030 new cancer cases and 563,700 cancer-related deaths in the United States (Ries, Eisner, Kosary, et al., 2004). Cancer is a leading cause of death, accounting for 23% of all deaths in 2001. Among persons age 65 and older in 2001, cancer was the second leading cause of death, accounting for 390,214 deaths. Further, cancer is the leading cause of death for Americans between the ages of 60 and 79, and is the second leading cause of death for persons over the age of 80 (Freid, Prager, MacKay, et al., 2004). Of the approximately one half million persons dying from cancer each year, about 80% are over the age of 60 (Jemal, Thomas, Murray, et al., 2002). The risk of developing cancers increases significantly with age. From the ages of birth to 39, 1 in 64 American males and 1 in 51 females will develop cancer. From the ages of 60 to 79, 1 in 3 males and 1 in 4 females will develop cancer (ACS, 2001).

Given the cancer incidence among elders, the disease is expensive for the Medicare program although it has been difficult to develop broadly accepted estimates. Using linked Medicare and Surveillance Epidemiology and End Results (SEER) data for 1984-1990, Riley and colleagues (1995) found total costs of cancer care from diagnosis to death vary by clinical stage of the disease at diagnosis. As expressed in 1990 dollars, the average Medicare cost from diagnosis to death per case of lung cancer is $29,184; for female breast cancer, $50,448; for prostate cancer, $48,684; for colorectal cancer, $51,865 (Riley, Potosky, Lubitz, et al., 1995). Estimates of costs for specific diagnoses are complicated by ongoing methodological refinements (Brown, Riley, Potosky, et al., 1999; Etzioni, Riley, Ramsey, et al., 2002, Hogan, Lunney, Gabel, et al., 2001). The most difficult issues relate to attributing costs other than those for primary cancer diagnostic and treatments to cancer or other co-morbid conditions. Accounting for some of these challenges, Brown et al. (2002) report on annual prevalence costs for the 13 most common cancers for 1996. They estimate the total expenditures for persons aged 65 and over for these 13 cancers combined at $41 billion dollars. Average first year after diagnosis Medicare costs for the five most common cancers range from $8,869 for prostate cancer to $21,608 for colorectal cancer in 1996 (Brown et al., 2002). These estimates do not include all costs associated with cancer care, cancer screening, and co-morbid conditions, yet they provide a clear sense of the role of cancer in total Medicare expenditures.

The 2000 Census found 35 million persons age 65 and older, and indicated that this elder population had grown rapidly and become more diverse. Continued increases in the US population of elders of color are anticipated based on the growing diversity of younger cohorts. The current federal racial/ethnicity categories are white, African American (AA), Asian American, Native Hawaiian/Other Pacific Islander (NHOPI), and American Indian/Alaskan Native (AI/AN). Moreover, Hispanic/ Latinos are included as a separate category that cuts across racial groups. It is, however, difficult to accurately assess the population growth for elders of color between 1990 and 2000, because of R/E classification and other changes for the 2000 count. Among these were the placement of the 'Hispanic' question prior to the 'Race' question, splitting the Asian/Pacific Islander groups into Asian and NHOPI, and allowing respondents to select multiple racial categories. Despite the challenges in assessing the actual0 growth of elders of color in the US, demographic projections show, for example, that Latino elders will make up almost 20% of the elderly population by 2050 (Day, 1996).

The burden of cancer is not borne equally across this diverse land, although the patterns of disproportionate impact vary by cancer site. The 2003, National Healthcare Disparities Report (DHHS/AHRQ, 2003) repeatedly points to differences by R/E, age, gender, social class, residential location, and region in cancer prevalence and outcomes as indicators of unequal health and healthcare. For example, 9.1% of Black males between the ages of 60 and 79, as compared to 7.5% of white males will develop cancer.[1] From age 70 to 79, 15.3% of Blacks versus 13.9% of whites will develop cancer. For females the burden is reversed, with white females from 60-79 developing cancer at greater rates than AA females (Mariotto, Gigli, Capocaccia, et al., 2002). Although older Black females develop cancer at lower rates than their white counterparts, Black survival rates are significantly lower. Five-year relative survival rates for AA males are also lower. Five-year survival rates for white males, ages 65-74, are 66.7%, for AAs of the same age, 61.8%. Five-year survival rates for white females, aged 65-74 are 58.9%, versus 44.2% for AA women of the same age (NCI, 2002c).

Table 1.1 provides a broader view of racial/ethnic group differences in cancer-related mortality by summarizing Federal accumulations of state death records, on all deaths and death rates for the 6 cancers that are responsible for the greater share of all cancer mortality: lung, colorectal, breast (female), and prostate (male). The table shows a consistent pattern: AA men have the highest relative risk of dying from cancer; followed by white men, AA women, and white women. Men and women in Latino, AI/AN, and API groups have much lower rates of cancer. But lower cancer prevalence or mortality rates overall do not imply better cancer survival. Singh, Miller, Hankey, et al., (2003) show that even after accounting for area economic status, men or women or both in each of the traditionally underserved R/E groups have notably lower rates of 5-year survival. Further, a focus on the largest causes of death among AAs and whites may mask other R/E disparities. For example, stomach and liver cancer among Asian Americans, colorectal cancer among Alaskan Natives, and colon and cervical cancer among Hispanic and Vietnamese-American women are notably higher than in other groups (Haynes & Smedley, 1999). For Korean men, stomach cancer replaced prostate as the most frequently diagnosed cancer; and for Vietnamese men liver cancer replaced colorectal as one of the most frequently diagnosed cancers. Stomach cancer rates among Korean men (48.9 per 100,000) and liver cancer rates among Vietnamese men (41.8 per 100,000) were higher than those for any other

---

1 Throughout the text, a preference has been given to reporting racial/ethnic categories using the current Census groupings and definitions. When source documents, however, adopt different labels or categories, the language of the source document is used.

Table 1.1 Mortality rates by site and race/ethnicity, 1996-2000*

	White	African American	Asian American and Pacific Islander	American Indian and Alaska Native	Hispanic/ Latino
All Sites					
Male	249.5	356.2	154.8	172.3	176.7
Female	166.9	198.6	102.0	115.9	112.4
Breast (female)	27.2	35.9	12.5	14.9	17.9
Colorectal					
Male	25.3	34.6	15.8	18.5	18.4
Female	17.5	24.6	11.0	12.1	11.4
Lung					
Male	78.1	107.0	40.9	52.9	40.7
Female	41.5	40.0	19.1	26.2	15.1
Prostate	30.2	73.0	13.9	21.9	24.1
Stomach					
Male	6.1	14.0	12.5	7.0	9.9
Female	2.9	6.5	7.4	4.2	5.3
Cervix	2.7	5.9	2.9	2.9	3.7

* Per 100,000 age-adjusted to the 2000 US standard population. Hispanic/Latinos are not mutually exclusive from other racial/ethnic groups.

Source: Ries et al., (eds). *SEER Cancer Statistics Review, 1975-2001*, National Cancer Institute. Bethesda, MD, http://seer.cancer.gov/csr/1975_2001/, 2004.

racial or ethnic group (Parker, Davis, Wingo, et al., 1998). Cancer rates for Native Americans living in urban environments are increasing while white urbanites are experiencing a decline in prevalence (Forquera, 2001).

Nonetheless, cancer and R/E differences observed in death records and SEER data must be viewed with caution, since both sources may underestimate mortality for Latino, AI/AN, Asian, and NHOPI populations because of inaccurate or missing coding of R/E group (Blustein, 1994; Izquierdo & Schoenbach, 2000; Becker, Bettles, Lapidus, et al., 2002). Further, the SEER data may not be fully representative of the health care experiences of persons of color in the United States because it is based on selected service areas. For example, 69% of the Hispanic SEER program population lives in California, and Mexican-Americans account for the majority of the Hispanic population in that area. Current representation for SEER of AAs in rural areas is limited primarily to the 10 rural counties in Georgia. Although new SEER sites and upgraded state registries are starting to come on line, available data is still subject to prior concerns (Haynes and Smedley, 1999).

Reports on Cancer, Race/Ethnicity, and Preventive Care

R/E and correlated socio-economic healthcare and health outcome disparities have been identified as a policy and program challenge for US healthcare systems for many years. National health priorities, as expressed by Federal statements such as Healthy People 2000 and Health People 2010 National Health Promotion and Disease Prevention Objectives (Keppel, Pearcy, and Wagener, 2002), have highlighted the reduction of such disparities as a central goal. There is a tendency in the United States to view health as primarily a function of genes and personal choices and healthcare as a commodity subject to market forces. Nonetheless, a consensus seems to have emerged that the persistence of R/E disparities is both inconsistent with our national valuing of individual opportunity and indicative of important failings in the quality and continuity of health services. Federally sponsored and private assessments of healthcare policies and programs reflect this emerging consensus by focusing new attention on health disparities and potential Medicare initiatives. These reports established R/E cancer disparities as a critical policy challenge, while highlighting the central roles that Medicare and other health insurers can play in addressing health disparities.

The Unequal Burden of Cancer

This assessment of The National Cancer Institute (NCI) research and programs for ethnic minorities and the medically underserved (Haynes and Smedley, 2000) highlighted the broad differences by R/E and socio-economic groups in cancer prevalence, morbidity, survivorship, and quality of life. The report recommends a shift in research focus to socially defined ethnicity and its correlates rather than race as a biological construct and the need for new research on behavioral interventions to manage risks for cancer across R/E and socio-economic groups. Another major recommendation was for CMS to participate in clinical trials that address the additional diagnostic and therapeutic costs associated with prevention initiatives.

Voices of a Broken System: Real People, Real Problems

The report from the President's Cancer Panel (Freeman and Reuben, 2001) drew upon evidence reviews and testimony by diverse individuals around the country. The report concluded 'most people in America receive neither the most appropriate care when faced with a cancer diagnosis, nor adequate cancer prevention and detection services' (p.1). The findings point to several determinants of inadequate access to cancer control services for many, including system of care barriers such as fragmentation of providers and limitations on benefits, financial barriers even for those with Medicare, and lack of accessibility of care for rural residents. Among the recommendations of this report are: immediate medical coverage for uninsured persons upon a diagnosis of cancer to ensure that no person with disease goes untreated, insurance coverage for anti-cancer agents and supportive medications regardless of method of administration, and reimbursement for non-physician personnel to assist with cancer screening and case management.

Unequal Treatment: Confronting Racial and Ethnic Disparities in Health Care

The Institute of Medicine's Board on Health Sciences Policy (Smedley, Stith, and Nelson, 2002) reviewed literature and commissioned expert analyses to understand how racial and ethnic minorities receive lower quality health services even when insurance-status, income and other access-related factors are controlled. The report considers how clinical encounters and the contexts in which these encounters occur can result in less than standard care. The study emphasizes the roles of Medicare and Medicaid financing and administrative systems in increasing access barriers while decreasing practitioner incentives for appropriate care for persons who rely primarily on public insurance. The report calls for numerous changes at multiple levels to address this problem, including: equal-access to high-quality financing and delivery service systems that limit fragmentation, encourage stronger, more stable patient-practitioner relationships in publicly-funded programs, enhanced financial support for interpreter services, and reimbursement for community health workers.

Reducing Disparities in Health Outcomes: Effective and Promising Outpatient Interventions with Underserved Populations

As part of the CMS Quality Improvement Organizations' (QIO) efforts to improve care quality and address health disparities for Medicare beneficiaries, this compendium report (Center for Health Care Quality, 2002) highlights health promotion interventions that have the potential to reduce health disparities. Among the 33 published studies reviewed were 12 breast and cervical cancer control projects. Several features of potentially effective programs noted in this review were: being evidence-based, formative approach leading to socio-cultural relevance, grass roots outreach, community advisory boards and partnerships, community health workers, small group educational approaches, physician engagement, and avoidance of attrition. The report recommends that all quality improvement efforts aimed at underserved Medicare recipients build on the experiences of these programs.

In addition to the reports that establish R/E cancer disparities as a challenge for Medicare, several other recent initiatives highlight healthcare program factors that need to be considered in addressing this challenge. First, the CMS Healthy Aging project completed comprehensive meta-analyses of interventions to support smoking cessation, interventions to increase use of selected Medicare preventive services (including breast, cervical, and colon cancer screening), and health risk assessment. Though these assessments of the literature do not focus on elders from traditionally underserved R/E groups, they underscore the dearth of studies focused on special populations among elders. The preventive services report concludes that appropriate preventive service use can be stimulated by health care organizations making theory-based changes in staffing and clinical procedures that also encourage patient self-management through financial incentives and reminders. Second, the Institute on Medicine led a review of prevention strategies from the social and behavioral sciences (Smedley and Syme, 2000) while the Task Force on

Community Preventive Services (TFCPS) is conducting systematic review of community preventive services (Zaza, Aguero, Briss, et al., 2000; Carande-Kulis, Maciosek, Briss, et al., 2000). Both initiatives provide important perspectives on consensus assessments of the efficacy of specific preventive services and the characteristics of effective approaches.

Overview of Methods

The evidence report sought to provide a comprehensive assessment of what is known about the causes and potential solutions for R/E cancer care and outcome disparities among Medicare beneficiaries. The work was organized with a conceptual framework that is outlined in Chapter 2. Using this framework, we sought a systematic assessment of the state of the science with respect to elders from traditionally excluded R/E groups and cancer prevention, detection, diagnosis, treatment and aftercare. We sought to develop an understanding of what leads to unequal care and unequal outcomes using epidemiological, medical science, and health service research studies. This evidence review drew upon three methods: systematic literature reviews, analyses of National Health Interview Survey data, and a survey and case studies of emerging models for addressing cancer disparities among elders. Specific elements of our methods are described in greater detail, as relevant, throughout this volume.

Systematic Literature Reviews

The literature reviews were organized around five areas of potential cancer prevention (physical exercise, nutrition/weight loss, smoking, drinking and supplemental insurance/usual source of care), the cancer sites with the greatest impacts on mortality and morbidity of Medicare patients (lung, breast, cervical, colon, and prostate), and several less prevalent cancer sites associated with notable R/E disparities (stomach, oral, pancreas, and leukemia). For the behavioral risk factors, evidence was sought for R/E differences in elder and lifetime exposure, interventions to change behavior among R/E elders, interventions to change behavior among R/E adult populations, and interventions to change behavior in elder populations. In this context, behavior change interventions with elders of color that included quantitative measures of impact in a controlled design were highlighted. Because there were few appropriate studies, we examined prior reviews and original papers that offered hints on effective program components for elders of color based on research with other population groups. For the major and less prevalent anatomical cancer sites; evidence was sought for R/E differences in prevalence, incidence, severity of disease, established risk factors and survival; R/E differences in risk factors, consensus on screening, diagnostic and treatment approaches; R/E differences in use of screening, timely diagnosis; treatments, and interventions to reduce R/E differences in screening, timely diagnosis, treatment, and aftercare. Literature on quality of life and survivorship were reviewed when they could further elucidate central questions in R/E disparities in treatment access and outcomes.

For both prevention and cancer site reviews, literature was identified using multiple strategies, including: electronic data base searches in Medline, PsychLit, CancerLit, and Cochrane group reviews; backwards searching using Social Science Citations Index/Web of Science to identify studies that had cited relevant papers; manual review of bibliographies in relevant papers; search of selected government and private websites; search in NCI, AHRQ and other Federal cancer and related funded project data bases; recommendations of consultant experts on each topic; and reports identified by screening interview/case study participants. The study focused on identifying published studies and widely disseminated reports, but in several cases, unpublished reports cited in prior reviews were obtained. In all cases, after review of abstracts suggested relevance to the project, full text articles were obtained and reviewed. In those few cases where sufficient numbers and consistency of available studies could support quantitative syntheses, standardized effect sizes were computed and assessments of heterogeneity of effect and potential moderator variables were performed.

Analysis of 2000 National Health Interview Survey (NHIS)

Because we found lacunae in basic descriptive data on health-related behaviors among elders, an analysis of the un-weighted results of the National Center for Health Studies 2000 NHIS was performed. We examined relationships between R/E group membership, behavioral risk factors, and self-reported screening participation.

Case Studies of Emerging Models

It seemed likely that many potentially efficacious and effective interventions to reduce R/E disparities in cancer care and outcomes for Medicare beneficiaries are currently operational and not yet the subject of published reports. Further, published studies on many interventions do not provide sufficient operational and organizational detail to address demonstration design and implementation questions. For these reasons, the study drew on multiple sources to identify emerging models for increasing participation of elders of color in cancer prevention and screening activities and/or increasing their access to appropriate and timely diagnostic, treatment and aftercare services. Outreach to multiple sources, including: federal agencies and federally-sponsored programs, health payer/delivery systems organizations, R/E identity and professional organizations, conference proceedings, foundation initiated programs, cancer centers, and mass distribution of requests for referrals were used to identify these programs. Screening interviews were conducted with 115 programs. Based on these interviews, an intentional heterogeneous sample of 25 sites was selected for case studies. Case studies were tailored to each site and were conducted by two-person teams that included an expert in cost-effectiveness issues. The case studies generally addressed questions such as: program history and theory of intervention, organizational and financing issues, perceptions of sources of disparities, intervention design and operations, measurement of program costs and outcomes, and findings with regard to volume of services and impacts. Not all case study sites could provide data on all issues. Case study reports were developed and reviewed by site representatives.

In addition to the case studies, we conducted a series of interviews with Indian Health Service and other AI/AN population experts, and explored the intersections of Medicare fee-for-service programming with the financing and delivery of health care for these groups. We also received detailed feedback on our reviews and recommendations from a national expert panel and this report reflects their corrections and recommendations. Our recommendations for new Medicare services were also presented to 25 diverse healthcare provider organizations, such as community health centers, safety net hospitals, comprehensive cancer centers, and public health agencies, and their perspectives have been taken into account.

Overview

The results of our evidence reviews and recommendations for Medicare demonstrations to reduce or eliminate R/E cancer care and outcome disparities among elders in the United States are presented in the chapters that follow. In Chapter 3, we present a conceptual framework for the evidence reviews. The conceptual framework builds on current thinking from health researchers and social scientists about how historic and current patterns of socio-economic inequalities create and sustain the importance of socially defined R/E groups for health and healthcare. In the context of cancer, health and healthcare use have typically been understood from a public health perspective that recognizes cancer control as involving a sequence of interventions at the population and individual level. Our framework integrates this concept of cancer control with new understandings of how R/E and correlated factors influence health outcomes.

Using this framework, Chapters 3 and 4 address the identification and management of potentially individually modifiable risk factors. In Chapter 2, we show that there is substantial evidence for R/E group differences among elders in risk factors such as smoking, obesity, lack of exercise, supplemental insurance, and lack of a usual, consistent source of primary care. Further, we find strong evidence from epidemiological studies for the importance of behavioral risks in cancer etiology and severity but almost no experimental evidence that altering behaviors influences cancer rates or outcomes. Such studies, of course, would be very difficult to implement because of the long lead times for many cancers and other challenges. Nonetheless, because there is evidence that behavioral risks can also influence both co-morbid conditions and treatment outcomes, it seems likely that some R/E disparities in cancer and health can be alleviated by increasing engagement of elders of color in management of behavioral risks and other modifiable determinants of health. In Chapter 4, we examine evidence about the capacity to alter these behavioral risk factors for elders in traditionally underserved R/E groups. We found almost no examples of proven behavior change strategies for R/E elders and evidence for real difficulties in engaging such persons in behavior change. There is sufficient evidence from studies with general aged populations and non-elderly adults of color, however, to suggest that elders of color could be engaged in a broad array of effective behavior change activities. Features of successful behavior change programming are described.

Chapters 5-7 examine R/E disparities in care and outcomes for breast, cervical, colorectal, lung, and prostate cancers. Although we sought to extend our reviews to other cancers, we did not find a sufficiently well developed literature on R/E and correlated socio-economic disparities among elders to support such reviews. Since the breast and cervical cancer literatures are notably larger with respect to both group differences and potential interventions, a separate chapter is devoted to each of these cancers. Chapter 7 examines the remaining three sites. We find notable R/E group differences in cancer prevalence, mortality, and survival among elders. But there were notable differences across anatomical sites in these patterns: in some cases, lower prevalence of cancer among R/E minority groups was starkly contrasted with higher survival for white elders. In other cases, mortality differences by R/E group outpaced differences in prevalence. In this context, strong differences across cancers in consensual views of appropriate screening, diagnostic, and treatment services are highlighted. Also highlighted is the interplay between cancer detection and prevalence estimates across social groups.

The reviews found extensive evidence for each of the cancers for Medicare R/E differences in use of detection, treatment, and aftercare services. We show evidence for factors at the individual, practitioner, financing, and service organization levels as potential causes of these differences in service use, although the literature both lacks adequate attention to specific R/E groups and cancer sites and needs new theory to accommodate the interactions among multiple patient, practitioner, and provider organizational determinants of use. Evidence for culturally tailored interventions for Medicare beneficiaries with respect to service use for most cancers was largely unavailable, and efforts to facilitate efficient progress through the phases of cancer treatment subsequent to suspicious screening results were generally not found. Nonetheless, an impressive set of studies that explored the use of culturally tailored approaches to breast and cervical cancer education and screening adherence was identified. Meta-analysis indicated significant average impacts of these interventions but considerable heterogeneity across projects.

In Chapter 8 we present a qualitative analysis of the theories of change and implementation experiences of emerging interventions to reduce or eliminate R/E disparities in cancer and health. The 25 case study sites were selected from a national sampling of emerging models that have not been comprehensively evaluated. The case study sites are based in diverse organizational settings and, target a range of R/E groups and cancer prevention, detection, and treatment goals. The programs address R/E cancer disparities by focusing on health risk management, screening education, screening adherence, and treatment management. Although programs used a variety of mechanisms for cultural tailoring, the most striking finding from the case studies was the predominance of the use of community members as project staff and communal planning and delivery of project activities. Using community health workers/promotoras de salud as cultural and linguistic translators to help patients navigate the health system was the primary mechanism for cultural tailoring in most of the case study sites. The chapter indicates that while community health workers are now viewed as an essential strategy for engaging elders of color in appropriate cancer care, that there is a tremendous opportunity to shape new expectations for the roles played by these workers and increase their effectiveness in influencing service use. In addition, programs that incorporated a management information system and decision-making support seemed to be effective in ensuring that community members, once motivated, actually received the services they required. Our findings suggest that multi-component interventions hold the greatest promise for addressing the disconnection between communities and the health system that programs perceived as playing a key role in R/E disparities in cancer control.

In Chapter 9, we provide a synthesis of the findings from all of these sources. We propose that a chronic disease conceptualization of cancer control may be required to address R/E and correlated socio-economic disparities in cancer. This approach reflects the changing nature of cancer control: a strong focus on prevention and periodic screening, complex, multi-component detection and treatment processes, and extended aftercare requirements. While a chronic care module may be helpful for all elders, it is more important for traditionally underserved elders because they have increased risks for some cancers and potential co-morbid conditions, face more practical barriers to adherence to medical care recommendations, and have increased likelihood for prior and ongoing experiences of mistrust, disrespect or disconnection from health care. Our evidence review highlighted the need for new kinds of human linkages between communities of color and health systems, including personnel with strong ties to targeted communities and new communal approaches to program planning and implementation. Based on these findings, the chapter outlines three possible Medicare demonstration services: health risk management (HRM), screening adherence and detection facilitation (SADF), and treatment and aftercare facilitation (TAF). We conclude by noting major challenges in implementing and evaluating demonstrations of these new services. By exploring the opportunities to reduce R/E cancer care and outcome disparities with modest incremental changes in Medicare would provide an important model for addressing other fundamental challenges to health services in this country.

References

ACS (2001, 2001). *Cancer facts & figures*, [Website]. American Cancer Society. Available: http://www.cancer.org [2001, 1/2001].

Becker, T., Bettles, J., Lapidus, J. et al. (2002). Improving cancer incidence estimates for American Indians and Alaskan Natives in the Pacific Northwest. *American Journal of Public Health*, 92(9): 1469-1471.

Blustein, J. (1994). The reliability of racial classifications in hospital discharge abstract data. *American Journal of Public Health*, 1994(6): 1018-1021.

Brown, M., Riley, G., Potosky, A. et al. (1999). Obtaining long-term disease specific costs of care: application to Medicare enrollees diagnosed with colorectal cancer. *Medical Care*, 37: 1249-1259.

Brown, M., Riley, G., Schussler, N. et al. (2002). Estimating health care costs related to cancer treatment from SEER-Medicare data. *Medical Care*, 40(8) IV-104-IV-117.

Capitman, J., Bhalotra, S., Calderon-Rosado,V. et al. (2004). *Cancer Prevention and Treatment Demonstrations for Ethnic and Racial Minorities: Evidence Report*. US Centers for Medicare and Medicaid, Baltimore, MD. http://www.cms.hhs.gov healthy aging/cancerprev.pdf.

Carande-Kulis, V., Maciosek, M., Briss, P. et al. J. (2000). Methods for systematic reviews of economic evaluations for the Guide to Community Preventive Services. Task Force on Community Preventive Services. *American Journal of Preventive Medicine*, 18(1 Suppl): 75-91.

Center for Health Care Quality, and Disadvantaged Area Support QIO – DASPRO. (2002). *Reducing Disparities in Health Outcomes: Effective and Promising Outpatient Interventions with Underserved Populations*. Memphis TN: Center for Healthcare Quality.

Day, J. (1996). *Population Projections of the United States by Age, Sex, Race and Hispanic origin: 1995-2050*. (Vol. P-25 #1130). Washington, DC.

Department of Health and Human Services; Agency for Healthcare Research and Quality. (2003). *National Healthcare Disparities Report*. http://www.qualitytools.ahrq.gov/ disparitiesreport/downloadreport.aspx.

Freeman, H. and Reuben, S. (2001). *Voices of a Broken System: Real People, Real Problems*. Bethesda, MD: President's Cancer Panel, National Cancer Program, National Cancer Institute, U.S. National Institutes of Health.

Freid, V., Prager, K., MacKay, A. et al. (2003). *United States, 2003: Chartbook on Trends in Health of Americans*. Hyattsville Md. National Center for Health Statistics. Updated tables as of 2/2004: http://www.cdc.gov/nchs/products/pubs/pubd/hus/updatedtables.html.

Forquera, R. (2001). *Urban Indian Health*. Washington, DC: Henry J Kaiser Foundation.

Haynes, M. and Smedley, B. (1999). *The Unequal Burden of Cancer: An Assessment of NIH Research and Programs for Ethnic Minorities and the Medically Underserved*. Washington, DC: Institute of Medicine, National Academy Press.

Hogan, C., Lunney, J., Gabel, J. et al. (2001). Medicare beneficiaries' costs of care in the last year of life. *Health Affairs*, 20(4): 188-195.

Izquierdo, J. and Schoenbach, V. (2000). The potential limitations of data from population-based state cancer registries. *American Journal of Public Health*, 90(5): 695-698.

Jemal, A., Thomas, A., Murray, T. et al. (2002). Cancer Statistics, 2002. *CA*, 52(1): 23-48.

Keppel, K., Pearcy, J., Wagener, D. (2002). *Trends in Racial and Ethnic-Specific Rates for Health Status Indicators: United States 1990-1998*. National Center for Health Statistics, Department of Health and Human Services, Hyattsville, MD. DHHS Publication No. (PHS_ 2002-1237 2-0025).

Mariotto, A., Gigli, A., Capocaccia, R. et al. (2002). *SEER Cancer Statistics Review 1973-1999: Complete and Limited Duration Cancer Prevalence Estimates*. Bethesda. MD: National Cancer Institute.

Parker, S., Davis, K., Wingo, P. et al. (1998). Cancers statistics by race and ethnicity. *CA: A Cancer Journal for Clinicians*, 48(1): 31-48.

Ries, L., Eisner, M., Kosary, C. et al. (eds) (2001). *SEER Cancer Statistics Review, 1975-2001*, National Cancer Institute. Bethesda, MD, http://seer.cancer.gov/csr/1975_2001/, 2004.

Riley, G., Potosky, A., Lubitz, J. et al. (1995). Medicare payments from diagnosis to death for elderly cancer patients by stage at diagnosis. *Medical Care*, 33(8): 828-841.

Singh, G., Miller, B., Hankey, B. et al. (2003). *Area Socioeconomic Variations in U.S. Cancer Incidence, Mortality, Stage, Treatment, and Survival, 1975-1999*. NCI Cancer Surveillance Monograph Series, Number 4. Bethesda, MD: National Cancer Institute, 2003. NIH Publication No. 03-5417.

Smedley, B. and Syme, S. (2000). *Promoting Health: Intervention Strategies from Social and Behavioral Research.* Washington, DC: National Academy Press.

Smedley, B., Stith, A., Nelson, A. (2003). *Unequal Treatment: Confronting Racial and Ethnic Disparities in Health Care.* Washington, DC: National Academy Press.

Zaza, S., Aguero, L., Briss, P. et al. (2000). Data collection instrument and procedure for systematic reviews. *Guide to Community Preventive Services, American Journal of Preventive Medicine,* 18(1S): 44-47.

Chapter 2

Racial/Ethnic Cancer Disparities: Conceptual Frameworks

Given increasing evidence for racial/ethnic and socio-economic disparities in health in the United States, recent years have seen an unparalleled level of attention to understanding the reasons why elders of color among other groups face shortened lives and greater burdens of disease and disability. Many analysts have concluded that racial ethnic (R/E) and social class differences in health are the products of unequal opportunities closely linked with historic and current political, economic and cultural exclusion. Differential access to health care and unequal quality and continuity of this care are frequently cited as two major factors in health inequity. In order to provide a context and conceptual framework for our review of evidence around causes and solutions for cancer disparities, this chapter examines theories for explaining racial/ethnic differences in health outcomes, explores general accounts for health care disparities, and suggests how these perspectives can be integrated with current concepts in cancer control.

An Emerging Consensus on Race/Ethnicity and Health

There is considerable evidence for R/E differences in mortality and morbidity in the United States. The most recent mortality data is for 2001 and reported in updated tables by Freid, Prager, MacKay, et al. (2004). Comparing whites and African Americans (AAs) born in 2001, men could anticipate an additional 7 years of life, and women an additional 5 years. For those turning age 65 in 2001, both male and female whites could anticipate about two additional years compared to their AA counterparts. Further, the age adjusted mortality rate for whites was 55% of the African American rate. For American Indian/Alaska Natives (AI/AN) mortality rates were higher than for whites in all states where estimates could be made, except Colorado and Nevada. Compared to whites, overall age adjusted death rates for Hispanic/Latino, Asian American, Native Hawaiian and other Pacific Islander groups (NHOPI) were notably lower in 2001 but Freid et al. (2004) warn that these estimates must be viewed with extreme caution because of age adjustment, immigration effects, and racial classification procedures. Among the leading health indicators for which national targets have been established, such as perinatal mortality, infant mortality, tuberculosis, work-related injury or death, or living in a community with poor air quality, R/E disparities that favored whites over other groups were noted for all indicators. Disparities appeared to be increasing for many of these measures (Keppel, Pearcy, and Wagener, 2002). Cancer disparities contributed to these trends. Jemal, Tiwari, Murray, et al. (2004) present the most recent data from the National Cancer Institute (NCI) and find that AA men and women have 40% and 20% higher death rates from all cancers combined than do white men and women, respectively. Further, while death rates for other R/E groups are lower overall than for whites, these groups face higher mortality from stomach, liver, and cervical cancers and experience later stages at diagnoses and shorter survival periods than do whites.

Although Federal health data systems provide consistent evidence that persons of color have more health problems and lose more years of productive life to cancer and other leading causes of death and disability than do whites, these comparisons are subject to considerable controversy (Oppenheimer, 2001; Mays, Ponce, Washington, 2003; Kreiger, 2000; Kittles & Weiss, 2003.) The classifications of race/ethnicity used in national health reporting correspond to categories in the US Census. Census data are the source for population denominators for health indicators. Changes in the US Census 2000 questions about race and ethnicity allowed for persons to describe themselves with respect to multiple 'racial' categories and Hispanic/Latino' ethnicity. But several of these racial categories reference country of origin or pan-ethnic groups (Asian, American Indian/Alaska Native, Asian Indian) that have questionable shared historical or cultural features. These changes made comparisons to prior periods difficult and created inconsistencies between population estimates and data derived from health data systems such as NCI's Surveillance, Epidemiology and End Results (SEER). They also once again show how 'race' and 'ethnicity' are contested categories.

Racial categories have long been debated and their meanings in health and social science contexts are difficult to define because they develop meaning from a historically fluid process of social, economic and political domination by majority groups rather than fixed and intrinsic features of individuals (Lott, 1998; Kaufman and Cooper, 1999; Bonilla-Silva, 1996). The terms remain important to health and social research because of the historic legacies and ongoing consequences of these multifaceted processes of oppression (Young, 1990; Guinier and Torres, 2002). In epidemiological studies from 1996-2000, for example, over 77% of articles referred to 'race' or 'ethnicity,' but most failed to provide theoretical or operational definitions (Comstock, Castillo, & Linday, 2004). Noting such difficulties, the Institute of Medicine at one point recommended replacing the term 'race' with the term 'ethnicity' in health studies, but this does not offer a way out of these debates because ethnicity is at least as controversial a term that is derived from the same history of political, social and ideological conflict (Oppenheimer, 2001). In our presentations, the terms 'race/ethnicity' and 'racial/ethnic' are used to refer to groups defined by these historical and current social, economic, and political patterns of domination and subordination that may also share cultural features such as worldviews, preferred styles of communication, and health-related attitudes or beliefs associated with group experiences in a racialized society.

In considering R/E disparities in cancer, evidence for group differences in cancer incidence or prevalence has lead to a popular concept that genetic predispositions associated with racial/ethnic groups may be central to cancer etiology. Two sets of findings suggest that this understanding is probably incorrect. First, genetic research played a key role in the redefinition of R/E as a social rather than biological construct since the early 1970s by showing that social race categories are not associated with human genetic variation and that such variation is continuous, complexly structured, constantly changing, and highly variable within social race categories (Goodman, 2000; Kittles & Weiss, 2003). Nonetheless, persons within small, homogenous communities who share parentage and environments may also share disease-relevant genetic predispositions but genetic variability within socially defined R/E groups indicates that this is most likely for health conditions linked to a single gene or gene series (Brawley, 2003). Further, within the United States and other countries that have experienced historical immigration from multiple locales, internal migration, and high levels of inter-marriage, there have emerged complicated patterns of ethnogenetic layering. Layering has made the genetic features of individuals within socially defined R/E categories extremely diverse and variable across regions and communities (Jackson, 2000). Second, emerging understandings of carcinogenesis suggest that it is a multistage process associated with complex interactions among genes (Sarasin, 2003; Mucci, Wedren, Tamimi, et al., 2001), interactions between multiple genetic and environmental factors (Malats, 2001; Greaves, 2002), and associated with stochastic influences of environmental factors on gene expression (Jaenisch & Bird, 2003; Jakobisiak, Lasek, & Golab, 2003; Oyonogo, 2002). In other words, recent developments in genetic understandings of race/ethnicity and carcinogenesis indicate that socially defined R/E groups are unlikely to be sufficiently homogenous with respect to disease predispositions or biological responses to environmental exposures to support a primarily biological account of group differences in the prevalence or course of cancer.

A number of theorists have proposed alternative explanations for how socially defined R/E groups come to exhibit differences in the prevalence or course of cancer and other health conditions. Kreiger (2003) summarizes these accounts by identifying six pathways from historical and current patterns of R/E domination and subordination to worse health for members of traditionally excluded R/E groups in comparison to whites in more affluent communities: a) economic and social deprivation, b) toxic substances and hazardous conditions in physical environments, c) socially inflicted traumas (mental, physical, and sexual from verbal threats to violent acts), d) targeted marketing of commodities that can harm health such as junk foods and psychoactive substances (cigarettes, alcohol, and other licit and illicit drugs), e) inadequate or degrading medical care, and f) psychological or physical responses to experiences of discrimination. Implicit in this account is that potentially individually modifiable health-related behaviors (tobacco and alcohol use, physical activities, unhealthy diets etc.) that have received the most attention as the proximal determinants of poor health are taken on by individuals not through lack of will or moral failings but as products of macro-individual factors (Tesh, 1988). For elders of color in particular, both current and cumulative lifetime exposure to potentially individually modifiable risk behaviors and environmental risk factors not subject to individual modification may be important determinants of poor health outcomes (Kelley-Moore & Ferraro,

2004; Wong, Shapiro, Boscardin, et al., 2003; Kingston & Smith, 1997; Ferraro & Farmer, 1996). Other writers have emphasized that historical and current patterns of exclusion may be associated with reduced social capital expressed as less adequate systems of social support and neighborhood cohesion that in turn reduce the resources that individuals have to overcome the effects of socio-economic deprivation (Lochner, Kawachi, Brennan, et al., 2003; Sretzer & Woolcock, 2002). Further, in societies troubled by R/E conflict, there may be less investment at the community level in creating health promoting opportunities and providing health and social services (Kaufman and Cooper, 2000; Reidpath, 2003). For example, Freeman and Reuben (2001) found many who reported enormous distances and other barriers to accessing cancer-related health services. Inadequate community and provider resources for cancer prevention, detection, and treatment were frequently emphasized by informants from traditionally excluded communities nationwide.

Unequal Health Care and Racial/Ethnic Disparities

A series of high-profile reports in the United States have emphasized the roles of R/E differences in the accessibility and quality of care (DHHS/AHRQ 2003; Smedley, Smith & Nelson, 2002; Lillie-Blanton, Rushing, Ruiz, et al., 2002; Kressin & Petersen, 2001). These reports conclude that R/E minorities and other traditionally undervalued socio-economic groups face difficulties accessing the health care system because of absent or inadequate health insurance and other financial and non-financial barriers. The roles of public and private health insurance policies and markets have often been cited as major determinants of these access barriers (Stark, 1999; Stevens, 1996). For older people in particular who face mounting costs for uncovered services, the Medicare and Medicaid programs are insufficient to overcome financial barriers to care and thus create notable group differences in use of a range of covered services (Crystal, Johnson, Sambamoorthi, et al., 2000; Stewart, 2004; Christensen and Shinogle. 1997; Pezzin & Kasper, 2002; Potosky, Breen, Graubard, et al., 1998). But the recent reports bring together overwhelming evidence that even among persons with adequate insurance who are receiving health care services there are still R/E disparities in the quality and continuity of care. These inequalities in care are expressed as: reduced receipt of primary and preventive services, greater use of avoidable but costly emergency services and invasive procedures, and less use of advanced technologies in acute treatment and chronic disease management. Both the Institute of Medicine (IOM) and the National Healthcare Disparities Report conclude that these patterns of unequal care are among the primary determinants of racial/ethnic health disparities that may be influenced by public financing and regulatory policies (DHHS/AHRQ 2003; Smedley et al., 2002).

The IOM report offered a range of possible explanations for unequal care across R/E groups, citing factors as diverse as patient expectations and the incentives faced by provider organizations under current financing arrangements (Smedley et al., 2002). Most notably, the report hypothesized that the primary mechanism that might link social inequality to health care use is practitioners' unintended behavior. It highlighted a psychological process by which practitioners' lack of familiarity with negotiating R/E differences compound the uncertainties of medical encounters. In this context, practitioners rely too heavily on stereotypes or simply forget to address all issues. Some of the best evidence for the idea that unintentional practitioner bias emerges in the high-pressure context of medical encounters leads to unequal care comes from work by Van Ryn and colleagues (Van, Ryn & Burke, 2000; Van Ryn & Su, 2003) that found that practitioners carry negative views of AA and low SES patients and this leads to less time and fewer actions in these encounters. While these accounts begin to explain how well intended professionals may act in ways that sustain R/E inequalities, they lack attention to explaining how bias clouds practitioners' judgments in multicultural contexts. Batts (1998), Bobo (1999) and others have offered social psychological accounts of R/E prejudice that focus on interactions between cognitive and affective responses to differences. Even professionals cognitively committed to just health care have grown up in a racialized society and so typically have few positive alternative routines for negotiating R/E differences. They thus have learned negative affective responses (fear, anger, sadness) towards members of other groups that can interrupt decision-making because it does not conform to their thinking in these situations. This negative affect may be further stimulated by actions of elders from underserved R/E groups who based on prior experiences of discrimination, unintentionally communicate a sense of distrust or disconnection.

A related – and perhaps, less controversial – approach focuses more on respect for cultural differences than on the unintended consequences of unexplored biases by practitioners. Evidence is growing for diverse cultural health-related beliefs and preferences for how health services are delivered. For example, Blackhall, Murphy, Frank, et al. (1995) surveyed culturally diverse senior center participants in the Los Angeles and found that unlike AA and white elders, those of Mexican or Korean heritage preferred that their families be told first about cancer or other life-threatening conditions and given the option as to how to inform the patient. Since US healthcare professional training and medical privacy laws value individual autonomy and practitioners prefer to speak with only one person, their behavior may be unintentionally disrespectful. Similarly, Baker, Hayes, and Fortier (1998) found that Spanish speaking primary care patients who used trained professionals or family members as interpreters were less satisfied with the interpersonal aspects of care and less likely to follow-up on physician recommendations. Based on these and similar findings, many have called for training of practitioners in cultural competence and/or cultural humility in order to improve their capacities to communicate effectively with patients from other racial/ethnic groups (Tervalon and Murray-Garcia, 1998; Brach and Frazer, 2000; Betancourt, Green, Carrillo, et al., 2003). No published studies have established, however, the impacts of cultural competence training for practitioners in reducing R/E care disparities. Some analysts have suggested that in order for such training to achieve its long-term goals, there must also be organizational attention to creating practice and care environments that embrace multiculturalism, provide incentives for practitioners to devote time and effort to patients with heightened needs because of broader social influences, and hold practitioners accountable for providing evidence-based and coordinated care (Weech-Maldonado, 2002).

A Conceptual Framework for Racial/Ethnic Disparities and Cancer Control

Although these general frameworks offer important clues for understanding R/E disparities in health and health care, they do not offer a specific framework for organizing an assessment of current knowledge in cancer control or developing proposals for reducing cancer care and outcome disparities among older people. The National Cancer Institute (NCI) has promoted a public health framework for cancer control that focuses on conducting '... basic and applied research in the behavioral, social, and population sciences to create or enhance interventions that, independently or in combination with biomedical approaches, reduce cancer risk, incidence, morbidity and mortality, and improve quality of life ...'(NCI, 2004). Similarly, the Trans-Health and Human Services Cancer Health Disparities Progress Review Group conceptualized the challenges in racial/ethnic cancer disparities in terms of discovery, development, and delivery of interventions that might alleviate the unequal burden of cancer by focusing on prevention, detection, treatment and aftercare (Department of Health and Human Services, 2004). These reports reflect the consensus that cancer control involves primary, secondary, and tertiary disease prevention. From this perspective, cancer control efforts include: reducing cancer incidence and prevalence by managing known risk factors at the individual and population levels, engaging populations and individuals in efficacious cancer screening programs, targeting services to detect cancer through diagnostic procedures to individuals with suspicious screening findings and those who are at high risk for cancers where screening programs have not been developed, offering appropriate primary and secondary treatments to persons diagnosed with cancer, and carefully monitoring individuals to detect cancer relapse and address complications of treatment. It seems reasonable to hypothesize that in a racialized society, R/E disparities can be created, sustained or managed by public health and health care interventions at each stage in the cancer control process.

Because cancer control differs at least to some extent by cancer site, the potential exists that R/E disparities arise in different ways and at different points in the process across R/E groups and cancer sites. This means that rather than examining prior science and potential strategies globally across all cancer sites and groups, it is important to explore the evidence base for new strategies using a disease-specific approach. For example, in the case of breast cancer, disparities might arise in management of health risks, screening participation, timely and correct diagnoses, primary treatment planning and delivery, secondary treatment planning and delivery, and relapse monitoring. In the case of lung cancer, by comparison, screening is not currently recommended by consensus panels or performed widely and there has been less call for secondary treatments. This

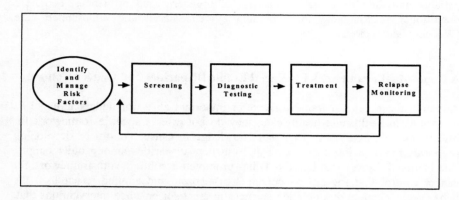

Figure 2.1 Sequential model of cancer control

difference in available treatment technology suggests the possibility of different strategies to reduce inequalities in treatment and outcome across these diseases.

Further, it is possible that different R/E groups among the US aged population experience barriers to appropriate care at different phases in the process. Because of these possibilities, we developed and refined sequential models for each cancer throughout the evidence review process. Figure 2.1 provides an example of a generic sequential model. Table 2.1 provides illustrative examples of the kinds of services or issues that might be associated with each step in the process for several cancer sites.

Table 2.1 Sequential model elements for four cancer sites*

	Lung	Breast	Prostate	Colon
Identify and Manage Risks	Smoking Cessation	Increase Exercise Genetic History	Weight Loss	Remove Polyps
Screening	No consensus	BSE/CBE Mammography	DRE PSA	Colonoscopy FOBT
Diagnosis	Chest X-ray Bronchoscopy Bronchial biopsy	Mammography Fine needle biopsy	Fine needle biopsy MRI	Colonscopy Angiography Biopsy
Primary and Secondary Treatments	Pulmonary resection Radiation Chemotherapy	Lumpectomy Auxillary node dissection Chemotherapy	Prostatectomy Radiation Chemotherapy	Segmental resection Radiation Chemotherapy
Monitor Relapse and Address Complications	Re-screening Radiology studies	Re-screening Hematoma	Re-screening Biopsy Incontinence	Colonoscopy Bowel Block Perforation

*Note: This table provides selected examples of elements considered in sequential models.

The sequential model of cancer control is generally more complex than indicated by the figure. It involves developing and applying knowledge aimed at populations, communities, and individuals to different extents at each phase. The work of developing and applying this knowledge occurs within diverse potential influences on cancer prevention, detection, and treatment disparities that need to be considered in reviewing evidence and exploring solutions. An emerging consensus notes that these potential determinants of health inequalities are inter-related and parts of larger social processes that extend well beyond health care (Mutaner, 1999):

- Individual and cultural factors: Cultural norms within R/E groups may lead individuals to adopt a range of health-related beliefs and behaviors that increase their risks of disease and reduce appropriate use of health services (Suarez, 1994; Thomas, Fox, Leake, et al., 1996). R/E groups also differ in education, income, wealth and other socioeconomic factors that influence how individuals participate in disease prevention and self-care activities as well as use of screening, treatment, and after-care services.
- Practitioner factors: Physicians and other health care practitioners may lack adequate cultural competence or face other barriers to addressing the care needs of R/E populations (Hannan, van Ryn, Burke, et al., 1999; Hawley, Earp, O'Malley, et al., 2000). Speaking in a second language or using interpreter services may limit their effectiveness (Kravitz, Helms, Azari, et al., 2000).
- Provider organizational factors: Health care provider organizations may not adopt care delivery and quality assurance systems that are responsive to R/E differences in health needs and use patterns. Providers serving low-income communities may lack adequate resources, operational systems, and inter-agency linkages to ensure continuity of care.
- System of care and financing factors: Some preventive and treatment services may not be covered, available, or accessible to R/E minorities (Potosky, Breen, Graubard, et al., 1998; Schoen, Lyons, Rowland, et al., 1997). Health care financing and quality assurance systems may not provide adequate information, incentives/sanctions, or reimbursement to promote targeting services to R/E minorities. Barriers to health care professional entry for R/E group members and lacunae in biological and medical care research may have limited the development of prevention/treatment options with optimal impacts on R/E group members.
- Community factors: The physical and social environments faced by R/E groups may include specific health risks (pollution, marketing of potential harmful products). Formal and informal organizations within these communities may lack resources or interest to support individual and institutional health promoting activities.

While these dimensions are useful in identifying potential determinants of health and health care disparities, they do not highlight where changes in Medicare and other health policy enhancements might most cost-effectively reduce racial/ethnic disparities in elder cancer and health outcomes and cancer-related service use. Figure 2.2 presents a conceptual model of cancer care and outcome disparities that seeks to distinguish components potentially influenced by Medicare and related health policies. The figure summarizes five key concepts that guided the evidence review and development of recommendations:

1) *Race/ethnicity is framed by social and contextual variables.* We described an emerging consensus that R/E categories are socially constructed and historically specific. These categories have come to be associated with patterns of health, social-psychological, economic and political inequalities created and maintained through culture, institutions, interpersonal behavior, and personal beliefs and attitudes. Bonilla-Silva labeled this process 'racialization.' Average life chances – the typical length and quality of life – have come to vary by R/E groups in our society. Cancer disparities are only one component of this process. Individual Medicare beneficiaries who are of African, Hispanic/Latino, American-Indian/Alaska Native, Asian, or Native Hawaiian and Other Pacific Islander (NHOPI) descent have already experienced full lives that have been at least partially shaped by their groups' experiences of inequalities. The multiple factors that create and sustain the social and health significance of R/E for individuals are also associated with community and system of care factors, such as the accessibility of health care and the appropriateness of health care resources to community needs. Health care policies may mediate the effects of these historical and current patterns of oppression on cancer, but a larger set of political, economic and cultural changes would be required to eliminate them entirely.

2) *Race/ethnicity and other social factors are linked.* The influences on cancer care or outcomes of R/E group membership and other indicators of social location such as gender, age, education, socio-economic status (SES), and rural residence are inextricably inter-connected for individual Medicare beneficiaries. Elders in most R/E minority groups are more likely than their white peers to have low education, low income and assets, and to live in medically under-served urban and rural communities (Haber & Mitchell, 1999/2000; Freid et al., 2003). Each of these other social location factors is also associated with gradients in cancer risks and outcomes (Singh, Miller, Hankey, et al., 2003). Medicare beneficiaries currently experience and have already experienced a lifetime of unique combinations of these influences (Capitman, 2002). Studies that use R/E without sorting out the relative influence of cultural and socio-economic or community social capital correlates of these categories need to be viewed with particular caution. Rather than debating the relative importance of R/E and other social and economic determinants of cancer control, we focus as often as possible given current studies on identifying how these factors together influence care targeting, processes and outcomes.

3) *Race/ethnicity and other social factors are associated with lifetime exposure to behavioral and contextual risk.* For Medicare beneficiaries, R/E group and other social factors at least in part determine both current and cumulative lifetime exposures to engaging in behaviors (poor diet, physical inactivity,

tobacco use, alcohol use, and inconsistent primary care use) that have been identified as potential risk factors for cancer. In the same way, groups defined by R/E and other social factors often share current and cumulative lifetime exposure to contextual features (environmental pollutants, neighborhood violence, occupational exposures, and food additives) that have also been identified as potential risk factors for cancer. Research is largely absent for most cancers on the relative influence of current exposures, exposures at particular developmental periods, and cumulative lifetime exposures on cancer risks and outcomes: since most research focuses on identifying the roles of current exposures. Diverse public health initiatives and other public policies may influence both of these sets of factors at the population level in the future. In the short run, individuals with the assistance of health services or through public health initiatives may be able to modify behaviors but not social and environmental contexts. Health services, nonetheless may assist individuals in identification of contextual risks to ensure heightened attention to their potential influence on cancer. It seems likely, however, that some effects of risk exposures on cancer prevalence and outcome patterns will continue to be observed, even as health care systems adopt a perspective of heightened responsibility for addressing cancer risks associated with R/E group or similar dimensions of oppression. Thus Figure 2.2 indicates that in our society, elders in traditionally underserved R/E groups may enter the health systems with heightened needs for attention to primary and secondary cancer control activities, but that these same risks may also negatively influence their health outcomes independent of cancer control initiatives in individual health care contexts.

4) *Cancer control services in health care settings also determine racial/ethnic outcome disparities.* There is mounting evidence that unequal provision of cancer-related health services in the Medicare fee-for-service context influences R/E cancer-specific and broader health outcome disparities (Shavers & Brown, 2002; Bach, Cramer, Warren, et al., 2002). In prior reviews, some studies were conducted in so-called 'equal access and equal treatment' settings such as the Veteran's Administration Medical Centers or in clinical trials with independent that feature coverage for treatments. In these settings, there were few racial/ethnic differences in care process or outcomes, and these could be attributed to poorly managed co-morbid health conditions. Other reviews have concluded that health care systems directly contribute to R/E disparities and that Medicare and related policies can thus influence relevant dimensions of health care practice associated with outcome disparities. In Figure 2.2, the shaded area in the center focuses attention on cancer control services in health care settings as a key feature in disparities and the most apt target for Medicare and related health care financing policies. Public health related initiatives, such as information dissemination and reduction in production or marketing of toxic commodities with more of a population focus than a focus on individuals or a known set of enrollees, clearly have a central role in mediating the influences of social inequalities on health. Nonetheless, Medicare and other health insurers may be most influential on the programs and practices of individually focused health providers. At the same time, it should be noted that disparities in care are

themselves created and sustained by multiple factors outside of Medicare influence, such as: availability of health care professionals who are members of R/E groups, cultural/racial attitudes and cultural competence of health care professionals, mal-distribution of health care resources, and accessibility of safety net social services. Nonetheless, we expected that at least some of the components of the cancer control process that were under the influence of Medicare and other payer initiatives could also be directed to racial/ethnic cancer disparities for older people.

5) *Health care disparities care arise in each phase of the cancer control process.* The health care system and health service delivery are complex and they offer multiple opportunities to increase or decrease the likelihood of appropriate service use and positive health outcomes. With respect to cancer, that health care delivery occurs in multiple phases from prevention through treatment creates multiple opportunities to understand and influence cancer outcome disparities. As indicated in Figure 2.2, Medicare and other health policies that finance and regulate individual health care provision can influence cancer disparities in several ways. Health care disparities may occur with respect to primary care participation where there are opportunities to manage behavioral health risks and to identify and begin to manage any potential consequences of cumulative lifetime exposures to potentially disease-inducing social and physical environments. Primary care providers can also provide individual information, motivation and adherence support for cancer screening and follow-up services. Individuals at heightened risks for cancers without established screening programs need to received appropriate referrals for detection services, as do persons with suspicious screening results. This whole set of activities is potentially linked to early diagnosis of cancer, but the health system plays key roles in treatment planning, delivery of complete primary, secondary and adjuvant treatments, and engaging cancer survivors in ongoing aftercare programs of relapse monitoring and responding to co-morbid conditions. The report started with the hypothesis that there is a potential to both increase equitable access to appropriate care across R/E groups and reduce health care disparities at each phase in the prevention-detection-treatment – follow-up process. As such, the project recognized the potential for variation across cancer sites and R/E groups as to the phases in the cancer process where interventions might make the most cost-effective impact.

Although not indicated in Figure 2.2, our approach to racial/ethnic cancer disparities and Medicare policies adopted a focus on fee-for-service Medicare. A sizable minority of Medicare beneficiaries are members of managed care plans, but most elders use fee-for-service Medicare. Because of the contractual relationships with Medicare+ Choice plans, different mechanisms would be required for altering service use and outcome patterns for elder R/E group members than in fee-for-service Medicare. CMS determined that a focus on the fee-for-service context would afford an opportunity to explore care continuity and quality assurance issues that may also need to be addressed in managed care settings in diverse community settings.

Summarizing the major themes that organized our approach to racial/ethnic cancer disparities among elders as displayed in Figure 2.2, we began from the perspective that broader historical, socio-economic and cultural factors both determine the complex and inter-related meanings of social location (race/ethnicity, gender, social class, region and community) and shape the resources and environments of cancer control. Individual social locations are associated with lifetime cumulative and current effects of multiple potentially individually modifiable health-related behaviors and risks associated with physical and social environments. These factors have independent influences on R/E health outcome disparities. These same differences in risk profiles also create heightened demands on cancer control programming in the context of health care settings. This programming can be viewed as the central target of public policies to reduce cancer care disparities and may also have profound impacts on cancer outcomes. Finally, the cancer control activities of individually oriented health services provider organizations needs to be viewed from a perspective that recognizes that disparities are most likely produced through complex interactions among multiple actors and forces in these settings.

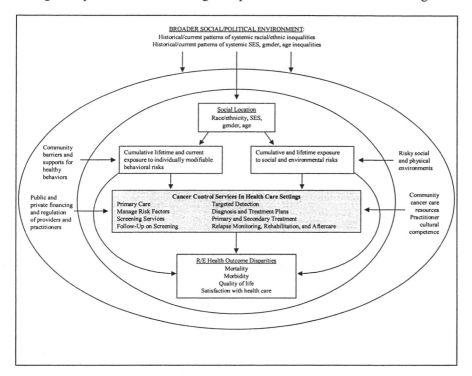

Figure 2.2 Conceptual model of cancer care and outcome disparities

Using the framework in Figure 2.2, the evidence reviews featured in this book were primarily focused on the shaded area in the figure: cancer control services in health care settings. One exception is our research on potentially modifiable individual health related behaviors and cancer risks. We found that much of the thinking and research about cancer disparities has been directed to the links between health-related behaviors such as maintaining a usual source of medical care and adopting health promoting behaviors, that it seemed important to review this literature to highlight to what extent cancer disparities are linked to behaviors and what can be done. Understanding the status of evidence for the influence of these factors on cancer also seemed essential for the design of primary care and other interventions to address and manage risk factors. While the evidence for the roles of individual health-related behaviors was more modest and contradictory than anticipated, there was much more epidemiological than behavior-change research available to assess, particularly as we turned attention to behavioral change interventions focused on elders of color. Moving beyond cancer prevention and primary care roles, the remaining chapters look primarily at initiatives around screening, detections, treatment, and aftercare for breast, cervical, colorectal, lung and prostate cancers because they have the most inclusive literatures. As shown in these chapters, the available research does not provide consistent coverage across cancer sites, R/E groups, or phases in the cancer control process. Even in Chapter 9, when we consider case studies of emerging programs, specific disease and population targets seem to be receiving variable research and demonstration attention that is not closely linked to the extent of documented disparities. Nonetheless, throughout our work, using this conceptual frame allowed a focus for the evidence reviews on issues most directly linked to how health care practitioners, and provider organizations create, sustain, and reduce or eliminate racial/ethnic disparities in cancer control and outcomes.

References

Bach, P., Cramer, L., Warren, J. et al. (1999). Racial differences in the treatment of early-stage lung cancer. *New England Journal of Medicine*, 341(16): 1198-1205.

Baker, D., Hayes, R., Fortier J. (1998). Interpreter use and satisfaction with interpersonal aspects of care for Spanish-speaking patients. *Medical Care*, 36(10): 1461-1470.

Batts, V. (1998). *Modern Racism: New Melody for the Same Old Tune.* Cambridge, Mass: Episcopal Divinity School, p. 16.

Betancourt, J., Green, A., Carrillo, J. et al. (2003). Defining cultural competence: a practical framework for addressing racial/ethnic disparities in health and health care. *Public Health Reports*, 118(4): 293-302

Blackhall, L., Murphy, S., Frank, G. et al. (1995). Ethnicity and attitudes toward patient autonomy. *Journal of the American Medical Association*, 274(10): 820-825.

Bobo, L. (1999). Prejudice as group position: Micro-foundations of relations. *Journal of Social Issues*, 55(3): 445-472.

Brawley, O. (2003). Population categorization and cancer statistics. *Cancer and Metastasis Reviews*, 22(1): 111-119.

Brach, C. and Fraser, I. (2000). Can cultural competency reduce racial and ethnic health disparities: a review and conceptual model. *Medical Care Research and Review*, 57(Sup.1): 181-217.

Capitman, J. (2002). Defining diversity: A primer and review. *Generations*, Fall: 8-15.

Christensen, S. and Shinogle, J. (1997). Effects of supplemental coverage on use of services by Medicare enrollees. *Health Care Financing Review*, 19(1): 5-17.

Coburn, D. (2000). Income inequality, social cohesion and the health status of populations: the role of neo-liberalism. *Social Science and Medicine*, (51): 135-146.

Comstock, R., Castillo, E. and Lindsay, S. (2004). Four-year review of the use of race and ethnicity in epidemiologic and public health research. *American Journal of Epidemiology*, 159(6): 611-619.

Crystal, S., Johnson, R. and Sambamoorthi, U. et al. (2000). Out-of-pocket health care costs among older Americans. *Journals of Gerontology Series: B Psychological Sciences Social Science*, 55(1): S51-62.

Department of Health and Human Services; Agency for Healthcare Research and Quality. (2003). National Healthcare Disparities Report. http://www.qualitytools.ahrq.gov/ disparitiesreport/downloadreport.aspx.

Department of Health and Human Services. (2004). *Making Cancer Health Disparities History: Report of the Trans-HHS Cancer Health Disparities Progress Review Group*, http://www.chdprg.omhrc.gov/pdf/chdprg.pdf.

Ferraro, K. and Farmer, M. (1996). Double jeopardy, aging as leveler, or persistent health inequity? A longitudinal analysis of white and black Americans. *Journal of Gerontology B: Psychological Sciences and Sociological Sciences*, 51(6): S19-328.

Freeman, H. and Reuben, S. (2001). *Voices of a Broken System: Real People, Real Problems*. Bethesda, MD: President's Cancer Panel, National Cancer Program, National Cancer Institute, U.S. National Institutes of Health.

Freid, V., Prager, K., MacKay, A. et al. (2003). *United States, 2003: Chartbook on Trends in health of Americans.* Hyattsville Md. National Center for Health Statistics. 2003. Updated tables as of 2/2004: http://www.cdc.gov/nchs/products/pubs/pubd/hus/updated tables.html.

Greaves, M. (2002). Cancer causation: the Darwinian downside of past success? *Lancet of Oncology*, 3(4): 244-251.

Goodman, A. 2000. Why genes don't count (for racial differences in health). *American Journal of Public Health*, 90(11): 1699-1702.

Haber, S. and Mitchell, J. (1999/2000). Access to physician's services for vulnerable Medicare beneficiaries, *Inquiry*, 36 (Winter): 445-460.

Hannan, E., van Ryn, M., Burke, J. et al. (1999). Access to coronary artery bypass surgery by race/ethnicity and gender among patients who are appropriate for surgery. *Medical Care*, 37(1): 68-77.

Hawley, S., Earp, J., O'Malley, M. et al. (2000). The role of physician recommendation in women's mammography use: is it a 2-stage process? *Medical Care*, 38(4): 392-403.

Jackson, F. (2000). Anthropological measurement: the mis-measure of African Americans. *Annals of the American Academy of Political and Social Sciences*, 568: 154-170

Jaenisch, R. and Bird, A. (2003). Epigenetics regulation of gene expression: How the genome integrates intrinsic and environmental signal. *Nature Genetics*, 33 (Sup.): 245-254.

Jakobisiak, M., Lasek, W. and Golab, J. (2003). Natural mechanisms protecting against cancer. *Immunology Letters*, 90(2-3): 103-122.

Jemal, A., Tiwari, R., Murray, T. et al. (2004). Cancer Statistics. (2004). *Cancer: A Cancer Journal for Clinicians*, 54(1): 8-29.

Kelley-Moore, J. and Ferraro, K. (2004). The Black/White disability gap: Persistent inequality in later life? *Journal of Gerontology: Social Science*, 598 (1): S34-S43.

Kittles, R. and Weiss, K. (2003). Race, ancestry, and genes: implications for defining disease risk. *Annual Review of Genomics and Human Genetics*, 4: 33-67.

Kingston, R. and Smith, J. (1997). Socioeconomic status and racial ethnic differences in functional status associated with chronic diseases. *American Journal of Public Health*, 87(5): 805-810.

Kravitz, R., Helms, L., Azari, R. et al. (2000). Comparing the use of physician time and health care resources among patients speaking English, Spanish, and Russian. *Medical Care*, 38(7): 728-738.

Kressin, N. and Petersen, L. (2001). The racial differences in the use of invasive cardiovascular procedures: Review of the literature and prescription for future research. *Annals of Internal Medicine*, 135(5): 352-366.

Lillie-Blanton, M., Rushing, O., Ruiz, S. et al. (2002). *Racial/Ethnic Differences in Cardiac Care: The Weight of the Evidence*. The Henry J Kaiser Foundation, Menlo Park. CA. http://www.kff.org/whythedifference/6040summary.pdf.

Lochner, K., Kawachi, I., Brennan R. et al. (2003). Social capital and neighborhood mortality in Chicago. *Social Science and Medicine*, 56: 1797-1805.

Mays, V., Ponce, N. and Washington, D. (2003). Classification of race and ethnicity: implications for public health. *Annual Review of Public Health*, 24: 83-110.

Malats, M. (2001). Gene-environment interactions in pancreatic cancer. *Pancreatology*, 1(5): 472-476.

Mucci, L., Wedren, S., Tamimi, R. et al. (2001). The role of gene-environment interaction in the etiology of human cancers: examples from cancers of the large bowel, lung, and breast. *Journal of Internal Medicine*, 249(6): 477-493.

Mutaner, C. (1999). Invited commentary: social mechanisms, race, and social epidemiology. *American Journal of Epidemiology*, 150(2): 121-126.

National Cancer Institute, (2004). Division of Cancer Control and Population Sciences: Overview and Highlights, http://cancercontrol.cancer.gov/bb/2004.pdf.

Oppenheimer, G. (2001). Paradigm lost: race, ethnicity, and the search for a new population taxonomy. *American Journal of Public Health*, 91(7): 1049-1055.

Oyongo, P. (2002). Genomics and oncology. *Current Opinion in Oncology*, 14(1): 79-85.

Pezzin, L. and Kasper, J. (2002). Medicaid enrollment among elderly Medicare beneficiaries: Individual determinants, effects of state policy, and impact on service use. *Health Services Research*, 37(4): 827-847.

Potosky, A., Breen, N., Graubard, B. et al. (1998). The association between health care coverage and the use of cancer screening tests. Results from the 1992 National Health Interview Survey. *Medical Care*, 36(3): 257-270.

Reidpath, D. (2003). Love thy neighbor – it's good for your health: A study of racial homogeneity, mortality and social cohesion in the United States. *Social Science and Medicine*, 57: 253-261.

Sarasin, A. (2003). An overview of the mechanisms of mutagenesis and carcinogenesis. *Mutation Research*, 544(2-3): 99-106.

Schoen, C., Lyons, B., Rowland, D. et al. (1997). Insurance matters for low-income adults: results from a five-state survey. *Health Affairs*, 16(5): 163-171.

Shavers, V. and Brown, M. (2002). Racial and ethnic disparities in the receipt of cancer treatment. *Journal of the National Cancer Institute*, 94(5): 334-357.

Singh, G., Miller, B., Hankey, B. et al. (2003). *Area Socioeconomic Variations in U.S. Cancer Incidence, Mortality, Stage, Treatment, and Survival, 1975-1999*. NCI Cancer Surveillance Monograph Series, Number 4. Bethesda, MD: National Cancer Institute, 2003. NIH Publication No. 03-5417.

Smedley, B., Stith, A. and Nelson, A. (2002). *Unequal Treatment: Confronting Racial and Ethnic Disparities in Health Care.* Washington, DC: Institute of Medicine, National Academy Press.

Sretzer, S. and Woolcock, M. (2002). Health by association: Social capital, social theory, and the political economy of public health. Von Hugel Institute Working Paper, WP2002-13.

Stark, F. (1999). History versus ideology: the Medicare reform debate. *Health Affairs*, 18(3): 265-267.

Stevens, R. (1996). Health care in the early 1960s. *Health Care Financing Review*, 18(2): 11-22.

Stewart, S. (2004). Do out-of-pocket health expenditures rise with age among older Americans? *The Gerontologist*, 44(1): 48-57.

Suarez, L. (1994). Pap smear and mammogram screening in Mexican-American women: the effects of acculturation. *American Journal of Public Health*, 84(5): 742-746.

Tervalon, M. and J. Murray-Garcia. (1998). Cultural humility versus cultural competence: a critical distinction in defining physician training outcomes in multicultural education. *Journal of Health Care for the Poor and Underserved*, 9(2): 117-125.

Tesh, S. (1988). Hidden Arguments. New Brunswick: Rutgers University Press.

Thomas, L., Fox, S., Leake, B. et al. (1996). The effects of health beliefs on screening mammography utilization among a diverse sample of older women. *Women's Health*, 24(3): 77-94.

Van Ryn, M. and Burke, J. (2000). The effect patient race and socio-economic status on physician's perceptions of patients. *Social Science and Medicine*, 50: 813-828.

Van Ryn, M. and Su, L. (2003). Paved with good intentions: do public health and human services providers contribute to racial/ethnic disparities in health? *American Journal of Public Health*, 93(2): 248-255.

Weech-Maldonado, R. (2002). Racial/ethnic diversity management and cultural competency: The case of Pennsylvania hospitals. *Journal of Healthcare Management*, 47(2): 111-126.

Wong, M., Shapiro, M., Boscardin, J. et al. (2002). Contribution of major diseases to disparities in mortality. *New England Journal of Medicine*, 347: 1585-159.

Chapter 3

Cancer Risk Factors and Racial/Ethnic Disparities

Public health experts have long proposed that modifiable risk factors such as smoking, diet, physical activity levels and excessive alcohol consumption are associated with increased risk of carcinogenesis and thus the incidence of cancer (McGinnis and Foege, 1993; Colditz and Gortmaker, 1995.) Increasingly, analyses of causal pathways for cancer have come to include an assessment of the potentiality of these modifiable risk factors and lack of a usual source of care. But the direct and interactive effects of environmental and behavioral factors with genetic or other biological factors in initiation, progression, and reversal of carcinogenesis are less clear for specific anatomical sites. If prevalence of potentially modifiable behavioral risk factors varies by racial/ethnic (R/E) group, then these differences may have an influence on cancer incidence rates. Thus, it is important to assess what is known about differentials in modifiable risk prevalence. This chapter also addresses the issue of the presence of risk factors that are not modifiable but signal need for heightened monitoring or diagnostic testing even if no screening exists or is performed. In this chapter we explore two related questions: (1) Among elders, do R/E groups differ in modifiable risk behaviors? (2) Are potentially individually modifiable behavioral risk factors associated with cancer for elders in traditionally underserved R/E groups?

To explore whether there are differences in the prevalence of behavioral risks across R/E groups, we conducted electronic searches of Medline and PsychInfo from 1985 to 2002, supplemented by citation search using Social Science Citation Index/Web of Science for selected papers. All searches used the following key words to locate studies of elders of color: minority elderly, elders of color, elders, minority, older adults, adults, African-American, Blacks, Hispanic, Latinos, American Indians/Native Americans, Pacific Islanders, and Asian American. We also conducted an analysis of the public use files of the 1999/2000 National Health Interview Survey (NHIS) and Cancer Control Supplement. The analysis selected only respondents age 65 or older and classified them by R/E groups – Hispanic of any racial group, African American or other African descent (AA), American Indian/Alaskan Native (AI/AN), Asian, Other. Both the Asian and Other categories were heterogeneous and included some persons of Native Hawaiian and Other Pacific Island (NHOPI) heritage, since the public use NHIS 1999/2000 data do not currently support use of the Census 2000 racial categories. Further, since the 'other' sample size was so small for elders, it was dropped from the analysis presented. With un-weighted data, we cross-tabulated R/E groups and selected modifiable risk behavior variables. Chapters 4-7 provide numerous examples of evidence for the argument recently posed by Bach, Cramer, Warren, et al., (2002) that differentials in cancer survival that cannot be attributed to access to care or quality/completeness of care, can be attributed to R/E differences in co-morbid conditions. Therefore, the focus in this review was on these potentially modifiable conditions.

Racial/Ethnic Differences in Major Behavioral Risks

Table 3.1 shows that risky behaviors appear to differ by R/E group. A caveat is that this reflects current behavior rather than cumulative lifetime exposure. It seems likely that the incidence of cancer is influenced by lifetime behavior, even if cancer progression and response to treatment are influenced by current behavior. No current methods or data to assess lifetime exposures have been identified, and thus current rates of smoking may not accurately reflect smoking-related risks for lung cancer. Furthermore, because the statistics relating to AI/AN are sparse, they should be interpreted with caution.

Physical Activity

AI/AN elders were least likely to report participation in moderate physical activity, and Asians were most likely. Men were somewhat more likely than women to be active in all groups. Across all R/E groups, notably small proportions of elders engaged in daily moderate exercise, the level that may be required for positive effect. These patterns are also reflected in other studies. For example, in a national survey of 2912 US women aged 40 and older from various racial/ethnic groups, over half the sample were currently in regular exercise, 25% in the pre-contemplative stage, and 15% in the contemplative stage (Seefeldt, Malina, and Clark, 2002). AA women were significantly less likely to be in the active stage even when age, BMI, education and smoking were controlled.

Obesity

Rates of being overweight were highest among AI/AN and AA, and lowest among Asians. Since weight and exercise are related, this may be a reflection of the increased rate of exercise among the latter, but it may also reflect dietary practices and genetic influences on metabolism. In all groups, but especially among Hispanic, AA, and AI/AN elders, women were more likely to be overweight than men. Similarly, according to information collected through the BRFSS in 1997, over one-quarter of AA, and AI/AN women were obese (Bolen, Rhodes, Powell-Griner, et al., 2000).

Table 3.1 Modifiable risk factors by race (NHIS 1999/2000, persons age 65 and over)

	White	AA	AI/AN	Asian	Hispanic	Total
Sample Size (N)	4807	696	16	71	573	6180
Gender (% Female)	62.68%	64.66%	56.25%	52.52%	59.34%	62.39%
Smoking	10.1%	12.6%	6.3%	7.0%	9.8%	10.3%
Moderate physical activity (1+/week)	46.7%	27.2%	6.3%	63.4%	33.2%	43.4%
>20% Overweight	32.4%	45.4%	56.3%	5.6%	34.6%	33.8%
Current Drinker	42.5%	22.3%	31.3%	28.2%	31.1%	39.0%
Source of sick care:						
• Clinic	10.6%	13.9%	18.8%	9.9%	18.3%	11.7%
• Doctor's office	82.7%	72.7%	68.8%	84.5%	69.8%	80.3%
Could not afford prescription drugs in last 12 months	3.7%	7.9%	6.3%	4.2%	5.6%	4.3%
Spoken to doctor in last 12 months	92.3%	90.8%	81.3%	94.4%	89.2%	91.9%

Tobacco Use

In NHIS as in other survey, AA elders reported the highest rate of tobacco use and Asian, AI/AN had the lowest rates. The pattern of smoking among younger AI/AN cohorts suggests that this pattern may be changing. Across all R/E groups, male elders are more likely to smoke than females, and this is especially true for the diverse Hispanic populations, where older men have among the highest smoking levels while older women have among the lowest.

R/E group differences in smoking may be more complex than indicated by the NHIS analysis. A growing literature indicates that among women, there are R/E, age, education or SES interactions in determining smoking patterns. For example, in one study (MacDowell, Guo, and Short, 2002) using the 1998 Ohio Family Health Survey, the authors assessed health behaviors and health of college educated and non-college educated African American and white women. The authors found that college educated AA women were less likely to have smoked over 100 cigarettes in their life time as compared with non-college educated AA women. However, among women who smoked over 100 cigarettes during their lifetime, current rates of smoking were higher among college educated than non-college educated AA women.

Alcohol Use

White elders in the NHIS were most likely to report being current drinkers, and AAs were least likely to be so. These results, however, may not adequately account for quantity and frequency of alcohol use or other life problems associated with drinking. For example, while AI/AN elders were less likely to be current drinkers than whites, personal accounts rendered by health care workers and noted in several of the case studies summarized in Chapter 4 suggest that the binge pattern of drinking engaged in by AI/ANs results in earlier mortality, with fewer active drinkers surviving to age 65 and beyond.

There is a growing literature describing low income and underserved R/E group elder drinking patterns in both institutional (Booth, Blow, Cook, et al., 1992) and community settings (Gomberg and Nelson, 1995; Bucholz, Sheline, and Helzer, 1995; Jackson, Williams, and Gomberg, 1998; Gomberg, 1999). All report R/E group differences in alcohol consumption (with non-white elders having higher prevalence rates of lifetime problem drinking and alcohol disorders) and corresponding adverse alcohol related health consequences. For example, in their review of epidemiological studies, Bucholz et al., (1995) note that in general AA elders were less likely to be drinkers than their white peers. However, the lifetime prevalence of alcohol dependence among AA male elders was much higher (21.6 %) than white male elders (12.5%). In a similar review, Jackson, et al., (1998) report AA male elders have much higher lifetime prevalence of alcohol disorders (24%) compared to white male elders (13%). In a small study (n= 169) examining the consequences of such lifetime abusive drinking patterns, Gomberg and Nelson (1995) report that AA male elders (69.6%) have significantly more self-reported alcohol-related health problems than their white peers (41.7%). In one of the few published studies to include Latino and Asian elders as comparison groups (Lubben, Weiler, and Chi, 1989), there do not appear to be significant differences between Latino elders and whites in either current or lifetime drinking patterns. However, Asian elders were less likely to have either a history of drinking or be current drinkers than either their AA, Latino or white peers (Lubben et al, 1989).

Usual Source of Care

Ease of access to primary care is a critical predictor of receiving preventive services, and minorities experience greater difficulties in accessing primary care, which results in differential rates of preventive screenings. AA, AI/AN and Hispanic elder NHIS respondents were most likely to report usually receiving health care at a clinic, while white and Asian elders were most likely to report usually receiving care at a doctor's office. These NHIS data point to a number of important, inter-related patterns in health care insurance coverage, access to care, and receipt of health promotion and cancer detection services. R/E minority elders are more likely to report delaying care because of cost, less likely to have private supplemental Medicare coverage, less likely to have a usual source of care, and as a result, are less likely to receive preventive treatments. For example, Dunlop, Manheim, Song, et al., (2002), examined the effect of economic access barriers on the 2-year utilization of 6,512 men and women for Hispanic, AA, and white ethnic/racial groups aged 70 or older using longitudinal data from the Asset and Health Dynamics Among the Oldest Old (AHEAD) survey. They found significant gender and R/E disparities in the use of physician, hospital, outpatient, home health, and nursing home care, with adjustment for economic access factors doing little to reduce these disparities, except for outpatient surgery differences. Compared with non-Hispanic white men and controlling for predisposing factors and measures of need, AA men had significantly fewer contact with physicians. In this same context, women of all R/E groups used fewer hospital or outpatient surgery services than men and men of color also used less outpatient surgery than white men.

Supplemental Coverage

One reason for the lower likelihood of having a physician's office as usual source of care for R/E minority elders and having higher rates of financial difficulties accessing care may be differences in supplemental insurance coverage. Using data from the 1996 Medicare Current Beneficiary Survey (MCBS), Pourat, Rice, Kominski, et al., (2000), report that R/E minority status consistently and significantly determine supplemental coverage. Although many cancer detection services are not subject to Medicare co-payments, having a supplemental policy may impact an individual's access to primary care and cancer diagnostic or treatment services. Medicare beneficiaries of AA, Latino, and Asian descent have much smaller odds of possessing any supplemental coverage compared to whites. Nine percent of whites have Medicaid as their only supplemental coverage as compared to 27% of AA, 16% of Latino, and 17 % of Asian elders. Pezzin and Kasper (2002) extend these analyses of the 1996 MCBS data, showing that less than 50% of very low income Medicare beneficiaries living in the community were enrolled in Medicaid, and that enrollment rates varied by as much as 18% between states with high and low investment in community care. Controlling for other factors, Latino elders were more likely to be dual enrolled than others. Across all groups, having Medicaid as a supplement to Medicare was associated with greater service use and expenditures for non-institutionalized elders. Another analysis of the 1996 MCBS by Janes, Blackman, Bolen, et al., (1999), also reveals that racial/ethnic minority elders are almost twice as likely to report cost as a factor in delaying care than whites.

Thus, in general, we found evidence of higher prevalence of major behavioral risk in under-served racial/ethnic elders. Next, we discuss whether there is evidence that links the higher prevalence of risk behaviors to specific anatomical cancer sites.

Racial/Ethnic Cancer Disparities and Modifiable Health Risks

In this section, we review the evidence for the roles of specific modifiable behavioral risk factors in breast, cervical, prostate, lung, colorectal, stomach, head/neck and pancreatic cancer incidence. We examine whether or not the epidemiological associations between specific behaviors and cancer incidence are sufficiently strong to justify Medicare reimbursement for behavior change interventions as one strategy to reduce R/E cancer disparities. Because much of the literature on behavioral factors and cancer has shied away from the aged population and because some current older adults under age 65 persons will join the Medicare rolls over the next few years, studies that include persons age 50 and older were considered in these reviews. With the exception of tobacco use studies, there is little available evidence focusing on cumulative exposures to these factors as distinct from the current behaviors of older people. Cumulative exposure presents conceptual difficulties, and there is uncertainty whether or not dose-response relationships between current behavior and incidence reflect threshold responses to current behavior or cumulative effects. This review is primarily focused on evidence for current behavior and cancer incidence, but notes evidence for cumulative effects when possible. In a similar vein, the bulk of the literature reviewed, points to the roles of behavioral risk factors for elders in general or specific R/E groups, and there is much less evidence for interactions between R/E group and specific behaviors in cancer incidence. Again with a few and somewhat speculative exceptions, there is little reason to believe that R/E group differences in cancer incidence by site reflect differential biological response to behavior rather than differences in behavior. Thus, we conclude that there are known modifiable risks for many cancers, arguing for enhanced monitoring and detection of high-risk, under-served groups. A major strategy for achieving this is to enhance access to primary care.

Table 3.2 provides a summary of the relationships of lifestyle factors and cancer incidence among elders. There is no risk factor that has not been definitively linked to at least one type of cancer. Of all risk factors, tobacco is overwhelmingly shown to be associated with the most types of cancers. This table cannot of course capture the synergistic action of several types of risky behavior acting in tandem.

Table 3.2 Summary of evidence for modifiable risk factors and type of cancer*

	Tobacco	Alcohol	Physical Exercise	Obesity	Diet
Breast	No	Mixed	Mixed	Mixed	Mixed
Cervix	Mixed	Mixed	No	No	Mixed
Prostate	Yes	No	Mixed	Yes	Mixed
Lung	Yes	No	No	No	Mixed
Colorectal	Mixed	No	Yes	Yes	Yes
Stomach	Yes	No	No	No	Yes
Head/Neck	Yes	Yes	No	No	Yes
Pancreas	Yes	No	Mixed	Yes	Mixed

* Based on prior research syntheses and this review, each potential risk factor is coded: 'Yes' if the bulk of evidence supports its association with cancers at the site; 'Mixed' if there is contradictory evidence, active debate, inconclusive evidence on the association with cancers at the site; and 'No' if the bulk of evidence indicates little or no association with cancers at the site.

Breast Cancer Risk Factors

Breast cancer is a major public health problem for all five R/E groups. Although the profile (the range) of known risk factors is the same for all women irrespective of R/E, incidence rates vary widely by R/E group. For example, for the period between 1992-1998, the reported incidence rates for breast cancer were highest for white women and lowest for Asians/Pacific Islanders (API): 115.5 for white women, 101.5 for AA women, 78 for Hispanic women, 68.5 AI/AN women, and 50.5 API women. Risk estimates based on these incidence rates vary similarly by age and R/E. For example, Morris, Wright, and Schlag (2001), used life tables and 1973-1997 incidence rates from the California Cancer registry to obtain risk estimates by R/E, for women currently aged 50 and over. They found 10-year risk estimates to be 2.9% (1 in 34) for white women, 2.3% (1 in 43) for AA women, 2.0% (1 in 51) for API women, 1.6% (1 in 63) for Hispanic women. Five-year risk estimates varied similarly ranged from 1.3% (1 in 75) among white and 0.8% (1 in 133) among Hispanic women (Morris et al., 2001). This wide variation in incidence or 10 year risks can be explained partly by differences in access to screening and partly by differences in exposure to lifestyle and environment risk factors. The risk is higher among older women, women who have a personal or family history of breast cancer (including breast cancer genes), biopsy-confirmed atypical hyperplasia, a long menstrual history (early menarche and late menopause), obesity after menopause, and recent use of oral contraceptives or post-menopausal estrogens and progestins, (hormone replacement therapy). It is also higher among women who have never had children or had their first child after age 30, who consume alcoholic beverages (ACS, cancer facts and figures, 2001), and who have higher breast density. R/E variation in breast cancer rates does not appear to arise from differential impact of these risk factors, but rather to differences in length of exposure and prevalence of these risk factors (Pathak, Osuch, and He, 2000; McTiernan, 2000; Hahn, Teutsch, Franks, et al., 1998). The variation in risk estimates by R/E despite similar risk factor profiles suggests that there are potentially modifiable risk factors. Thus both modifiable and non-modifiable factors have been shown to be associated with breast cancer, and it is difficult to determine exactly how the interaction of race/ethnicity precipitates cancer. Thus, in the following section, we discuss only the evidence for the role of three modifiable risk factors.

This section discusses the evidence regarding the association between breast cancer and three potentially modifiable risk factors among older adults – 1) *hormone replacement therapy* (HRT); 2) *nutrition/obesity*, diet low in fruits and vegetables, high fat diet, and high meat diet, 3) *health behavior* – alcohol consumption, tobacco, lack of physical activity. Genetic factors and environmental factors are excluded from this review because biological risk factors and genetic factors are currently not modifiable and except for radiation little is known about the role of environmental factors such as polycyclic hydrocarbons in the risk for breast cancer. Questions addressed in this section include: 1) Is there a significant association between breast cancer and (HRT); obesity, diet low in fruits and vegetables, high fat diet, high meat diet; excessive alcohol consumption and lack of physical activity? 2) Is there a differential impact by these risk factors on older R/E minority women compared to white women?

Hormone replacement therapy Overall the use of HRT is low (about 39%) with older white women being more likely to use HRT (about 60% more) than women of color (Connelly, Rusinak, Livingston, et al., 2000; MacDougall, Barzilag, and Helmic, 1999; MacLaren and Woods, 2001; Marsh, Brett, and Miller, 1999; Stafford, Saglam, Causino, et al., 1997; Stafford, Saglam, Causino, et al., 1998). Two studies suggest that more white women are recommended to use HRT than woman of color (Schneider, Davis, and Philips, 2000; Weng, McBride, Bosworth, et al., 2001). Past studies have shown that HRT poses a small to moderate risk of breast cancer (Pathak, Osuch, and He, 2000; Ross, Paganini-Hill, Gerkins, et al., 1980; Au, 2000; Neves-e-Castro, Samsioe, Doren, et al., 2002)). The risk however, is related to length of use (over 3 years) (Genazzani and Gambacciani, 1999; Bergkvist and Persson, 1996; Ross, Paganini-Hill, Wan, et al., 2000; Faiz and Fentiman, 1998), and the type of hormone used (Ross, Paganini-Hill, Wan, et al., 2000). Nonetheless, one study, found that the risk associated with HRT use was not distinguishable from that due to increasing age. Recent evidence from studies of the association of HRT and breast cancer have shown an increased risk of breast cancer with extended use of HRT (Kolata and Peterson, 2002). Other recent studies on other effects of long term HRT use such as cardiovascular disease have also shown unfavorable outcomes. For example, Chen, Weiss, Newcomb, et al., (2002), found that risk of breast cancer increased 60-85% for recent long-term users of HRT. Rates were increased whether the women had used estrogen or estrogen plus progestin therapy. They found that HRT use particularly increased the risk for lobular tumors.

In light of findings on the relationship between HRT and breast cancer Marsden, (2002) performed a review of the recent literature on the association of HRT and breast cancer. Marsden reviewed the Collaborative Group for Hormonal Factors in Breast Cancer (1997) reanalysis of 51 case-control studies of the association between HRT and breast cancer and concluded that long-term use (10+ years) of HRT does increase risk of breast cancer but that risk of breast cancer decreases with cessation of HRT. Studies published after 2001 were not included in Marsden's analysis.

The role of estrogen-progesterone combinations and their sequencing in the dosage is also controversial. Some studies suggest that addition of progesterone lowers the risk while others suggest that use of estrogen alone lowers the risk. Nonetheless, there is no evidence that HRT use increases mortality due to breast cancer. In contrast, breast cancer survival for women who use HRT is better than that for women who do not use HRT (Schairer, Gail, Byrne, et al., 1999; Gajdos, Tartter, and Babinszki, 2000; Bergkvist and Persson, 1996; Bonnier, Bessenay, Sasco, et al., 1998; Verhuel, Conelingh-Bennink, Kenemans, et al., 2000). This is partly because HRT use is associated with histologically favorable tumors, including smaller tumors, favorable histology, positive ER status and disease free survival, and early stage diagnosis (Bonnier, Romain, Giasalone, et al., 1995; Bonnier et al., 1998; Bonnier, Sakr, Bessenay, et al., 2000; Cobleigh, Narlock,

Oleske, et al., 1999; Delgado, Lin, and Coffey, 1995; Gajdos et al., 2000; Gapstur, Marrow, and Seller, 1999; Jones, Ingram, Mattes, et al., 1994; Magnusson, Homberg. Norden, et al., 1996; Manjer, Malina, Berglund, et al., 2001; Salmon, Ansquer, Asselain, et al., 1999).

Diet and breast cancer To determine the role of diet, articles that examined the cancer risks associated with dietary fat, fruits and vegetables, whole grain cereal and fiber, micronutrients, meat, poultry, and dairy foods, hormones in food and pesticides in food were included. Diets low in fat and high in fiber, fruits, vegetables, and grain products are associated with reduced risks for many cancers (Clifford, Ballard, Lanza, et al., 2001). Much of this evidence however, comes from country correlation and case control studies rather than from randomized controlled studies and may therefore require further research. Doll and Peto (1981) estimate that about 35 percent of cancer deaths may be related to dietary factors. Diets high in fat have been associated with increased risk of breast cancer (USDHHS, 1988; National Research Council, 1989). The association between fat and breast cancer has been more with total fat than with any specific type of fat. For example, Hursting and colleagues (1990) found a much stronger association between breast and total fat intake compared to the specific type of fat, i.e., saturated, monounsaturated, or polyunsaturated fat. A meta-analysis of 12 case-control studies showed a significant positive association between breast cancer risk and saturated fat intake in postmenopausal women (Howe, Hirohata, Haslop, et al., 1990), while other studies of the same population (Willett, Stampfer, Colditz, et al., 1990; Willett, Hunter, Stampfer, et al., 1992) reported that increased intake of total saturated and monounsaturated fats was associated with increased colon cancer but not breast cancer.

There is no consistent evidence regarding a protective role for fruits and vegetables. There is conflicting evidence regarding a protective effect of fiber against breast cancer (Cornell University BCERF, 2001; Jacobs, Marquart, and Slavin, 1998). Jacobs et al., (1998) performed an in-depth review and meta-analysis of 40 case-control studies that studied diets high in whole grains and cancer. They found that the case-control literature supported the hypothesis that whole grain intake protects against some cancers. Protective effects from fruits and vegetables have been reported for breast cancer. It is suggested that vitamins (especially carotenoids and vitamin A, alpha-tocopheral (vitamin E), vitamin C, vitamin D and minerals found in these foods may have a protective effect; however, the evidence is not strong (Wu, Helzlsouer, Comstock, et al., 1999). Other studies such as a prospective study of 61,463 women (Terry, Suzuki, Hu, et al., 2001), found no increased risk of breast cancer with a western style diet over one high in fruits and vegetables. Sellers, Kushi, Cerhan, et al., (2001), found a small increase in breast cancer rates amongst women with the lowest 10th percentile of folate intake as compared to those with >50th percentile of folate intakes. There is currently no strong evidence regarding risk or protective effect of Vitamins A and E, and Folic Acid (Wu et al., 1999). There is evidence for Vitamin C, D and B, particularly B12 and B6. Vitamin C is seems to be protective only in obese postmenopausal women but not in the general population (Levi, Pasche, Lucchini, et al., 2001; Michels, Holmberg, Bergkvist, et al., 2001).

There is no evidence regarding the association between breast cancer and a specific fat type. There is however evidence for the positive association of total fat on breast cancer (Barrett-Connor and Friendladen, 1993). According to a 1999 reviews by Cornell University, 25 cohort studies that looked at the effect of total fat were inconsistent, and only two of the studies reported that high fat diet was significantly associated with the risk of breast cancer. None of the cohort studies on the role of dietary fat reported an effect on breast cancer (Cornell University BCERF, 2001). But significant association between dietary fat and breast cancer has been consistently reported in about 95 animal models. The lack of association between dietary fat and breast cancer however may be due to measurement problems rather than the lack of effect (Cornell University BCERF, 2001). A review focused on elderly for this report also showed inconsistent evidence regarding the role of dietary fat and Vitamins A, E, and fiber. There is evidence regarding the risk of breast cancer and red meat but no evidence for poultry (chicken) and pork or fish (Cornell University BCERF, 2001). Thus, while there is substantial research into the question of diet and its role in breast cancer, much of it is still relatively general in nature.

Obesity and breast cancer   The literature reviewed shows strengthening evidence for obesity and weight gain as modifiable risk factors for breast cancer in older women. One critical question is: when in one's lifetime are obesity and weight gain risky for postmenopausal breast cancer? Three closely related measures of obesity – total weight, body mass index (defined as weight (in kg) divided by height in meter squared, (Kg/m^2), waist-to-hip ratio have been linked to breast cancer. Body weight captures both lean mass and body fat irrespective of distribution; body mass index is a standardized measure of body weight, adjusting for height, while waist to-hip ratio measures central fat deposits. It has been hypothesized that central fat deposit is also an indicator of hormonal disturbances (e.g. insulin resistance, decreases in sex hormone binding globulin, levels, androgen levels and conversion of androgen to estrogen) that have also been associated with breast cancer. In addition, increased body fat can store toxins and can serve as a continuous source of carcinogens (Friedenreich, 2001a).

The risk posed by obesity and weight gain depends on menopausal status. Although higher body weight and body mass index are protective in pre-menopausal white women they are positively associated with breast cancer in postmenopausal women. Adult weight gain and increases in central body fat, which commonly occur during menopause, have been associated consistently with an increased risk of postmenopausal breast cancer. Increased relative weight (compared to young adult weight) and weight gain after menopause have been associated with the largest increases in relative risks (Ballard-Barbash, Forman, and Kipnis, 1999).

The association of breast cancer with waist-to-hip ratio is stronger than that with body weight or with body mass index, perhaps because waist to hip ratio is more precise measure of body fat – particularly central adiposity. A population-based case-control study of white and black women in North Carolina from 1993-1996 showed that associations between BMI, waist-to-hip ratio, and breast cancer were similar for white and black women (Hall, Newman, Millikan, et al., 2000). The authors found a positive association between higher waist-to-hip ratio for all women when adjusted for BMI. Barnett and colleagues (2001), in a study of 106 healthy pre-menopausal African American women found that body fat distribution was a better marker of a hormonal pattern associated with increased breast cancer risk than was obesity.

The breast cancer risk from obesity seems greater for women after menopause and to increase with age (La Vecchia, Negri, Franceschi, et al., 1997). Maintaining a healthy adult weight (after age 20), regular exercise in young adulthood and after age 35, and avoiding weight gain around the menopausal period appear to reduce the risk of postmenopausal breast cancer. The most recent review by Friedenreich (2001) shows that inconsistencies in the literature are attributable to measurement errors (especially self reported measures), failure to account for changes in these measures that occur over one's lifetime, and differences in the definition and cut-off points for measures of obesity and central adiposity. There is currently compelling evidence from larger sample size, and designs using direct rather than self reported measures and ones that account for period in one's life when these measures were taken. There is also strong evidence from studies that pooled the original studies and applied uniform measures (Friedenreich, 2001). It should be pointed out, however, that the preventive effect of reduction in dietary fat has not been demonstrated, but two recent reviews have examined the weight loss as an adjuvant approach in women diagnosed with breast cancer (Chlebowski, 2002; Chlebowski, Aiello, and McTiernan, 2002).

Physical exercise and breast cancer   The evidence is also strengthening for the role of physical exercise in postmenopausal breast cancer risk. Much of this evidence however comes from observational studies. Few studies examine the role of race/ethnicity in this relationship. Most studies reviewed, both national and international, found significant inverse association between physical exercise and breast cancer in postmenopausal women (Adams-Campbell, Rosenberg, and Rao, 2001; Breslow, Ballard-Barbash, Munoz, et al., 2001; Carpenter, Ross, Paganini-Hill, et al., 1999; Drake, 2001; Friedenreich and Rohan, 1995; Friedenreich, Thune, Brinton, et al., 1998; Friedenreich, 2001a; Gammon, John, and Brotton, 1998; Gilliland, Li, Baumgartner, et al., 2001; Matthews, Shu, Jin, et al., 2001; Thune, Brenn, Lund, et al., 1997; Thune and Farberg, 2001; Verloop, Rookus, and van der Kooy, 2000). A few studies, however, did not find a significant association (Albanes, Blair, and Yaylar, 1989; Dorgan, Brown, Barrett, et al., 1994; Lee, Cook, Rexrode, et al., 2001; Luoto, Latikka, Pukkala, et al., 2000; Moore, Moore, Carrasco, et al., 2000). Postmenopausal women with high levels of physical activity have lower body and abdominal fat. And physically active women are less likely to gain body fat and abdominal fat after menopause than sedentary women (Astrup, 1999). But the findings from randomized controlled trials comparing exercise with no intervention, and diet with diet plus exercise allow neither a firm conclusion on the role of physical activity in limiting total fat and abdominal fat after menopause, (Astrup, 1999). Critical questions again include what type of exercise, how much exercise and when in one's life is it beneficial? Friedenreich, 2001b using a large population based case control study (N=1233 incident breast cancer cases, 1241 controls), measured the impact of lifelong occupational, household and recreation activities. The study found that occupational and household exercise of at least moderate intensity has an inverse relationship with breast cancer. Recreational exercise of any intensity had no relationship with breast cancer.

With regard to timing, exercise seems to be beneficial if done in young adulthood. For example, one study evaluated the association between physical exercise and the risk of breast cancer risk among 64,524 AA women age 21-69. They found that women who were exercising for seven or more hours per week (as compared to less than one hour) at age 21 had significantly reduced risk for breast cancer overall and pre-menopausal breast cancer, at age 30 for breast cancer overall, and at age 40 for postmenopausal breast cancer (Adams-Campbell et al., 2001). Lifetime exercise seems to be beneficial in women who do not gain considerable weight in adulthood. For example Carpenter 1999, found that exercise activity was not protective for women who gained considerable (> 17%) weight during adulthood. However, among women with more stable weight, breast cancer risk was substantially reduced for those who consistently exercised at high levels throughout their lifetime, those who exercised more than 4 hours per week for at least 12 years, and those who exercised vigorously during the most recent 10 years. Strenuous exercise appears to reduce breast cancer risk among post-menopausal women who do not gain sizable amounts of weight during adulthood.

Smoking Khuder, Mutgi, and Nugent (2001) performed a meta-analysis of peer-reviewed studies on the association of smoking and breast cancer published between 1984 and 2001. They found that relative risk (RR) for ever-smokers was 1.10. The authors found that the association between smoking and breast cancer was strongest amongst pre-menopausal women (RR 1.21). Based on their meta-analysis, Khuder et al. (2001) concluded that smoking was a weak risk factor for breast cancer with higher risk for pre-menopausal women and those who began smoking at an early age.

Alcohol Excessive alcohol consumption has been associated with increased risk of breast cancer (Schatzkin, Freedman, Dawsey, et al., 1994; Singletary and Gapstur, 2001; Terry et al., 2001; Stoll, 1999; Hiatt and Bawol, 1984; Hankinson and Willett, 1995(b); O'Connell, Hulka, Chambless, et al., 1987; Longnecker, Paganini-Hill, and Ross, 1995). Sellers et al. (2001), found increased risk of breast cancer amongst heavy drinkers who also had low folate intake (RR 1.59 95% CI 1.05-2.41). It is not established if the association between alcohol and breast cancer is causal in nature. Over 50 epidemiologic studies have found small to modest increases in risks of breast cancer associated with drinking alcoholic beverages (Schatzkin et al., 1994). The excess risk of breast cancer associated with alcohol varies by amount consumed, with 20-30% excess risk associated with consumption of about one drink per day and 60-70% excess risk associated with heavy drinking (Colditz, 1990; Garfinkel, Boffetta, and Stellman, 1988). Some studies, however have found no association between alcohol and breast cancer. Four of these studies were European studies (Ranstam and Olsson, 1995; Royo-Bordonada, Martin-Moreno, Guallar, et al., 1997; Sneyd, Paul, Spears, et al., 1991; Ferraroni, Decarli, Franceschi, et al., 1998) and two were US studies (Kinney, Millikan, Lin, et al., 2000; Zhang, Kreger, and Dorgan, 1999).

Cervical Cancer Risk Factors

When cancerous cells appear in the superficial layers of the cervix, it is known as noninvasive cervical cancer. When such cells penetrate the deeper layers of the cervix it is called invasive cervical cancer. The nomenclature can be somewhat confusing, as the staging a is based upon the level of penetration and the cell types involved. This topic is elaborated in Chapter 6.

HPV and cervical cancer   The major risk factor for uterine cervix cancer is the Human Papilloma virus (HPV) Women who are infected with HPV are at higher risk of developing cervical intraepithelial neoplasia (CIN) (a benign precursor of cervical cancer) as well as cervical cancer. Women infected with HPV are 10 or more times more likely to develop cervical cancer than are HPV-negative women (Koutsky and Galloway, 1988). Only the high risk, sexually transmitted HPV sub-types have been associated with abnormal growths related to cervical cancer (Schoell, Janicek, and Mirhashemi, 1999). Different strains of HPV may be more common and play a larger role in cancer risks in certain groups (MacLehose, Harpster, Lanier, et al., 1999). The type of HPV might also impact on prognosis for invasive cervical cancer (Schwartz, Daling, Shera, et al., 2001). An association between type of HPV and mortality from cervical cancer has also been found.

Several factors increase a woman's chance of contracting HPV. Among those are early age of sexual activity, multiple sexual partners, and male partner(s) having other multiple partners and having HIV (Miller, Kolonel, Bernstein, et al., 1996; NCI, 2002). Giuliano and colleagues (1999) studied the risk of HPV infection among Mexican-American women. They found that Mexican born women, despite fewer risk behaviors such as multiple partners and later age of first intercourse, were significantly more at risk of HPV infection than Mexican American women born in the United States. The authors' hypothesized that some unmeasured factor such as the sexual behavior of male partners might influence HPV risk (Giuliano, Papenfuss, Schneider, et al., 1999). Oral contraceptives may also increase the risk of HPV through the mechanism of progestins stimulating HPV gene expression (Smith, Cokkinides, Eschenbach, et al., 2002).

Although the link between HPV and uterine cervix cancer is obvious, studies that have tried to link high-risk sexual activity to cervical cancer have been inconsistent. This is perhaps partly because not all HPV leads to cervix cancer; only certain subtypes and most of the pre-cancerous lesions caused by low risk HPVs tend to regress (NCI Cervical cancer prevention PDQ, 2002). There are currently no commercially available tests that distinguish various sub types of HPV, although there is a test that has been approved by the Food and Drug administration that identifies the presence or absence of HPV. Given this technical limitation, it is not possible to ascertain R/E patterns for HPV subtypes. It is however, possible to ascertain R/E patterns in high-risk cytology (pre-cancerous lesions i.e. CIN 2-3). These are discussed under R/E patterns in detection rates in Chapter 6.

Other cervical cancer risks   Most women who contract HPV do not develop cancer. For this reason, it is commonly held that HPV alone is not capable of inducing cervical cancer. Exposures to cofactors seems to be important determinants of which HPV-infected women will develop the disease (NCI, 2002). Possible cofactors include 1) smoking (passive or active), 2) oral contraceptive use, 3) poor diet (poor nutrition), 4) parity (high parity), 5) other sexually transmitted diseases, including herpes simplex virus-2 (HSV-2) and immunological status such as infection with HIV. The evidence with respect to nutrition and smoking and cervical cancer are reviewed below.

Several studies of dietary factors and cervical cancer risk have been performed, but they provide relatively weak evidence for the potential to reduce cervical cancer in older women through dietary interventions. Nonetheless, an older comprehensive review of fruits and vegetable consumption and cancer did show some evidence (Block, Patterson, and Subar, 1992). In a case-control study of serum carotenoids and risk of CIN in American Indian women aged 18-45, Schiff, Patterson, Baumgartner, et al., (2001) found that increased carotenoid levels reduced the risk of CIN. HPV was found to be a significant risk factor for CIN. Low folate levels were found to increase risk of cervical cancer in a multiethnic case-control study of 150 cases and 179 controls aged 18-84 recruited from clinics in Oahu Hawaii between 1992 and 1996 (Goodman, McDuffie, Hernandez, et al., 2001).

The evidence for the roles of cigarette smoking and cervical cancer is also inconclusive: it has been studied both as independent determinant and as a co-factor along with HPV. Nonetheless, a review of the literature also cited several large studies that showed increased risk of cervical cancer with smoking in a dose dependent manner (Moore, Moore, Carrasco, et al., 2002). Cigarette smoking has also been reported to substantially elevate the death rates for cervical cancer. In a study by Wyatt and colleagues (2001) using 1997-1998 data from the Kentucky cancer registry, 61% of cases of invasive cervical cancer reported a history of smoking tobacco. A multi-center case-control study of the association between smoking and adenocarcinomas and squamous cell carcinomas of the uterine cervix by (Lacey, Frisch, Brinton, et al., 2001) found an inverse association between current smoking and adenocarcinoma, but a positive association between smoking and squamous cell carcinoma and a stronger association between smoking over one pack per day and squamous cell carcinoma. An interaction effect between smoking and HPV was found with regard to increased risk of high-grade cervical squamous intraepithelial lesion (HSIL) (Coker, Bond, Williams, et al., 2002). The authors looked at both active and passive smoking, their interaction with HPV and the development of SIL. Information on HPV and SIL were taken from pap smear samples. Analysis included only HPV positive women since the authors consider HPV to be a necessary cause of cervical carcinoma.

Thus, abundant evidence exists for the role of several modifiable risk factors and their role in cervical cancer. More than with most cancers, lack of regular access to preventive screening services constitutes a very significant risk factor.

Prostate Cancer Risk Factors

The precise etiology of prostate cancer is unknown but genetic and environmental factors have been pinpointed as playing important roles. Age is the most important risk factor. The probability of having a prostate cancer increases with age. Under the age of 40, it is a very rare event, being observed in 1 out of 10,000 men. In the 40-59 age group, the probability of developing this malignancy is 2.1%. The probability increases sharply for men in the 60-79 age group (12%), and is highest in men over 80, where 1 out of 6 develop clinical prostate cancer (Jemal, Thomas, Murray, et al., 2002). Men with a family history of prostate cancer have a higher risk of prostate cancer. A man with one or two first-degree family members with prostate cancer is twice and five times (respectively) as likely to develop prostate cancer than a man without family history (Office of Technology Assessment, 1995).

A recent systematic review analyzed the roles of vegetables, fruits and micro-nutrients in prostate cancer. Fruits do not appear correlated with prostate cancer risk. Vegetables, including tomatoes, beans and legumes could be inversely associated with prostate cancer. Beta-carotenes and vitamin E could have a protective effect on the risk of prostate cancer. However, beta-carotene intakes have been associated with a 25% risk increase of prostate cancer among cigarette smokers (Albanes, Heinonen, Huttunen, et al., 1995). In all cases, further research is needed for definitive evidence.

The relationship between dairy products and calcium intakes with prostate cancer was analyzed as part of the Physician's Health Study, with a cohort of 20,855 males followed for 11 years. The overall incidence of prostate cancer was 4.8%. Men who consumed more than 2.5 servings a day of dairy products had a 34% higher risk of developing prostate cancer than those who consumed less than half a daily serving. Similarly, men who consumed more than 600 mg a day of calcium experienced a 32% higher risk of cancer than those who consumed less than 151 mg of calcium a day. The group with high intakes of calcium from dairy products also had lower levels of 1.25-dihydroxyvitamin D3, a hormone that might have a protective effect against prostate cancer (Chan, 2001). R/E differences were not reported in this study. Men with low serum levels of selenium are twice as likely to develop prostate cancer as men with high serum levels of this element (Clark, Combs, Turnbull, et al., 1996). Race/ethnicity of participants was not reported in this study. In summary, more evidence is needed to establish the role of dietary factors on prostate cancer. A randomized clinical trial on the effect of vitamin E and selenium on prostate cancer risk is underway. This trial plans to enroll 32,400 healthy men and results are expected by 2013 (Klein, Thompson, Lippman, et al., 2001).

Racial/ethnic differences in prostate cancer risk Men of African descent are at a higher risk of developing prostate cancer, with risks among AA men 30-60% higher than non-AA men. This higher risk occurs even at earlier ages. In the 50 to 54 age group, AA men are twice as likely to develop this cancer than whites (Office of Technology Assessment, 1995).

A literature review suggests genetic factors as possible explanations for R/E differences in risk of prostate cancer with two potential types of R/E variation identified: differences in prevalence of some alleles of specific genes and differences in rare germline mutations. The former, potentially responsible for differences in serum levels of androgens or their metabolites, might be associated with a small risk increase of cancer, and could account for the largest proportion of the ethnic differences in that risk. By contrast, rare germline mutations appear to be associated with a significant risk increase, and yet might account for only a small fraction of those ethnic differences in prostate cancer risk (Shibata and Whittemore, 1997). Families with high risk of prostate cancer have linkage of a marker, HPC11, with a gene in Chromosome 1. Among families with at least three members with prostate cancer, the prevalence of this marker has been greater in AA compared to white men (over 50% vs. 34%). This could explain in part the high incidence of this cancer among AAs (Powell and Meyskens, 2001).

Androgens influence both the development and progression of prostate cancer. AAs have testosterone levels higher than any other ethnic group. A gene, the CYP17, plays a key role in the biosynthesis of androgens. Differences in its genotypes have been reported to be associated with prostate cancer. AAs with prostate cancer are 2.8 times more likely to have a genotype homozygous for the C allele in CYP17 than healthy controls of the same R/E. When this genotype is present in patients with prostate cancer, there is a 700% greater likelihood for higher-grade lesions. This finding could also explain part of the more aggressive histology observed in this R/E group (Kittles, Panguluri, Chen, et al., 2001). Other genetic variations, such as those observed in the HSD3B2 gene, could be a risk factor for prostate cancer and explain part of the R/E variation in this cancer risk (Devgan, Henderson, Yu, et al., 1997). High-grade prostatic intraepithelial neoplasia (PIN) is considered the most predictive precursor of invasive prostate cancer. AAs have a higher prevalence and greater extent of PIN, which could explain more rapid progression of this cancer for this group (Montironi, Mazzucchelli, Marshall, et al., 1999).

Modifiable factors, such as diet and physical activity have not been conclusively shown as risk or preventive factors of prostate cancer. If their role in prostate cancer is established, they could explain why AA men seem more vulnerable to the development of this cancer. This ethnic group is likely to eat fewer vegetables and more saturated fat than whites, potentially increasing their risk for prostate cancer. However, AA groups consume fewer dairy products than whites, which could provide them a protective factor against prostate cancer (Basiotis and Rajen, 1998).

The relationships of fat and total calorie intake with prostate cancer have been studied in animal experiments and epidemiological studies in humans. Resulting evidence is contradictory and far from being conclusive (Bosland, Oakley-Girvan, and Whittemore, 1999). One of the epidemiological studies that has shown an association between total saturated fat intake and risk of prostate cancer in all of the ethnic groups studied (Blacks, Whites, Chinese-Americans and Japanese-Americans), estimated that saturated fat intake could explain about 10% of the differences in the incidence of prostate cancer between Blacks and whites (Whittemore, Wu. Kolonel, et al., 1995).

Results from a cohort of 5377 men, followed for an average of 15 years by the National Health and Nutrition Examination Survey, show that AA men, with a daily low level of non-recreational physical activity, have a risk of prostate cancer 3.7 times higher than AA men who report being very active. This study failed to show however, a similar significant correlation among whites, or any significant correlation between exercise (recreational activity) and cancer. Moreover, there were no significant correlations between anthropometric measurements, (height, elbow width, body mass index, weight, or skinfold thickness), and prostate cancer in either R/E group (Clarke and Whittemore, 2000).

Current smoking status was associated with a 30% increase in death risk from prostate cancer among 348,874 men screened for this cancer and followed for an average of 16 years. The same cohort study showed that Blacks had a 2.7 times higher risk of prostate cancer-specific death than non-Blacks (Coughlin, Neaton, and Sengupta, 1996). A potential interaction effect between race and smoking was not reported in this study.

Colorectal Cancer Risk Factors

Colorectal cancer is the second most common cause of cancer-related deaths in the United States. While it has relatively high incidence and is fatal when diagnosed at later stages, it typically emerges after an extended pre-cancerous stage. Prevention of colorectal cancer is possible through detection and screening of pre-cancerous adenomatous polyps. A large body of literature has documented that the transition from normal colonic mucosa to adenomatous polyps to adenocarcinoma is a gradual process that can take decades and offers multiple opportunities for intervention (Alberts, 2002). The key molecular events in this process have been characterized (Schulmann, Reiser, and Schmiegel, 2002). Although much of the research has focused on the relatively rare polyposis syndromes, the US Preventive Services Task Force concludes that detection and removal of polyps, even in asymptomatic persons is as an effective colorectal cancer prevention strategy (Pignone and Levin, 2002).

There have been numerous efforts to address the chemoprevention of polyp development and progression to invasive cancer. Clinical trials have addressed both calcium and fiber as dietary supplements in patients who have already had polyps. Asano and McLeod (2002), Pignone and Levin (2002) and other reviewers have concluded that the five relevant clinical trials, involving over 4349 subjects, provide no evidence that increased dietary fiber intake reduces the incidence or recurrence of polyps within a 2-4 year period. By contrast, Pignone and Levin (2002) and Schulmann et al. (2002) conclude that the clinical trials do suggest that calcium may be effective in preventing reoccurrence of adenomatous polyps. More recently, attention has focused on aspirin and other non-steroidal anti-inflammatory drugs (NSAIDs) as prevention agents. One possibility is that these drugs inhibit the expression of cyclooxygenase-2 (COX-2). COX-2 has been associated with tumor progression in animal models. As a result, attention has been focused more recently on selective COX-2 inhibitors such as celecobrix, and these drugs have been recently approved for the management of familial polyposis syndromes and are being studied as potential mechanisms for management of sporadic colorectal polyps (Alberts, 2002).

While the removal of polyps and their relationships with NSAIDS and COX-2 inhibitors are the primary current targets of colorectal cancer prevention initiatives, there is compelling evidence for potentially modifiable health behaviors in the development and progression of this disease. The primary known and modifiable risk factors for colorectal cancer are physical inactivity, obesity, and diet. A review of published studies estimated that risk of colon cancer could be attributed to being physically inactive (13%), eating a Western-style diet (12%), and having a first-degree relative with the disease (8%) (Slattery, 2000). Regarding physical inactivity, an analysis of prospective longitudinal data from over 80,000 participants in the nurses' health study found that the relative risk of colon cancer was 0.54 for women who expended 21 metabolic equivalents (METs) per week versus women who expended 2 MET-hours/week (Martinez, Giovannucci, Spiegelman, et al., 1997). Similarly, a prospective study of 47,723 male health professionals age 40 to 75 found that physical activity was inversely associated with risk for colon cancer in a six-year follow-up for high versus low quintiles in terms of expenditure of energy on leisure activities (Giovannucci, Ascherio, Rimm, et al., 1995). Another study by White, Jacobs, and Daling, (1996) compared physical activity twelve to two years prior to the diagnoses of colon cancer and found that men and women who had moderate to intensive recreational or work activity two or more times a week were 0.7 times as likely to have colon cancer as those who did not exercise. Slattery and Potter (2002) found that higher levels of exercise maintained independent importance, but prediction was improved by interactions of activity with other variables. Also, high vegetable diets were much more protective in sedentary populations than active ones.

Obesity is an independent risk factor for colorectal cancer, but it appears that physical activity can offset the risk. The American Cancer Society's Cancer Prevention Study II (496,239 women and 379,167 men) found that, after controlling for multiple covariates, men with BMI 32.5 were 1.90 times as likely to die from colon cancer as men with BMI of 22.0-23.5 and among women, the groups with BMI of 30.0-32.4 had higher relative risk (1.37) than the 22.0-23.5 BMI group (Murphy, Calle, Rodriguez, et al., 2000). Slattery, Potter, Caan, et al., (1997) found that both men and women were at higher risk if they had relatively large body mass index (BMI), low lifetime activity intensity, or high calorie diets. Being in the higher risk category on all three domains increased the odds ratio to 3.35. However, high physical activity was found to offset being in the high-risk diet and

BMI groups. Another case-control study of 1,983 colon cancer cases and 2,400 age and gender-matched controls found that the third of the cases with the highest BMI compared to the third with the lowest were at higher risk for both men and women (Caan, Coates, Slattery, et al., 1998). A family history of colorectal cancer greatly increased these odds. Two of the studies of activity levels in the previous section also showed independent risks for obesity: Martinez and colleagues (1997) found that women with a BMI   29 were at 1.45 times the risk of colon cancer as women with BMI   21. Giovannucci and colleagues (1995) found the OR for colon cancer was 2.56 for men with waists of 43 inches or more compared to those with waists of 35 inches or less.

Diet is also a well-established risk factor for colorectal cancer. A six-year prospective study of 32,051 non-Hispanic whites found that food intake characteristic of a 'Western-style' diet is associated with colon cancer (Singh and Fraser, 1998). Those eating red or white meat once or more a week had risk ratios of 1.90 and 3.29 respectively compared to those with no meat intake. An inverse risk was found with legume intake. Another study of the multi-center case control cancer study cited under exercise found that colon cancer patients with a mutation of the p53 tumor suppressor gene were more likely to eat a Western-style diet compared to controls (OR 2.03) (Slattery and Potter, 2002). There is one study that associates risk for CRC with poverty. A study of 1,219 CRC patients in the Connecticut tumor registry found that patients who came from census tracts with a poverty rate of 20% or higher had the highest risk of death. The study controlled for age, stage or disease, and comorbidity (Polednak, 2001). The evidence for smoking as a risk factor for colorectal cancer is mixed, not recent, and inconclusive (Sandler, Sandler, Comstock, et al., 1988; Longnecker, Clapp, and Sheahan, 1989).

Lung Cancer Risk Factors

Modifiable risks for lung cancer include smoking, second hand smoke, and occupational exposures to asbestos, radon, and other carcinogens. Lung cancer risk is associated with the number of cigarettes smoked, number of years of smoking, the age smoking began, tar content, and depth of smoke inhalation. 1 out of 10 smokers will develop lung cancer. Smoking cessation lowers the risk but the risk ratio is 1.5 after 10-15 years of abstinence. Approximately 3000 deaths from lung cancer per year are attributable to exposure to second-hand-smoke. Variables in exposure include the size of the room, ventilation, and concentration of smoke (Chandy, Lesser, and Rashid,, 2001). Jemal et al., (2002) stated that cigarette smoking accounts for 80% of lung cancer cases in men and 70% of lung cancer cases in women. (ACS, 2002a). Stewart (2001) reported that menthol cigarettes also may increase lung cancer risk. Menthol combustion produces benzo-a-pyrenes, which are a powerful carcinogen and that menthol cigarettes have higher tar content than regular cigarettes.

Pope and colleagues (2002), in a longitudinal study of 1.2 million adults from 1982 to 1998, found that long-term exposure to fine particulates was a risk factor for cardiopulmonary and lung cancer mortality. Their study involved linking air pollution data for metropolitan areas with vital statistics data. Because more people of color reside in urban areas as compared to whites, fine particulate air pollution may be an increased risk factor for lung cancer for those individuals.

Stomach Cancer Risk Factors

Stomach cancers arise in several anatomic locations and are now viewed as distinct conditions with distinct histological features. Evidence is emerging for differentials across R/E groups in the US and abroad in the incidence of these different forms. Distinct etiological processes across the different forms of stomach cancer are also being described. There are a number of known modifiable risk factors. Foremost of these is diet. Diets high in fresh fruits and vegetables reduce risk while diets high in salt, nitrates and preservatives, and smoked foods increase stomach cancer risk (ACS 2002b). Individuals with low socioeconomic status are twice as likely to develop stomach cancer than those of higher socioeconomic status. A literature review on animal and in vitro studies of the anticarcinogenic effect of garlic on stomach and other cancers by Fleischauer and Arab (2001) found case control studies of stomach cancer that point to a protective effect of a high intake of cooked or raw garlic. Garlic supplements did not seem to lower stomach cancer risk, however. There is some evidence that tomatoes may play a protective role (Giovanucci, 1999).

Stomach surgery for benign causes is thought to be a risk factor. Fisher, Davis, Nelson, et al., (1993) found a significantly increased risk of stomach cancer up to 20 years following stomach surgery, beginning in year two. The risk was greatest for those treated by gastrectomy for ulcers. In another study comparing subjects with and without stomach cancer and 89,082 subjects without stomach cancer, Molloy and Sonnenberg (1997) found that old age, male sex, non-white ethnicity, history of gastric ulcers, and gastric resection were risk factors for stomach cancer. Griem, Kleinerman, Boice, et al., (1994) found that gastric ulcers increased the risk of stomach cancer. Radiation therapy combined with surgery, or given to treat a gastric ulcer, increased the risk of stomach cancer ten times. An increased risk for stomach cancer in individuals who had a family history of the Ewing's Sarcoma family of tumors was also found (Novakovic, Goldstein, Wexler, et al., 1994).

The World Health Organization has classified Helicobacter pylori as a carcinogen for gastric cancer. Imrie, Rowland, Bourke, et al., (2001) reviewed the literature on Helicobacter pylori in an attempt to determine the association between H. pylori in childhood and the development of distal gastric adenocarcinoma in adulthood. The major risk factor in incidence of H. pylori is poor socioeconomic conditions in childhood. The authors did find an association between H. pylori and gastric cancer. Alexander, and Brawley (2000), in a review of the literature, cited that several U.S. studies had found highest frequencies of stomach cancer in areas with the highest rates of helicobacter pylori infections in the population. They also reported that H. pylori infection was highly prevalent in black and Hispanic populations.

Racial/Ethnic differences in stomach cancer risks Wu, Wan, and Bernstein, (2001) conducted a population-based study in Los Angeles County of whites, blacks, Hispanics, and Asian Americans with esophageal and gastric cancers to determine if alcohol, smoking, and being overweight were risk factors. They found that current cigarette smoking was a risk factor for all gastric cancers. Alcohol was not a risk factor for any of the tumor types. High body-mass index (BMI) was significantly associated with esophageal and gastric cardia adenocarcinomas. Burns and Swanson (1995) conducted a population-based case control study of risk for stomach cancer among blacks and whites. Black men and black and white women had increased odds of stomach cancer if they had ever smoked. Occupations that increased risk of stomach cancer were: agricultural jobs, driver sales, assemblers, mechanics, and material movers, black women working as assemblers, and white women working as food workers. They found no association between occupations with heavy dust exposure and stomach cancer.

Theuer (2000) found notable differences in Asian versus non-Asian patients with regard to gastric adenocarcinoma. Asians were more likely to be diagnosed before age 60. They were less likely to have distant metastases and were more likely to undergo surgery than other racial groups. Three-year survival rates were significantly higher than those for non-Asians. The authors attributed greater survival rates for Asians with regional disease to higher rates of surgery. They also hypothesized that Asians had a less aggressive tumor biology than non-Asians.

Oral Cancers Risk Factors

Oral cancers are between 4 and 5 times more common in men than women (Yang, Thomas, Daling, et al., 1989). These cancers also are more common in people over 60 years of age, usually because they take many years to develop (American Cancer Society [ACS], 2001). Use of tobacco and alcohol abuse are the major modifiable risk factors for the development of head and neck cancers (ACS, 2001; Williams and Horn, 1977). A recent study shows that among the US veterans, the risk for laryngeal and pharyngeal cancers is increased in the presence of Gastroesophageal Reflux Disease (GERD), independent of age, gender, smoking, and alcohol intake (El-Serag, Hepworth, Lee, et al., 2001). Poor nutrition is considered responsible for approximately one-third of all cancers, including oral cancers (Long, 1999). In fact, a systematic review of the literature regarding nutrition and laryngeal cancer shows that the risk seems to increase with low intake of vitamin C, beta-carotene and vitamin E (Long, 1999; Riboli, Kaaks, and Esteve, 1996). Similarly, increased consumption of fruits and vegetables, and of vegetable oils and fish was associated with lower risk (Riboli et al., 1996).

There is some evidence that poor oral health is associated with increased risk of oral cancer (ACS, 2001; Rubright, Hoffman, Lynch, et al., 1996). Individuals with oral cancer, evidently, show high prevalence of painful or ill-fitting dentures (Rosenberg, 1990) due to anatomical changes of the oral cavity. In fact, for males, increased risk of oral cancer is associated with painful or ill-fitting dentures. Whether these associations are causal or due to the lack of detection and treatment of precursors lesions in persons with poor or no dental care is unclear. It is well established that leukoplakias – pre-cancerous lesions in the mouth – are amenable to early detection and treatment (Schwartz, 2000). Thus uncertainty about the role of denture fit in oral cancer parallels the age and stage patterning of cervical cancer in that current data does not permit distinguishing differences in disease process from differences in treatment quality and access. Age is a non-modifiable risk of oral cancer. Individuals diagnosed with late-stage oral cancers tend to be older (ACS, 2001; Rubright et al., 1996) screening or examination. A 1999-2000 analysis of Medicare coverage for 'medically necessary dental services' suggested policy changes to allow Medicare coverage of dental services related to surgery, chemotherapy and radiation in head and neck cancers and in leukemia (Patton, White, Field, 2001).

Cancers of the larynx and hypopharynx are about 50% more common among AA patients than among whites (Muir and Weiland, 1995; Shiboski, Shiboski, and Silverman Jr., 2000). These differences are mainly attributed to higher smoking rates among AAs (Roach, Alexander, and Coleman, 1992). Studies show that survival rates are lower for AA, as compared to whites (Arbes and Slade, 1996; Moore, Moore, Carrasco, et al., 2001). The greatest racial disparity in mortality is observed among individuals under 60 years of age, and in AA men compared to white males (Moore et al., 2001). Whites and individuals younger than 65 are more likely to have an oral cancer examination in the past year than other R/E and age groups (Horowitz and Nourjah, 1996; Martin, Bouquot, Wingo, et al., 1996). A dental visit is one of the most advocated settings to screen and diagnose oral cancers, however, older people, particularly racial/ethnic minority elders, report not having seen a dentist in the past year (Yellowitz, Goodman, and Farooq, 1997). Medicare does not cover many basic dental care services (e.g., treatment, filling, removal or replacement of teeth).

Pancreatic Cancer Risk Factors

Pancreatic cancer affects more men than women in all R/E groups. Regarding modifiable risk factors for pancreatic cancer, cigarette smoking has been constantly recognized as an important risk one (Chiu, Lynch, Cerhan, et al., 2001; Miller et al., 1996; Stolzenberg-Solomon, Pietinen, Barrett, et al., 2001). Other risk factors which have been suggested include: elevated BMI and caloric intake (Michaud, Giovannucci, Willett, et al., 2001b; Silverman, 2001), high fat diets, low folate intake (Silverman, 2001), low levels of physical activity (Michaud et al., 2001b), diabetes mellitus, peptic ulcer surgery (Tascilar, van Rees, Sturm, et al., 2002) and some occupations. Two prospective studies conducted in the US show no association between drinking coffee and alcohol and risk of developing pancreatic cancer (Michaud et al., 2001a).

Both incidence and mortality rates are higher for AA males and females, compared to their white counterparts. Native Hawaiians show slightly higher incidence rates than whites, whereas rates for Hispanics and the Asian-American groups are generally lower (Miller et al., 1996). A recent study using SEER data from 1973-1995 in Hawaii, San Francisco and Seattle showed no racial differences in survival after adjusting for age (Longnecker, Karagas, Tosteson, et al., 2000).

Overall, pancreatic cancer risk increases with age particularly among African Americans and Japanese.

Summary of Findings

The major findings from our review of reports on cancer risk factors and, R/E differences in modifiable risks, are summarized below. We find that there is epidemiological evidence linking one or more of the behavioral risks to each of the cancers. Some evidence exists that R/E differences in behavioral risk factors do explain some of the R/E differences in cancer. However, available epidemiological studies do not differentiate cumulative lifetime exposure to behavioral risks from current behaviors as influences on cancers. Thus, we find strong evidence from epidemiological studies for the importance of behavioral risks in cancer etiology and severity but almost no experimental evidence that altering behaviors influences cancer rates or outcomes. This is most obviously a function of lead-time biases and other challenges for such studies). Importantly, we find substantial evidence for health care system risk factors, such as lack of access to primary care. Their impact is particularly grievous in cancers where early detection is preventive in nature (cervical cancer and colorectal cancer). Furthermore, the evidence is missing that conclusively links race/ethnicity to genetic features associated with most cancers.

These findings need to be interpreted within a broader understanding of the changing demographics and epidemiological profile in the U.S. The US population has aged significantly and technological advances have changed the length and nature of the aging process. Chronic, disabling illnesses dominate the landscape of health care services and a delivery system devoted to acute care. The etiology of the leading causes of morbidity and mortality, such as heart disease, cancer, cerebrovascular disease, chronic lung disease, diabetes, and chronic liver disease, can be traced in large part to modifiable risk factors. These include the abuse of tobacco, alcohol, and drugs; inattention to diet and physical activity; and the misuse of toxic agents, firearms, sexual behavior, and motor vehicles (McGinnis and Foege, 1993). Yet our efforts at intervention begin only once the clinical conditions manifest themselves, usually as people age, rather than forestalling their occurrence through prevention. Furthermore, once chronic conditions become apparent, we fail to make use of continuing prevention efforts to slow progression and improve the functioning of older adults. While this is true for the aging population in general, factors leading to the underutilization of preventive measures, self-care, and the promotion of healthy behaviors are exacerbated in the case of underserved populations.

References

ACS – American Cancer Society. (2001). *Cancer Facts and Figures 2001*. Atlanta, GA: American Cancer Society.

ACS – American Cancer Society. (2002a). *Cancer Facts and Figures for African Americans 2000-2001*. Atlanta, Georgia: ACS.

ACS – American Cancer Society. (2002b). *Cancer Facts and Figures*, [Website]. Available: http://www.cancer.org [2002, 11/2002].

Adams-Campbell, L.L., Rosenberg, L. and Rao, R.S. (2001). Strenuous physical activity and breast cancer risk in African-American women. *Journal of the National Medical Association*, 93(7-8): 267-275.

Albanes, D., Blair, A. and Taylor, P.R. (1989). Physical activity and risk of cancer in the NHANES I population. *American Journal of Public Health*, 79(6): 744-750.

Albanes, D., Heinonen, O.P., Huttunen, J.K., et al. (1995). Effects of atocopherol and b-carotene supplements on cancer incidence in the Alpha-Tocopherol Beta-Carotene Study. *The American Journal of Clinical Nutrition*, 62(6): 1427S.

Alberts, D.S. (2002). Reducing the risk of colorectal cancer by intervening in the process of carcinogenesis: A status report. *Cancer Journal*, 8(3): 208-221.

Alexander, G. and Brawley, O. (2000). Association of Helicobacter Pylori Infection with Gastric Cancer. *Military Medicine*, 165(1): 21-27.

Arbes, S.J. and Slade, G.D. (1996). Racial differences in stage at diagnosis of screenable oral cancers in North Carolina. *Journal of Public Health Dentistry*, 56(6): 352-354.

Asano, T. and McLeod, R.S. (2002). Dietary fibre for the prevention of colorectal adenomas and carcinomas. *Cochrane Database Systems Review*, 2.

Astrup, A. (1999). Physical activity and weight gain and fat distribution changes with menopause: current evidence and research issues. *Medical Science Sports Exercise*, 31(11 Suppl): S564-7.

Au, G.K. (2000). Evaluation of the benefits and risks of hormone replacement therapy. *Hong Kong Medical Journal*, 6(4): 381-389.

Bach, P., Schrag, D., Brawley, O. et al. (2002). Survival of Blacks and Whites after a cancer diagnosis. *Journal of the American Medical Association*, 287(16): 2106-2113.

Ballard-Barbash, R., Forman, M.R. and Kipnis, V. (1999). Dietary fat, serum estrogen levels, and breast cancer risk: a multifaceted story. *Journal National Cancer Institute*, 91(6): 492-494.

Barnett, J.B., Woods, M.N., Rosner, B et al. (2001). Sex hormone levels in premenopausal African-American women with upper and lower body fat phenotypes. *Nutrition and Cancer*, 41(1-2): 47-56.

Barrett-Connor, E. and Friedlander, N.J. (1993). Dietary fat, calories, and the risk of breast cancer in postmenopausal women: a prospective population-based study. *Journal of the American College of Nutritionists*, 12(4): 390-399.

Basiotis, M.L. and Rajen, S.A. (1998). Report card on the diet of African Americans. *Family Economics and Nutrition Review*, 11(3): 61.

Bergkvist, L. and Persson, I. (1996). Hormone replacement therapy and breast cancer: A review of current knowledge. *Drug Safety*, 15(5), 360-370.

Berkel, H.J., Turbat-Herrera, E.A., Shi, R. et al. (2001). Expression of the translation initiation factor eIF4E in the polyp-cancer sequence in the colon. *Cancer Epidemiology, Biomarkers and Prevention*, 10(6): 663-666.

Block, G., Patterson, B. and Subar, A. (1992). Fruit, vegetables, and cancer prevention: a review of the epidemiological evidence. *Nutrition and Cancer*. 18(1): 1-29.

Bolen, J.C., Rhodes, L., Powell-Griner, E.E. et al. (2000). State-specific prevalence of selected health behaviors, by race and ethnicity: Behavioral Risk Factor Surveillance System, 1997. *Morbidity, Mortality Weekly Report: CDC Surveillance Summary*, 49(2): 1-60.

Bonnier, P., Romain, S., Giacalone, P.L. et al. (1995). Clinical and biological prognostic factors in breast cancer diagnosed during postmenopausal hormone replacement therapy. *Obstetrical Gynecology*, 85(1): 11-17.

Bonnier, P., Bessenay, F., Sasco, A.J. et al. (1998). Impact of menopausal hormone-replacement therapy on clinical and laboratory characteristics of breast cancer. *International Journal of Cancer*, 79(3): 278-282.

Bonnier, P., Sakr, R., Bessenay, F. et al. (2000). Effects of hormone replacement therapy for menopause on prognostic factors of breast cancer. *Gynecological and Obstetrical Fertilization*, 28(10): 745-753.

Booth, B.M., Blow, F.C., Cook, C.A. et al. (1992). Age and ethnicity among hospitalized alcoholics: A nationwide study. *Journal of Alcohol Clinical Experimental Research*, 16(6): 1029-1034.

Bosland, M.C., Oakley-Girvan, I. and Whittemore, A.S. (1999). Dietary fat, calories, and prostate cancer risk. *Journal of the National Cancer Institute*, 91(6): 489-491.

Breslow, R.A., Ballard-Barbash, R., Munoz, K et al. (2001). Long-term recreational physical activity and breast cancer in the National Health and Nutrition Examination Survey I epidemiologic follow-up study. *Cancer Epidemiology, Biomarkers and Prevention*, 10(7): 805-808.

Bucholz, K., Sheline, Y. and Helzer, J. (1995). The Epidemiology of Alcohol Use, Problems, and Dependence in Elders: A Review, in T. Beresford and E. Gomberg (eds), *Alcohol and Aging*, New York: Oxford University Press.

Burns, P. and Swanson, G. (1995). Stomach cancer risk among black and white men and women: the role of occupation and cigarette smoking. *Journal of Occupational and Environmental Medicine*, 37(10): 1218-1223.

Caan, B.J., Coates, A.O., Slattery, M.L. et al. (1998). Body size and the risk of colon cancer in a large case-control study. *International Journal of Obesity Related Metabolic Disorders*, 22(2): 178-184.

Carpenter, C.L., Ross, R.K., Paganini-Hill, A. et al. (1999). Lifetime exercise activity and breast cancer risk among post-menopausal women. *British Journal of Cancer*, 80(11): 1852-1858.

Chan, E.C. (2001). Promoting informed decision making about prostate cancer screening. *Comprehensive Therapy*, 27(3): 195-201.

Chandy, D., Lesser, M. and Rashid, A. (2001). Lung cancer: early intervention is the key. *Patient Care*, 35(20): 12.

Chen, C.L., Weiss, N.S., Newcomb, P. et al. (2002). Hormone replacement therapy in relation to breast cancer. *Journal of the American Medical Association*, 287(6): 734-741.

Chlebowski, R.T., Aiello, E. and McTiernan, A. (2002). Weight loss in breast cancer patient management. *Journal of Clinical Oncology*, 20(4): 1128-1143.

Chlebowski, R.T. (2002). Breast cancer risk reduction: strategies for women at increased risk. *Annual Review of Medicine*, 53: 519-540.

Chiu, B.C., Lynch, C.F., Cerhan, J.R. et al. (2001). Cigarette smoking and risk of bladder, pancreas, kidney, and colorectal cancers in Iowa. *Annual Epidemiology*, 11(1): 28-37.

Clark, L., Combs, G.F., Turnbull, B.W. et al. (1996). Effects of selenium supplementation for cancer prevention in patients with carcinoma of the skin: A randomized controlled trial. *Journal of the American Medical Association*, 276(24): 1957-1963.

Clarke, G. and Whittemore, A.S. (2000). Prostate cancer risk in relation to anthropometry and physical activity: the National Health and Nutrition Examination Survey I Epidemiological Follow-Up Study. *Cancer Epidemiology, Biomarkers and Prevention*, 9(9): 875-881.

Clifford, C., Ballard, R.B., Lanza, E. et al. (2001). *Diet and Cancer Risk*. NCI – National Cancer Institute: Washington, DC.

Cobleigh, M.A., Norlock, F.E., Oleske, D.M. et al. (1999). Hormone replacement therapy and high S phase in breast cancer. *Journal of the American Medical Association*, 281(16): 1528-1530.

Coker, A.L., Bond, S.M., Williams, A. et al. (2002). Active and passive smoking, high-risk human papillomaviruses and cervical neoplasia. *Cancer Detection and Prevention*, 26(2): 121-128.

Colditz, G. (1990). A prospective assessment of moderate alcohol intake and major chronic diseases. *Annals of Epidemiology*, 1: 167-177.

Colditz, G.A. and Gortmaker, S.L. (1995). Cancer prevention strategies for the future: risk identification and preventive intervention. *Milbank Quarterly*, 73(4): 621-651.

Connelly, M.T., Richardson, M. and Platt, R. (2000). Prevalence and duration of postmenopausal hormone replacement therapy use in a managed care organization, 1990-1995. *Journal of General Internal Medicine*, 15(8): 542-550.

Connelly, M.T., Rusinak, D., Livingston, W. et al. (2000). Patient knowledge about hormone replacement therapy: implications for treatment. *Menopause*, 7(4), 266-272.

Cornell University, (2001). Cornell University Program on Breast cancer an environmental Risk factors in New York. *Url: http//www.cfe.cornell.edu/bcerf/, Revised July, 2001.*

Coughlin, S.S., Neaton, J.D. and Sengupta, A. (1996). Cigarette smoking as a predictor of death from prostate cancer in 348,874 men screened for the Multiple Risk Factor Intervention Trial. *American Journal of Epidemiology*, 143(10): 1002-1006.

Delgado, D.J., Lin, W.Y. and Coffey, M. (1995). The role of Hispanic race/ethnicity and poverty in breast cancer survival. *Puerto Rico Health Sciences Journal*, 14(2): 103-116.

Devgan, S.A., Henderson, B.E., Yu, M.C. et al. (1997). Genetic variation of 3b-hydroxysteroid dehydrogenase type II in three racial/ethnic groups: Implications for prostate cancer risk. *The Prostate*, 33(1): 9-12.

Doll, R. and Peto, R. (1981). The causes of cancer: Quantitative estimates of avoidable risks of cancer in the United States today. *Journal of the National Cancer Institute*, 66: 1191-1308.

Dorgan, J.F., Brown, C., Barrett, M. et al. (1994). Physical activity and risk of breast cancer in the Framingham Heart Study. *American Journal of Epidemiology*, 139(7): 662-669.

Drake, D.A. (2001). A longitudinal study of physical activity and breast cancer prediction. *Cancer Nursing*, 24(5): 371-377.

Dunlop, D.D., Manheim, L.M., Song, J. et al. (2002). Gender and ethnic/racial disparities in health care utilization among older adults. *Journal of Gerontology: Series B: Psychological and Sciences and Social Sciences*, 57(4): S221-233.

El-Serag, H.B., Hepworth, E.J., Lee, P. et al. (2001). Gastroesophageal reflux disease is a risk factor for laryngeal and pharyngeal cancer. *American Journal of Gastroenterology*, 96(7): 2013-2018.

Faiz, O. and Fentiman, I.S. (1998). Hormone replacement therapy and breast cancer. *International Journal of Clinical Practice*, 52(2): 98-101

Ferraroni, M., Decarli, A., Franceschi, S. et al. (1998). Alcohol consumption and risk of breast cancer: a multicentre Italian case-control study. *European Journal of Cancer*, 34(9): 1403-1409.

Fisher, S.G., Davis, F., Nelson, R. et al. (1993). A cohort study of stomach cancer risk in men after gastric surgery for benign disease. *Journal of the National Cancer Institute*, 85: 1303-1310.

Fleischauer, A. and Arab, L. (2001). Garlic and cancer: A critical review of the epidemiologic literature. *The Journal of Nutrition*, 131(3S): 1032s-1040s.

Friedenreich, C.M. and Rohan, T.E. (1995). Physical activity and risk of breast cancer. *European Journal of Cancer Prevention*, 4(2): 145-151.

Friedenreich, C.M., Thune, I., Brinton, L.A. et al. (1998). Epidemiologic issues related to the association between physical activity and breast cancer. *Cancer*, 83(3Supp): 600-610.

Friedenreich, C.M. (2001a). Review of anthropometric factors and breast cancer risk. *European Journal of Cancer Prevention*, 10(1): 15-32.

Friedenreich, CM Courneya, KS Bryant, WE. (2001b). Relationship between intensity of physical activity and breast cancer risk reduction. *Medical Science and Sports Exercise*, 37(9): 1538-1545.

Gammon, M.D., John, E.M. and Britton, J.A. (1998). Recreational and occupational physical activities and risk of breast cancer. *Journal of the National Cancer Institute*, 90(2): 100-117.

Garfinkel, L., Boffetta, P. and Stellman, S.D. (1988). Alcohol and breast cancer: A cohort study. *Preventive Medicine*, 17: 686-693.

Gapstur, S.M., Morrow, M. and Sellers, T.A. (1999). Hormone replacement therapy and risk of breast cancer with a favorable histology: results of the Iowa Woman's Health Study. *Journal of the American Medical Association*, 281(22): 2091-2097.

Gajdos, C., Tartter, P.I. and Babinszki, A. (2000). Breast cancer diagnosed during hormone replacement therapy. *Obstetrical Gynecology*, 95(4): 513-518.

Genazzani, A.R. and Gambacciani, M. (1999). Hormone replacement therapy: the perspectives for the 21st century. *Maturitas*, 32(1): 11-17.

Gilliland, F.D., Li, Y.F., Baumgartner, K. et al. (2001). Physical activity and breast cancer risk in hispanic and non-hispanic white women. *American Journal of Epidemiology*, 154(5): 442-50.

Giovannucci, E., Ascherio, A., Rimm, E.B. et al. (1995). Physical activity, obesity, and risk for colon cancer and adenoma in men. *Annals of Internal Medicine*, 122(5): 327-334.

Giovannucci, E. (1999). Tomatoes, tomato-based products, lycopene, and cancer: review of the epidemiologic literature. *Journal of the National Cancer Institute*, 91: 317-331.

Giuliano, A.R., Papenfuss, M., Schneider, A. et al. (1999). Risk factors for high-risk type human papillomavirus infection among Mexican-American women. *Cancer Epidemiology, Biomarkers and Prevention*, 8(7): 615-620.

Gomberg, E. and Nelson, B. (1995). Black and white older men alcohol use and abuse. In T. Beresford and E.S. Gomberg (eds), *Alcohol and Aging*. New York: Oxford University Press.

Gomberg, E. (1999). Substance abuse in elderly. In P. Ott, R. Tarter, and R. Ammerman (Eds.), *Source Book on Substance Abuse*. Boston, MA: Allyn–Bacon.

Goodman, M.T., McDuffie, K., Hernandez, B. et al. (2001). Association of methyllene-tetrahydrofolate reductase polymorphism C677T and dietary folate with the risk of cervical dysplasia. *Cancer Epidemiology Biomarkers and Prevention*, 10(12): 1275-80.

Griem, M.L., Kleinerman, R.A., Boice, J.D. et al. (1994). Cancer following radiotherapy for peptic ulcer. *Journal of the National Cancer Institute*, 86: 842-849.

Hahn, R.A., Teutsch, S.M., Franks, A.L. et al. (1998). The prevalence of risk factors among women in the United States by race and age, 1992-1994: Opportunities for primary and secondary prevention. *Journal of the American Medical Women's Association*, 53(2): 96-104, 107.

Hall, I.J., Newman, B., Millikan, R.C. and Moorman, P.G. (2000). Body size and breast cancer risk in black women and white women: the Carolina Breast Cancer Study. *American Journal of Epidemiology*, 151(8): 754-764.

Hankinson, S.E. (1999). Waist circumference, waist: hip ratio, and risk of breast cancer in the Nurses Health Study. *American Journal of Epidemiology*, 150(12): 1316-1324.

Hankinson, S.E. and Willett, W.C. (1995). Alcohol and breast cancer: is there a conclusion? *Nutrition*, 11: 320-321.

Hiatt, R.A. and Bawol, R.D. (1984). Alcoholic beverage consumption and breast cancer incidence. *American Journal of Epidemiology*, 120(5): 676-683.

Horowitz, A.M. and Nourjah, P.A. (1996). Factors associated with having oral cancer examinations among US adults 40 years of age or older. *Journal of Public Health Dentistry*, 56(6): 331-335.

Howe, G.R., Hirohata, T., Hislop, T.G. et al. (1990). Dietary factors and risk of breast cancer: combined analysis of 12 case-control studies. *Journal of the National Cancer Institute*, 82(7): 561-569.

Hursting, S.D., Thornquis, M. and Henderson, M.M. (1990). Types of dietary fat and the incidence of cancer at five sites. *Preventive Medicine*, 19: 242-253.

Imrie, C., Rowland, M., Bourke, B. et al. (2001). Is helicobacter pylori infection in childhood a risk factor for gastric cancer? *Pediatrics*, 1007: 373-380.

Jackson, J.S., Williams, D.R. and Gomberg, E.S. (1998). Aging and Alcohol Use and Abuse Among African Americans: A Life-Course Perspective. In E. Gomberg, A. M. Hegedus, and R.A. Zucker (Eds.), *Alcohol Problems and Aging*, Bethesda, MD: National Institute on Alcohol Abuse and Alcoholism.

Jacobs Jr., D.R., Marquart, L. and Slavin, J. (1998). Whole-grain intake and cancer: an expanded review and meta-analysis. *Nutrition and Cancer*, 30(2): 85-96.

Janes, G.R., Blackman, D.K., Bolen, J.C. et al. (1999). Surveillance for use of preventive health care services by older adults, 1995-1997. *MMWR – Morbidity and Mortality Weekly Report*, 48(SS-8): 51-88.

Jemal, A., Thomas, A., Murray, T. et al. (2002). Cancer Statistics, 2002. *CA: A Cancer Journal for Clinicians*, 52(1): 23-48.

Jones, C., Ingram, D., Mattes, E. et al. (1994). The effect of hormone replacement therapy on prognostic indices in women with breast cancer. *Medical Journal of Australia*, 161(2): 106-110.

Kinney, A.Y., Millikan, R.C., Lin, Y.H. et al. (2000). Alcohol consumption and breast cancer among black and white women in North Carolina (United States). *Cancer Causes Control*, 11(4): 345-357.

Kittles, R.A., Panguluri, R.K., Chen, W. et al. (2001). Cyp17 promoter variant associated with prostate cancer aggressiveness in African Americans. *Cancer Epidemiology Biomarkers and Prevention*, 10(9): 943-947.

Klein, E., Thompson, L.M., Lippman, S.M. et al. (2001). SELECT: the next prostate cancer prevention trial. *The Journal of Urology*, 166(4): 1311-1315.

Kolata, G. and Petersen, M. (2002, July 10). Hormone replacement study a shock to the medical system. *The New York Times*.

Koutsky, L.A. and Galloway, D.A. (1988). Holmes KK Epidemiology of genital human papillomavirus infection. *Epidemiological Reviews*, 1: 122-163.

Khuder, S.A., Mutgi, A.B. and Nugent, S. (2001). Smoking and breast cancer: a meta-analysis. *Reviews on Environmental Health*, 16(4): 253-261.

Lacey Jr., J.V., Frisch, M., Brinton, L.A. et al. (2001). Associations between smoking and adenocarcinomas and squamous cell carcinomas of the uterine cervix (United States). *Cancer Causes Control*, 12(2): 153-161.

La Vecchia, C., Negri, E., Franceschi, S. et al. (1997). Body mass index and post-menopausal breast cancer: an age-specific analysis. *British Journal of Cancer*, 75(3): 441-444.

Lee, I.M., Cook, N.R., Rexrode, K.M. et al. (2001). Lifetime physical activity and risk of breast cancer. *British Journal of Cancer*, 85(7): 962-965.

Levi, F., Pasche, C., Lucchini, F. et al. (2001). Dietary intake of selected micronutrients and breast-cancer risk. *International Journal of Cancer*, 91(2): 260-263.

Long, S.A. (1999). The use of antioxidant nutrients to prevent and treat cancers of the aerodigestive tract. *Dental Hygiene*, 73(2): 93-98.

Longnecker, M.P., Clapp, R.W. and Sheahan, K. (1989). Associations between smoking status and stage of colorectal cancer at diagnosis in Massachusetts between 1982 and 1987. *Cancer*, 64(6): 1372-1374.

Longnecker, M.P., Paganini-Hill, A. and Ross, R.K. (1995). Lifetime alcohol consumption and breast cancer risk among postmenopausal women in Los Angeles. Cancer *Epidemiology, Biomarkers and Prevention*, 4(7): 721-725.

Longnecker, D.S., Karagas, M.R., Tosteson, T.D. et al. (2000). Racial differences in pancreatic cancer: comparison of survival and histologic types of pancreatic carcinoma in Asians, blacks, and whites in the United States. *Pancreas*, 21(4): 338-343.

Lubben, J.E., Weiler, P.G. and Chi, I. (1989). Gender and ethnic differences in the health practices of the elderly poor. *Journal of Clinical Epidemiology*, 42(6): 725-733.

Luoto, R., Latikka, P., Pukkala, E. et al. (2000). The effect of physical activity on breast cancer risk: a cohort study of 30,548 women. *European Journal of Epidemiology*, 16(10): 973-980.

MacDougall, L.A., Barzilay, J.I. and Helmick, C.G. (1999). Hormone replacement therapy awareness in a biracial cohort of women aged 50-54 years. *Menopause*, 6(3): 251-256.

MacDougall, L.A., Barzilay, J.I. and Helmick, C.G. (1999). The role of personal health concerns and knowledge of the health effects of hormone replacement therapy (HRT) on the ever use of HRT by menopausal women, aged 50-54 years. *Journal of Women's Health and Gender Based Medicine*, 8(9): 1203-1211.

MacDowell, M., Guo, L. and Short, A. (2002). Preventive health services use, lifestyle health behavior risks, and self-reported health status of women in Ohio by ethnicity and completed education status. *Women's Health Issues*, 12(2): 96-102.

McGinnis, J. and Foege, W. (1993). Actual causes of death in the United States. *Journal of the American Medical Association*, 270(18): 2207-2212

MacLaren, A. and Woods, N.F. (2001). Midlife women making hormone therapy decisions. *Women's Health Issues*, 11(3): 216-230.

MacLehose, R.F., Harpster, A., Lanier, A.P. et al. (1999). Risk factors for cervical intraepithelial neoplasm in Alaska Native women: a pilot study. *Alaska Medicine*, 41(4): 76-85.

Magnusson, C., Homberg, L., Norden, T. et al. (1996). Prognostic characteristics in breast cancers after hormone replacement therapy. *Breast Cancer Research Treatment*, 38(3): 325-334.

Manjer, J., Malina, J., Berglund, G. et al. (2001). Increased incidence of small and well-differentiated breast tumours in post-menopausal women following hormone replacement therapy. *International Journal of Cancer*, 92(6): 919-922.

Marsden, J. (2002). Hormone-replacement therapy and breast cancer. *Lancet Oncology*, 3(5): 303-311.

Marsh, J.V., Brett, K.M. and Miller, L.C. (1999). Racial differences in hormone replacement therapy prescriptions. *Obstetrical Gynecology*, 93(6): 999-1003.

Martin, L.M., Bouquot, J.E., Wingo, P.A. et al. (1996). Cancer prevention in the dental practice: oral cancer screening and tobacco cessation advice. *Journal of Public Health Dentistry*, 56(6): 336-340.

Martinez, M.E., Giovannucci, E., Spiegelman, D. et al. (1997). Leisure-time physical activity, body size, and colon cancer in women. Nurses' Health Study Research Group. *Journal of the National Cancer Institute*, 89(13): 948-955.

Matthews, C.E., Shu, X.O., Jin, F. et al. (2001). Lifetime physical activity and breast cancer risk in the Shanghai Breast Cancer Study. *British Journal of Cancer*, 84(7): 994-1001.

McTiernan, A. (2000). Associations between energy balance and body mass index and risk of breast carcinoma in women from diverse racial and ethnic backgrounds in the U.S. *Cancer*, 88 (5 Suppl): 1248-1255.

Michaud, D.S., Giovannucci, E., Willett, W.C. et al. (2001a). Coffee and alcohol consumption and the risk of pancreatic cancer in two prospective United States cohorts. *Cancer Epidemiology, Biomarkers and Prevention*, 10(5): 429-437.

Michaud, D.S., Giovannucci, E., Willett, W.C. et al. (2001b). Physical activity, obesity, height, and the risk of pancreatic cancer. *Journal of the American Medical Association*, 286(8): 921-929.

Michels, K.B., Holmberg, L., Bergkvist, L. et al. (2001). Dietary antioxidant vitamins, retinol, and breast cancer incidence in a cohort of Swedish women. *International Journal of Cancer*, 91(4): 563-567.

Miller, B., Kolonel, L.N., Bernstein Jr., L.Y. et al. (1996). *Racial/Ethnic Patterns of Cancer in the United States 1988-1992: Cervix Uteri Cancer – U.S. Racial/Ethnic Cancer Patterns*, Bethesda, MD: National Cancer Institute.

Miller, B.A., Kolonel, L.N., Bernstein Jr., L. et al. (1996). *Racial/Ethnic Patterns of Cancer in the United States 1988-1992*. (Vol. NIH Pub. No. 96-4104). Bethesda, MD: National Cancer Institute.

Molloy, R. and Sonnenberg, A. (1997). Relation between gastric cancer and previous peptic ulcer disease. *Gut*, 40(2): 247-252.

Montironi, R., Mazzucchelli, R., Marshall, J.R. et al. (1999). Prostate cancer prevention: review of target populations, pathological biomarkers, and chemopreventive agents. *Journal of Clinical Pathology*, 52(11): 793-803.

Moore, D.B., Folsom, A.R., Mink, P.J. et al. (2000). Physical activity and incidence of post-menopausal breast cancer. *Epidemiology*, 11(3): 292-296.

Moore, T.O., Moore, A.Y., Carrasco, D. et al. (2001). Human papillomavirus, smoking, and cancer. *Journal of Cutaneous Medicine and Surgery*, 5(4): 323-328.

Morris, C.R., Cohen, R., Schlag, R. et al. (2000). Increasing trends in the use of breast-conserving surgery in California. *American Journal of Public Health*, 90(2): 281-284.

Morris, C.R., Wright, W.E. and Schlag, R.D. (2001). The risk of developing breast cancer within the next 5, 10, or 20 years of a woman's life. *American Journal of Preventive Medicine*, 20(3): 214-218.

Muir, C. and Weiland, L. (1995). Upper aerodigestive tract cancers. *Cancer*, 75(1 Suppl): 147-153.

Murphy, T.K., Calle, E.E., Rodriguez, C. et al. (2000). Body mass index and colon cancer mortality in a large prospective study. *American Journal of Epidemiology*, 152(9): 847-854.

NRC. (1989). *National Research Council, Committee on Diet and Health, Food and Nutrition Board, Commission on Life Sciences. Diet and Health: Implications for Reducing Chronic Disease Risk.* Washington, DC: National Academy Press.

NCI. (2002). *Cervical Cancer Prevention*. NCI. Available: http://www.cancer.gov [2002, Date Last Modified: 07/2002].

Neves-e-Castro, M., Samsioe, G., Doren, M. et al. (2002). Results from WHI and HERS II: Implications for women and the prescriber of HRT. *Maturitas*, 42(4): 255.

Novakovic, B., Goldstein, A.M., Wexler, L.H. et al. (1994). Increased risk of neuroectodermal tumors and stomach cancer in relatives of patients with Ewing's Sarcoma family of tumors. *Journal of the National Cancer Institute*, 86: 1702-1706.

O'Connell, D.L., Hulka, B.S., Chambless, L.E. et al. (1987). Cigarette smoking, alcohol consumption, and breast cancer risk. *Journal of the National Cancer Institute*, 78(2): 229-234.

Office of Technology Assessment. (1995). *Costs and effectiveness of prostate cancer screening in elderly men.* Washington, D.C.: U.S. Congress.

Pathak, D.R., Osuch, J.R. and He, J. (2000). Breast carcinoma etiology: current knowledge and new insights into the effects of reproductive and hormonal risk factors in black and white populations. *Cancer*, 88(5 Suppl): 1230-1238.

Patton, L.L., White, B.A. and Field, M.J. (2001). Extending Medicare coverage to medically necessary dental care. *Journal of the American Dental Association*, 132(9): 1294-1299.

Pezzin, L. and Kasper, J. (2002). Medicaid enrollment among elderly Medicare beneficiaries: Individual determinants, effects of state policy, and impact on service use. *Health Services Research*, 37(4): 827-847.

Pignone, M. and Levin, B. (2002). Recent developments in colorectal cancer screening and prevention. *American Family Physician*, 66(2): 297-302.

Polednak, A.P. (2001). Poverty, comorbidity, and survival of colorectal cancer patients diagnosed in Connecticut. *Journal of Health Care for the Poor and Underserved*, 12(3): 302-310.

Pope, C.A.I., Burnett, R.T., Thun, M.J. et al. (2002). Lung cancer, cardiopulmonary mortality, and long-term exposure to fine particulate air pollution. *Journal of the American Medical Association*, 287(9): 1132-1141.

Powell, I.J. and Meyskens, F.L. (2001). African American men and hereditary/familial prostate cancer: Intermediate-risk populations for chemo-prevention trials. *Urology*, 57(4); 178-181.

Pourat, N., Rice, T., Kominski, G. et al. (2000). Socioeconomic differences in Medicare supplemental coverage. *Health Affairs*, 19(5), 186-196.

Ranstam, J. and Olsson, H. (1995). Alcohol, cigarette smoking, and the risk of breast cancer. *Cancer Detection and Prevention*, 19(6): 487-493.

Riboli, E., Kaaks, R. and Esteve, J. (1996). Nutrition and laryngeal cancer. *Cancer Causes and Control*, 7(1): 147-156.

Roach, M. 3rd, Alexander, M. and Coleman, J.L. (1992). The prognostic significance of race and survival from laryngeal carcinoma. *Journal of the National Medical Association*, 84(8): 668-674.

Rosenberg, S.W. (1990). Oral complications of cancer therapies. Chronic dental complications. *NCI Monograph*, 9: 173-178.

Ross, R.K., Paganini-Hill, A., Gerkins, V.R. et al. (1980). A case-control study of menopausal estrogen therapy and breast cancer. *Journal of the American Medical Association*, 243(16): 1635-1639.

Ross, R.K., Paganini-Hill, A., Wan, P.C. et al. (2000). Effect of hormone replacement therapy on breast cancer risk: estrogen versus estrogen plus progestin. *Journal of the National Cancer Institute*, 92(4): 328-332.

Royo-Bordonada, M.A., Martin-Moreno, J.M., Guallar, E. et al. (1997). Alcohol intake and risk of breast cancer: the euramic study. *Neoplasm*, 44(3): 150-156.

Rubright, W.C., Hoffman, H.T., Lynch, C.F. et al. (1996). Risk factors for advanced-stage oral cavity cancer. *Archives of Otolaryngology Head and Neck Surgery*, 122(6): 621-626.

Salmon, R.J., Ansquer, Y., Asselain, B. et al. (1999). Clinical and biological characteristics of breast cancers in post-menopausal women receiving hormone replacement therapy for menopause. *Oncology Report*, 6(3): 699-703.

Sandler, R.S., Sandler, D.P., Comstock, G.W, et al. (1988). Cigarette smoking and the risk of colorectal cancer in women. *Journal of the National Cancer Institute*, 80(16): 1329-1333.

Schatzkin, A., Freedman, L.S., Dawsey, S.M. et al. (1994). Interpreting precursor studies: what polyp trials tell us about large-bowel cancer. *Journal of the National Cancer Institute*, 86(14): 1053-1057.

Schairer, C., Gail, M., Byrne, C. et al. (1999). Estrogen replacement therapy and breast cancer survival in a large screening study. *Journal of the National Cancer Institute*, 91(3): 264-70.

Schiff, M.A., Patterson, R.E., Baumgartner, R.N. et al. (2001). Serum carotenoids and risk of cervical intraepithelial neoplasia in Southwestern American Indian women. *Epidemiology, Biomarkers and Prevention*, 10(11): 1219-1222.

Schneider, A.E., Davis, R.B. and Phillips, R.S. (2000). Discussion of hormone replacement therapy between physicians and their patients. *American Journal of Medical Quality*, 15(4): 143-147.

Schoell, W.M., Janicek, M.F. and Mirhashemi, R. (1999). Epidemiology and biology of cervical cancer. *Seminars in Surgical Oncology*, 16(3): 203-211.

Schulmann, K., Reiser, M. and Schmiegel, W. (2002). Colonic cancer and polyps. *Best Practice and Research. Clinical Gastroenterology*, 16(1): 91-114.

Schwartz, S.M., Daling, J.R., Shera, K.A. et al. (2001). Human papillomavirus and prognosis of invasive cervical cancer: a population-based study. *Journal of Clinical Oncology*, 19(7): 1906-1915.

Schwartz, J.L. (2000). Biomarkers and molecular epidemiology and chemoprevention of oral carcinogenesis. *Critical Review in Oral Biology and Medicine*, 11(1): 92-122.

Schulmann, K., Reiser, M. and Schmiegel, W. (2002). Colonic cancer and polyps. *Best Practices Research. Clinical Gastroenterology*, 16(1): 91-114.

Seefeldt, V., Malina, R.M. and Clark, M.A. (2002). Factors affecting levels of physical activity in adults. *Sports Medicine*, 32(3): 143-168.

Sellers, T.A., Kushi, L.H., Cerhan, J.R. et al. (2001). Dietary folate intake, alcohol, and risk of breast cancer in a prospective study of postmenopausal women. *Epidemiology*, 12(4): 420-428.

Shibata, A. and Whittemore, A.S. (1997). Genetic predisposition to prostate cancer: possible explanations for ethnic differences in risk. *The Prostate*, 32(1): 65-72.

Shiboski, C.H., Shiboski, S.C. and Silverman Jr., S. (2000). Trends in oral cancer rates in the United States, 1973-1996. *Community Dental Oral Epidemiology*, 28(4): 249-56.

Silverman, D.T. (2001). Risk factors for pancreatic cancer: a case-control study based on direct interviews. *Teratogenesis, Carcinogenesis, Mutagenesis*, 21(1): 7-25.

Singh, P.N. and Fraser, G.E. (1998). Dietary risk factors for colon cancer in a low-risk population. *American Journal of Epidemiology*, 148(8): 761-774.

Singletary, K.W. and Gapstur, S.M. (2001). Alcohol and breast cancer: review of epidemiologic and experimental evidence and potential mechanisms. *Journal of the American Medical Association*, 286(17): 2143-2151.

Slattery, M.L. (2000). Diet, lifestyle, and colon cancer. *Seminars in Gastrointestinal Disease*, 11(3): 142-146.

Slattery, M.L., Potter, J., Caan, B. et al. (1997). Energy balance and colon cancer – beyond physical activity. *Cancer Research*, 57(1): 75-80.

Slattery, M.L. and Potter, J.D. (2002). Physical activity and colon cancer: confounding or interaction? *Medical Science and Sports Exercise*, 34(6): 913-9.

Smith, R.A., Cokkinides, V., Eschenbach, A.C. et al. (2002). American Cancer Society guidelines for the early detection of cancer. *CA: A Cancer Journal for Clinicians*, 52(8): 8-23.

Sneyd, M.J., Paul, C., Spears, G.F. et al. (1991). Alcohol consumption and risk of breast cancer. *International Journal of Cancer*, 48(6): 812-815.

Stafford, R.S., Saglam, D. and Causino, N. (1997). Low rates of hormone replacement in visits to United States primary care physicians. *American Journal of Obstetrical Gynecology*, 177(2): 381-387.

Stafford, R.S., Saglam, D., Causino, N. et al. (1998). The declining impact of race and insurance status on hormone replacement therapy. *Menopause*, 5(3): 140-144.

Stewart, J.H.I. (2001). Lung Carcinoma in African Americans. *Cancer*, 91(12): 2476-2482.

Stoll, B.A. (1999). Alcohol intake and late-stage promotion of breast cancer. *European Journal of Cancer*, 35(12): 1653-1658.

Stolzenberg-Solomon, R.Z., Pietinen, P., Barrett, M.J. et al. (2001). Dietary and other methyl-group availability factors and pancreatic cancer risk in a cohort of male smokers. *American Journal of Epidemiology*, 153(7): 680-687.

Tascilar, M., van Rees, B.P., Sturm, P.D. et al. (2002). Pancreatic cancer after remote peptic ulcer surgery. *Journal of Clinical Pathology*, 55(5): 340-345.

Terry, P., Suzuki, R., Hu, F.B. et al. (2001). A prospective study of major dietary patterns and the risk of breast cancer. *Cancer Epidemiology, Biomarkers and Prevention*, 10(12): 1281-1285.

Theuer, C. (2000). Asian gastric cancer patients at a Southern California comprehensive cancer center are diagnosed with less advanced disease and have Superior Stage-Stratified Survival. *The American Surgeon*, 66(9): 821-826.

Thune, I., Brenn, T., Lund, E. et al. (1997). Physical activity and the risk of breast cancer. *New England Journal of Medicine*, 336(18): 1269-1275.

Thune, I. and Furberg, A.S. (2001). Physical activity and cancer risk: dose response and cancer, all sites and site-specific. *Medical Science and Sports Exercise*, 33(6): S530-550.

USDHHS. (1988). *U.S. Department of Health and Human Services: The Surgeon General's Report on Nutrition and Health, DHHS (PHS)*. Washington, DC: Department of Health and Human Services, Public Health Service.

Verheul, H.A., Conelingh-Bennink, H.J., Kenemans, P. et al. (2000). Effects of estrogens and hormone replacement therapy on breast cancer risk and on efficacy of breast cancer therapies. *Maturitas*, 36(1): 1-17.

Verloop, J., Rookus, M.A., van der Kooy, K. et al. (2000). Physical activity and breast cancer risk in women aged 20-54 years. *Journal of the National Cancer Institute*, 92(2): 128-135.

Weng, H.H., McBride, C.M., Bosworth, H.B. et al. (2001). Racial differences in physician recommendation of hormone replacement therapy. *Preventive Medicine*, 33(6): 668-673.

White, E., Jacobs, E.J. and Daling, J.R. (1996). Physical activity in relation to colon cancer in middle-aged men and women. *American Journal of Epidemiology*, 144(1): 42-50.

Whittemore, A.S., Wu, A.H., Kolonel, L.N., et al. (1995). Family history and prostate cancer risk in Black, White, and Asian Men in the United States and Canada. *American Journal of Epidemiology*, 141(8): 732-40.

Whittemore, A.S., Kolonel, L.N., Wu, A.H. et al. (1995). Prostate cancer in relation to diet, physical activity, and body size in Blacks, Whites and Asian in the United States and Canada. *Journal of the National Cancer Institute*, 87(9): 652-661.

Willett, W.C., Stampfer, M.J., Colditz, G.A. et al. (1990). Relation of meat, fat, and fiber intake to the risk of colon cancer in a prospective study among women. *New England Journal Medicine*, 323: 1664-1672.

Willett, W.C., Hunter, D.J., Stampfer, M.J. et al. (1992). Dietary fat and fiber in relation to risk of breast cancer. *Journal of the American Medical Association*, 268: 2037-2081.

Williams, R.R. and Horm, J.W. (1977). Association of cancer sites with tobacco and alcohol consumption and socioeconomic status of patients: interview study from the Third National Cancer Survey. *Journal of the National Cancer Institute*, 58(3): 525-547.

Wu, K., Helzlsouer, K.J., Comstock, G.W., et al. (1999). A prospective study on folate, B12, and pyridoxal 5'-phosphate (B6) and breast cancer. *Epidemiology, Biomarkers and Prevention*, 8(3): 209-217.

Wu, A., Wan, P. and Bernstein, L. (2001). A multiethnic population-based study of smoking, alcohol, and body size and risk for adenocarcinomas of the stomach and esophagus (United States). *Cancer Causes and Control*, 12(8): 721-732.

Wu, Z.H., Black, S.A. and Markides, K.S. (2001). Prevalence and associated factors of cancer screening: why are so many older Mexican American women never screened? *Preventive Medicine*, 33(4): 268-273.

Wyatt, S.W., Lancaster, M., Bottorff, D. et al. (2001). History of tobacco use among Kentucky women diagnosed with invasive cervical cancer: 1997-1998. *Journal of the Kentucky Medical Association*, 99(12): 537-539.

Yellowitz, J.A., Goodman, H.S. and Farooq, N.S. (1997). Knowledge, opinions, and practices related to oral cancer: results of three elderly racial groups. *Special Care Dentist*, 17(3): 100-104.

Young, T.B., Ford, C.N. and Brandenburg, J.H. (1986). An epidemiologic study of oral cancer in a state-wide network. *American Journal of Otolaryngology*, 7(3): 200-208.

Yang, P.C., Thomas, D.B., Daling, J.R. et al. (1989). Differences in the sex ratio of laryngeal cancer incidence rates by anatomic subsite. *Journal of Clinical Epidemiology*, 42(8): 755-758.

Zhang, Y., Kreger, B.E. and Dorgan, J.F. (1999). Alcohol consumption and risk of breast cancer: the Framingham Study revisited. *American Journal of Epidemiology*, 149(2): 93-101.

Chapter 4

Race/Ethnicity and Primary Prevention of Cancers in Elders

In 1979 McKeown noted, 'The role of individual medical care in preventing sickness and premature death is secondary to that of other influences; yet society's investment in health care is based on the premise that it is the major determinant. It is assumed that we are ill and made well, but it is nearer the truth that we are well and made ill ...' (McKeown, 1979). The important role of prevention is better recognized among younger populations and in the context of infectious disease. The role of prevention is considered almost paradoxical in older adults and chronic disease, because of the presumed cumulative negative effect of years of exposure to behavioral and environmental risks. There is, however, growing epidemiological and experimental evidence that prevention activities can have beneficial health effects along the continuum of aging, as well as in the presence of chronic disease. Smoking cessation, physical activity and exercise, a healthful diet, and alcohol use cessation or moderation have all been shown to be associated with improved cardiovascular and respiratory health as well as improved quality of life. Notwithstanding this emerging consensus, the care our health systems provide to older adults focuses primarily on the management of acute disease. The situation is exacerbated in the case of traditionally excluded elders of certain racial/ethnic (R/E) groups as systemic, provider organization, practitioner, and individual factors combine to create barriers to engagement and maintenance of behavior change.

This chapter asks the following question: Is there evidence to support the effectiveness of behavioral interventions addressing physical activity, nutrition, body mass, tobacco use, and alcohol use with African American (AA), American Indian/Alaska Native (AI/AN), Hispanic, Native Hawaiians and Other Pacific Island (NHOPI), and Asian American elders? After briefly discussing our evidence review strategy, attention turns first to studies of care access as a risk factor for inadequate engagement in primary prevention activities. Attention then turns to studies that address each of the major risk behavior change domains and summary conclusions.

Selection and Identification of Interventions

We conducted electronic searches of Medline and PsychInfo from 1985 to 2002, supplemented by backward search using Social Science Citation Index/Web of Science for selected papers. All searches used the following key words to locate studies of elders of color: minority elderly, elders of color, elders, minority, older adults, adults, AA, Hispanic, AI/AN, NHOPI, and Asian American. We used numerous keywords for the domains of behavioral interventions and also considered multiple keywords to identify roles of physicians and other practitioners in behavior changes. For example, for the search on physical activity interventions, additional key words included physical activity, exercise, exercise programs, and health promotion programs. Other sources of information were the RAND Healthy Aging reports for CMS (Shekelle, Stone, Maglioni, et al., 2000) and the Task Force on Community Preventive Services reviews (Zaza, Aguero, Briss, et al., 2002). In order to be considered for this review, source documents needed to (1) have a study population primarily composed of persons of AA, Latino, Asian, AI/AN, or NHOPI decent and/or separate analyses of intervention impact by R/E group; (2) have a study population primarily composed of persons age 50 and older and/or separate analyses for this age group; and (3) use a controlled design and offer at least pre- and post-test measures for a treatment group or treatment/control group post-test measure. In this literature, studies use both behavioral measures and clinical measures to assess outcomes, and we considered studies of both kinds. For example, with respect to nutrition and weight loss, we considered studies with behavioral measures such as consumption of dietary fat, fruits, vegetables, and fiber, as well as studies with clinical measures such as change in cholesterol level, weight, BMI, and blood pressure. We included both single component interventions, as well as programs that targeted multiple behaviors (multi-component models). All papers that appeared to meet these criteria based on abstracts were obtained in full text, and reviewed by at least two study team members for satisfaction of study criteria. Evidence tables were created for these studies only. As we note below, there were insufficient studies of behavior change with elders of color to support meta-analysis. For this reason, we subsequently expanded our searches to include behavior change in general elder populations and persons under age 65 in communities of color.

Behavior Change: The Role of the Health Care System Roles

Health Insurance

In order to receive primary care, having health insurance is a prerequisite. The association of insurance status and preventive service use may be largely a reflection of reduced access to a usual source of care among those with inadequate supplemental insurance. The link between preventive services and primary care is well established. For example, Christensen and Shinogle (1997) report that ambulatory visits among Medicare beneficiaries with supplemental coverage is seven to ten percent higher than among beneficiaries without supplemental coverage and that having a regular source of care can double the likelihood of a physician giving prevention advice on diet, tobacco cessation, and physical activity. Similarly, Gentry, Longo, Housseman, et al., (1999) report that patients were more likely to disclose behavioral risks for disease if they had a usual source of care. Ettner (1999) reports that respondents without a usual source of care report being one-third as likely to have a preventive medical visit during the year, and they have one half the likelihood of reporting behaviors related to substance abuse. AA, Hispanic, and Asian elders report worse experiences with primary care on seven of eight indicators studied in the 1997-1998 Medical Expenditure Panel Survey (Shi, 1999). AA elders were less likely to have a specific doctor they saw at a facility, potentially impoverishing their experience of primary care (Janes, Blackman, Bolen, et al., 1999).

Physicians/Primary Care Practitioners

Although these studies emphasize the importance of Medicare supplemental insurance and a usual source of primary care as strong determinants of access to preventive and cancer detection services, it is important to emphasize the roles of physicians and other medical practitioners in promoting behavior change. For example, there is accumulating evidence that physicians do not counsel all smokers to quit (Frank, Winkleby, Altman, et al., 1991; Goldstein, Niaura, Willey-Lessane, et al., 1997) and even successful smoking cessation interventions that meld physician referral with targeted paraprofessional interventions have been difficult to sustain without ongoing reimbursement and systemic supports. Similarly, lack of time and staff support for physical activity counseling continues to be a concern of physicians (King, 2001). In addition, lack of reimbursement, lack of skill and confidence in counseling for behavior modification is a common concern voiced by physicians for physical activity counseling. Using data from the 1995 National Health Interview Survey, Wee, McCarthy, Davis, (1999) found that only 34% of participants received counseling about physical activity from their physicians. Physicians were less likely to counsel those patients who were only moderately overweight and those from lower socioeconomic groups. Nonetheless, in one study, 40% of community-dwelling Medicare beneficiaries who initiated activity said that their physician was a very important influence (Burton, Shapiro, German, et al., 1999).

Primary care practitioners and elder patients need to be able to prioritize the many competing demands of both preventive care and those of chronic illness. Busy primary care settings cannot consistently implement disparate health behavior interventions; these interventions share common elements that can be combined under a common model (Eakin, 2001). For example, in the area of self-management of chronic illness, a common model has been identified to address health behavior change (Lorig, Sobel, Stewart; 1999, Leveille, Wagner, Davis, 1998; Von Korff, Gruman, Schaeffer, et al., 1997). It appears that supervised health promotion programs with an exercise and chronic disease self-management component with primary care collaboration, covering a variety of behavioral issues, and follow-up telephone counseling may potentially be extremely effective for elders since a large percentage have chronic disease.

Lack of time and staff support for counseling, lack of reimbursement, and lack of skill and confidence in counseling for behavior modification are common barriers to counseling expressed by physicians. For example, using data from the

1995 National Health Interview Survey, Wee and colleagues found that only 34% of participants received counseling about physical activity from their physicians. Physicians appeared to counsel as a form of secondary prevention and were less likely to counsel those patients who were moderately overweight and belonged to lower socioeconomic groups. Higher counseling rates were observed in obese patients or who had comorbid conditions (Wee, 1999). This is unfortunate, because considerable research exists for the effect of physician and other provider counseling on physical activity in adults. For example, a systematic review of the effect of physician counseling to promote physical activity in adults identified thirteen articles in the past 30 years out of which six were randomized controlled trials and seven were quasi-experimental studies (Petrella and Lattanzio, 2002). Most studies used strategies to address stage of change and found positive relationships between counseling for physical activity adoption, stage of change, and change in physical activity level but long-term effect of interventions were not established. Interventions that included written materials, considered behavior change strategies, and provided training and material for physicians effectively increased physical activity levels.

Race/Ethnicity, Elders and Behavioral Interventions

Two major themes arise from the literature on cancer and potentially modifiable risk factors. Epidemiological evidence indicates the importance of behavioral risk factors in many of the most prevalent cancers as well as co-morbid health conditions that influence cancer treatment and other health outcomes. At the same time, there is evidence that underserved R/E group elders sometimes experience greater cumulative lifetime or current exposure to these risks. The potential thus exists to reduce R/E disparities in cancer and health by increasing engagement of these elders in health risk management activities and lifestyle/behavior change programs. Because the literature proved so sparse in this area, we also examined a broader range of review and original papers on increasing engagement of elders, regardless of R/E, increasing engagement of adults of color, regardless of age, and increasing engagement by general adult populations in health risk management.

Physical Activity Interventions

We were unable to find general review articles on physical activity interventions and elders from traditionally excluded R/E groups. One paper focused on AA women (Young, Charleston, Felix-Aaron, 2001). The intervention was designed to optimize social support, group goals were incorporated, and class times were compatible with the church schedule. Sessions began with prayer and inspirational scripture messages. This paper did not report outcomes. Another paper by Baskin, Resnicow, Campbell, et al., (2001) discussed the benefits of public health organizations collaborating with black churches to conduct health promotion programs since the majority of AA adults regularly attend church. Although the paper discussed program examples, we rejected this paper, as it did not report physical activity outcomes.

Physical activity and multi-component programs   Three studies involved underserved R/E adults aged 50 years or greater and focused on physical activity and/or multi-component behavior change, (Kachevar, Smith, Bernard, et al., 2001, Damush, Stump, Saportio, et al., 2001; Agurs-Collins, Kumanyida, Ten Have, et al, 1997). Kachevar and colleagues (2001) conducted a pilot randomized controlled trial with AI/AN elders, aged 55-75 that demonstrated the efficacy of a community-based six-week exercise program in significantly improving self-perceived frequency in exercise participation. Damush et al., (2001), demonstrated how merging of primary care referral to a community-based physical activity program based on social-cognitive theory resulted in improved participation of physical activity in a sample of 500, primarily low-income, AA women, aged 50 or over. A randomized controlled trial of a culturally-sensitive community-based intervention with 64 AA women aged 55-79 years reported a significant mean physical activity score increase of 22 points at 3 months. However, no significant changes were found at 6 months (Agurs-Collins, et al., 1997).

Several reviews of physical activity and multi-component interventions and individual studies with a focus on physical activity in elders were identified. In a comprehensive systematic review, King, Rejeskim, Buchner (1998) identified 29 studies from 1985 to 1997 involving randomized controlled or quasi-experimental interventions to promote in physical activity by older adults. In this review, effective strategies targeting older adults used behavioral or cognitive-behavioral strategies rather than health education, exercise prescriptions, or instruction alone. The review reported increased physical activity participation rates but a relative lack of specific behavioral or program-based strategies aimed at promoting physical activity. A number of studies illustrated that structured group-based physical activity formats did result in short-term improvement (6 months or less), but may not have produced long-term changes in behavior. Studies of interventions using a combination of group and home-based formats found better activity adherence compared to programs that used a group format only. Face-to-face counseling, and structured exercise or home-exercise with ongoing telephone supervision was effective in improving adherence rates up to 2 years in 3 studies. Song, Lee, Lam, Bae, (2003) report on the results from 22 experimental subjects and 21 controls (older women with osteoarthritis) who completed pre- and post-test measures over a 12 week interval for a Tai Chi intervention. Subjects improved on measures of physical activity and functioning. Similarly, a study by Clark, Stump, Damush (2003) of an intervention for 72 mostly low-income, AA women 50 years and older showed that even sub-optimal adherence to moderate-intensity exercise yielded improvements in several outcome measures such as body weight, body mass index, waist circumference, and exercise self-esteem.

Physical activity programs and sites of delivery   Our search for controlled trials of physical activity interventions also revealed a church-based culturally-tailored intervention using the social learning theory, with 20 weekly sessions on physical activity and nutrition, taught by lay advisors. This program improved physical activity at one-year follow-up in AA adults (Yanek, Vecker, Joy, 2001). However, a six month culturally-tailored intervention using the social cognition theory in Mexican American women did not increase physical activity; possibly due to randomization failure (Carlos Poston, Haddock, Olvera, et al., 2001). In another study, an intervention emphasizing self-directed learning and culture was more effective in Pima Indians at preventing weight gain and glucose intolerance, than a more behavioral intervention which involved structured physical activity and nutritional recommendations (Narayan, Hoskin, Kozak, et al., 1998). Both groups reported significantly improved physical activity levels but neither intervention achieved weight loss on average. Thus, an indirect approach motivated from within the culture was more effective than the lifestyle intervention.

A review of 38 randomized controlled studies to determine the effectiveness of physical activity interventions for older adults from 1985 to 2000, identified three types of interventions: home-based, group-based/supervised, and educational (van der Bij, Laurant, et al., 2002). In 16 of the 17 studies reporting participants' ethnicity, samples were exclusively or predominantly white. Authors reported that all three interventions can result in increased physical activity but that changes were small and short-lived without clear evidence on the effectiveness of behavioral reinforcement strategies such as reminder telephone calls, social support, and buddy groups on the initiation and maintenance of physical activity. Only a minority of studies evaluated changes in physical activity levels, with group-based and education interventions effective in increasing physical activity in the short-term. Long-term education interventions were ineffective in improving physical activity levels and insufficient data were available on long-term effectiveness of group-based interventions. A review of the CHAMPS II model, a one-year behavior change program for seniors based on social cognitive theory, showed that 58% of the targeted group adopted a new physical activity and 35% maintained this activity (Stewart, Verboncocur, McLellan, et al., 2001). This study of 173 adults aged 65-90 years is important as it is based on the personal choice model and designed to increase moderate physical activity through utilization of existing community programs. But the sample was fairly well educated and did not include R/E minority elders. Programs like the CHAMPS II could be delivered by community agencies linked with primary care via physician referral with feedback to the physician or having the initial counseling session take place within the primary care setting.

Our review of physical activity interventions in adults included five randomized controlled lifestyle interventions, one pre-post study which included 70% minority adults, one randomized controlled study of minority adult women, one pre-post study of older adults (>65 years), and one randomized controlled study of older adults (>65 years), from 1995 to 1998. This review demonstrated that lifestyle physical activity interventions effectively increased and maintained levels of physical activity to levels that meet or exceed public health guidelines for physical activity using social cognitive theory, the trans-theoretical model, and social learning theory.

Future directions for physical activity programs   There is a need for more emphasis on the role of physician counseling to promote physical activity by elders in underserved R/E groups. Physician counseling on physical activity to ethnic minorities may be very effective, because of the esteem accorded physicians by elders of underprivileged groups. Physicians may believe that counseling patients with low socioeconomic status (SES) is less effective, but data demonstrate that low-income patients are actually more likely to attempt behavioral change based on physician advice (Taira, Safran, Seto, et al., 1997). Offering an option of a primary care referral to a home-based program may need to be looked into. Models using interventions by mail and telephone need to be tested and lifestyle approaches need to be tested in older individuals and those with chronic disease. More research is needed on long-term effectiveness of group-based interventions to promote physical activity and on behavioral interventions in elders with chronic disease.

Although we can not draw firm conclusions about effective and efficient program designs to promote physical activity programs for elders of color, the studies examined here offer evidence to confirm that interventions are effective with general elder populations, and that they can be effective among elders of color. Although social cognitive approaches to physical activity promotion in elders may have some applicability and can help focus the programs, alternatives to traditional group-based intervention may be more effective in promoting physical activity in older adults. These approaches allow older adults to have maximum flexibility in planning the activity and appear to recognize that older individuals are diverse in terms of what type of program will work for them. Successful behavioral interventions in R/E minority elders may require creating an environment of social support and resulting self-initiated behavior (Gregg and Narayan, 1998). Initial face-to-face contact and individualized personal physical activity delivered in traditional group formats, home-based activity programs, (or a combination), reinforced by repeated telephone contact appears essential. Telephone contact needs to be problem-solving oriented and motivational. This follow-up could be delivered by a number of community organizations linked with primary care via physician referral with regular reports sent back to the physician (Eakin, 2001). There is also evidence that linking primary care interventions (by physicians, nurses or paraprofessionals based in the primary care setting) with community-based resources existing outside the health care system can support physical activity for older adults (Leveille, 1998). This is essential for the initial engagement of the lifestyle change, tracking, and reinforcement and enhances the motivational and implementation support that is needed.

Dietary Interventions

There are few studies focusing on dietary interventions for R/E minority elders. Of the seven randomized controlled trials reviewed by Kumanyika, Espeland, and Bahnson (2002) that did focus on this population, five focused on AA elders, one included 41% AA elders, one included both white and AA elders, and only one study included Hispanic elders. Because these studies utilized diverse outcome measures, meta-analysis was inappropriate: for example, 4 studies included a weight loss or change in BMI measure while 3 offered data on fat consumption. Studies also varied with respect to time frames considered, with some considering only change from the beginning to end of the intervention and others considering longer-term outcomes. None considered outcomes over more than 18 months. Findings from these studies do suggest that an intervention including individualized counseling can result in improvements in both behavioral and clinical outcomes measured over the course of the study period for persons who enroll (Kumanyika, et al., 2002).

The Women's Health Trial Feasibility Study in Minority Populations examined 2,208 women ages 50-79 from multiple R/E groups. (Coates, Bowen, Krista, et al., 1999). It showed significant decreases in fat intake after 6 months among women who were assigned a personal fat gram goal and participated in group sessions for 18 months. The intervention was successful in maintaining an 80% participation rate at 18 months. The group sessions in this intervention included discussions of behavioral and nutritional change strategies. The results also showed that there were no significant differences in the results of the intervention between black women and white women. The study found, however, that the intervention was less effective for Hispanic participants. Resnicow, Jackson and Want (2001) conducted a randomized controlled trial with members of 14 AA churches with an intervention including motivational interviewing. In this study, churches, rather than individuals, were randomly assigned to 1) comparison group, 2) self-help intervention with 1 telephone cue call, or 3) self-help with 1 cue call and 3 counseling calls. The telephone counseling for the third group was based on motivational interviewing. The self-help portion of the intervention included a video, cookbook, printed health education materials, and several cues imprinted with project logos. The significant increase in consumption of fruits and vegetables among those receiving motivational interviews highlights the impact that an individual cognitive-emotional intervention can have on behavior change.

Other studies focusing on dietary interventions for R/E minority elders include a culturally tailored modification to the Duke University Rice Diet weight loss program by Ard, Rosati and Oddone (2000), in which 56 AA participants receiving the intervention lost an average of 14.8 pounds, had a decrease in BMI of 2.5kg/m^2, and a decrease in cholesterol of 13.7mg/dL. A recent study looked at 421 overweight white elders and 163 black elders with controlled hypertension (Kumanyika, 2002). Participants were randomized to counseling for weight loss, sodium reduction, both weight loss and sodium reduction, or to usual care which included the use of an anti-hypertensive drug. The combined programs resulted in weight loss for both R/E groups, with no R/E difference in effect.

Interventions targeting adults of color have found that diet interventions can successfully change behavior. For example, the Southeast Cholesterol Project (Keyserling, Ammerman, Davis, 1997) used the 'Food for Heart Program' consisting of dietary risk assessment, clinician counseling materials, and culturally specific patient education materials. Patients in 21 rural health centers (of whom 40% were aged over 50, and 40% were AA) were randomized to usual care or to the dietary intervention. Significant improvements were found for total serum cholesterol, LDL, and dietary change in the intervention group. At one-year follow-up, the reduction in cholesterol was 0.09 mmol/L greater for the intervention group compared to the control group.

Other weight loss interventions No review paper on weight loss interventions with adults of color was identified. Available studies of weight loss interventions in populations of color have focused on the under 65 population. For example, one study looked at physiological responses of inactive obese pre-menopausal AA and Caucasian women to a 13-week exercise training and behavior modification program (Glass, Miller, Szymanski, et al., 2002). The results of the study showed that there were similar outcomes across R/E group for number of exercise sessions completed, total minutes of exercise for the entire intervention, the average minutes of daily exercise, and total estimated exercise energy expenditure. Other results showed similar and statistically significant reductions in BMI, and girth measurements. These results indicate that the higher prevalence of obesity in AA women is not due to unique physiological responses to diet and exercise, and it seems reasonable that these findings may be generalized to elders. Agurs-Collins and colleagues conducted a weight loss intervention for 64 overweight African Americans with non-insulin dependent diabetes ages 55-79 (Agurs-Collins, et al., 1997). The intervention included twelve weekly group sessions, 1 individual session and 6 biweekly group sessions. There were two comparison 'usual care' groups in this study. The first received 1 individual session and 6 biweekly sessions. The second received 1 class and 2 informational mailings. At three months, there were statistically significant differences between the intervention and the usual care groups for weight, level of physical activity, dietary intake of fat, saturated fat, cholesterol, nutrition knowledge, and HbA1c. At six months statistically significant differences were found for weight and HbA1c.

A study of the effects of dietary counseling for fat and/or energy reduction and weight loss in 86 AA and white pre-menopausal women showed that a low-fat, low-energy diet resulted in similar, statistically significant decreases in BMI, percent body fat, and waist circumference in both R/E groups (Djuric, Lababidi, Heilbrun, et al., 2002). McMahon, Fujioka, Singh, et al, (2000) studied the efficacy of the use of sibutramine, a weight-loss drug, in obese white and African Americans patients with hypertension. The intervention group experienced weight loss within the first 6 months and maintained weight until the end of the 12-months period; changes in body weight were similar for both white and AA patients. Another study looked at the impact of motivational interviewing in improving adherence to behavioral weight-control programs for older, R/E diverse obese women with non-insulin dependent diabetes (Smith, Heckemeyer, Kratt, et al., 1997). Of the women participating women, 42% were AA. Participants were assigned to one of two groups. The first group was assigned to a standard 16-week behavioral weight-control program providing instruction in diet, exercise, and behavioral modification. The second group was assigned to the same group behavioral program with three individualized motivational interviewing sessions added. Outcome measures for this study included weight loss, attendance at group meetings, recording food diaries, and recording blood glucose levels. The results showed that those receiving the motivational interviews were more likely to: attend group meetings, complete food diaries, and record blood glucose levels. Members of both groups experienced weight loss, but there was not a statistically significant difference between the groups.

In a pre - and post - test one group study, 23 pre-menopausal AA women participated in a 32 week culturally tailored lifestyle enhancement awareness program of 16 weekly sessions on weight loss (setting goals, monitoring eating behavior and addressing factors influencing weight loss) and 16 weekly sessions on weight loss maintenance (addressing relapse); factors associated with both weight loss and weight loss maintenance were studied (Walcott-McQuigg, Chen, Davis, et al., 2002). Women completing the weight loss program showed significant reductions in BMI, percentage body fat, waist/hip ratio, and a significant increase in exercise activity, with weight loss being significantly correlated with attendance and dietary readiness to decrease emotional eating. Women who completed the weight maintenance program maintained a significant loss in BMI, and increased their HDL and dietary readiness to monitor hunger and eating cues.

Recruiting volunteers and maintaining participation for the entire course of dietary intervention studies has been identified as a critical issue in this literature. For example, in a study by Yanek and colleagues, churches, rather than individuals were assigned to treatment and controls. The researchers encountered difficulty in getting churches to agree to have their members be in the control group (Yanek, 2001). The problem with maintaining volunteer participation over a study is highlighted in this same study where, at one-year follow-up, only 56% of participants completed the biological measures of the study and only 38% completed the behavioral, diet, and physical activity measures. Another problem is that most of the dietary intervention literature has been targeted to the general adult population, not R/E minorities, and there is a wealth of information from major national interventions and smaller studies. The CDC's 5 A Day for Better Health Program is an example of a dietary intervention aimed at providing educational materials to individuals of all ages and races in order to increase their consumption of fruits and vegetables. For example, results of a pilot study of an educational intervention to increase fruit and vegetable consumption among callers to the Cancer Information Service found that a brief educational message using materials from the '5 A Day for Better Health Program' and reinforcement with follow-up mailings led to behavior change (Marcus, Morris, Rimer, 1998). The study also showed that after a 4-week follow-up subjects consumed an average of 0.75 additional servings per day compared to before the intervention.

Tilley, Glanz, Kristal (1999) report the results of the Next Step Trial worksite dietary intervention. This randomized control trial included 5,042 employees, 66% were over age 50, and 97% were male. The intervention included classes, mailed self-help materials, and personalized dietary feedback. At one-year follow-up, there was a statistically significant 0.9% decrease in fat consumption, a 0.5g/1,000 kcal increase in fiber consumption, and a 0.2 serving/day increase in the consumption of fruits and vegetables. At two years, these results were significant for fiber only. Miller conducted a meta-analysis of weight loss research over twenty-five years comparing the effects of diet only, exercise only, and diet plus exercise (Miller, Koceja, Hamilton, 1997). The results show that the weight loss over a 15-week period for a middle-aged population from each of these methods was 10.7 +/- 0.5, 2.9 +/- 0.4, and 11.0 +/- 0.6 kg, respectively. However, the results at one-year follow up indicate that diet plus exercise was the most effective method of weight loss. Another meta-analysis looked at effect of a low-fat diet on weight loss (Astrup, Gurnwald, G., and Melanson, 2000). The authors found that the low-fat intervention produced a mean fat reduction of 10.2% (8.1-12.3). The low-fat intervention group also had greater weight loss compared to controls.

A recent literature review of dietary intervention and disease prevention highlights the impact that diet can have on preventing cancer, heart disease, stroke, and non-insulin dependent diabetes (Bowen and Beresford, 2002). This work synthesizes the results of interventions aimed at individuals, families, and those delivered through providers and through other community channels such as worksites, churches, and grocery stores. Most of the studies reviewed did not focus on interventions for R/E groups but taken together, these studies give some indication of the effectiveness of interventions in the general population. The results of this literature review indicate that most individual intervention studies have been geared toward individuals with existing risk factors and to individuals who were motivated to change behavior in some way. Because highly motivated individuals are more likely to engage fully in the interventions, this leads to the conclusion that more intense interventions can result in larger effect sizes. For this reason, self-selection of volunteers plays an important part in the outcome of a study, and building more evidence on the determinants of engagement arises as a central concern. A similar finding was reported in an Evidence Report from the Agency for Healthcare Research and Quality entitled 'Efficacy of Interventions To Modify Dietary Behavior Related to Cancer Risk.' (AHRQ, 2000) This report found that in a review of studies on fruit intake, all six studies that were conducted in high-risk populations reported significant intervention effects compared to only eight out of fourteen studies conducted among general-risk populations. This is not, however, direct evidence that fruitful intervention strategies can be effectively adapted to use by Medicare beneficiaries of color in need of such services.

In its review of 92 studies on the impact of interventions on dietary fat intake and consumption fruits and vegetables the AHRQ Evidence Report concludes that there are several dietary interventions that appear to be effective in modifying diet (AHRQ, 2000). These include interventions involving social support, goal setting, small groups, food-related activities such as cooking, and interventions with a family component. Of seven studies reviewed that used social support as part of the intervention, all seven reported a significant intervention effect for total fat intake. This report also emphasizes the need for future dietary intervention research to follow participants for more than one year in order to learn more about the long term effects of dietary intervention, the maintenance of change, and the prevention of relapse over time.

Tobacco Use Reduction Interventions

Literature reviews reveal almost no published studies of tobacco use reduction interventions conducted with elders, irrespective of R/E group. Elders have been included in general populations studies of a wide range of tobacco use reduction interventions (clinical treatment, community-based interventions and mass media programs) and in studies of culturally-tailored programs directed at specific R/E communities. There appear to be no published studies that report separate impact findings for R/E minority elders of behavioral, NRT, or anti-depressant interventions. The Public Health Service guideline, *Treating Tobacco Use and Dependence* (Fiore, Bailey, Cohen, et al, 2000) identifies effective treatments and specific responsibilities for clinical practice sites, for cessation specialists and for health care systems. Notwithstanding the potential differences in the ways in which some racial/ethnic groups might absorb and metabolize constituents of tobacco smoke, dose-related counseling for R/E minority elders will be effective as will pharmacotherapy; and health care systems must support the continuing clinical treatment of tobacco use.

The other theme is that strategies for tobacco use reduction among underserved R/E group elders require cultural tailoring. In the general population, only a fraction of current smokers seek out assistance in tobacco cessation. Engaging the current smoker in treatment is a formidable challenge across all populations; and since smokers in communities of color may respond to mass media and tobacco cessation messages differently from whites (Warnecke, Flay, Kviz, et al., 1991), specific cultural tailoring of programs, and promotion of those programs, can assist in engaging these elders. Research conducted by the NCI-funded *Programa Latino Para Dejar de Fumar*, for example, on the attitudes, expectancies and values of Hispanic smokers led to strategies that incorporate familism (the normative and behavioral influence of relatives) and *simpatía* (a social mandate for positive social relationships) (Perez-/Stable et al. 1993, Marin and Perez-Stable, Marina, 1995). The self-help manual developed in this program was just one example cited in a 1998 Surgeon General's report on tobacco use among R/E minority groups (US National Center for Chronic Disease Prevention and Health Promotion, 1998). It should be noted, however, that emerging research and theory on cultural factors and decision-making suggests that building programs that effectively engage these values requires greater attention to context and competing motivation (Briley, Morris, and Simonson, 2000). Other examples included programs for American Indian, Chinese, and Vietnamese communities. Similarly, the Massachusetts Tobacco Control Program has developed tobacco media campaigns for minority populations. These culturally-tailored interventions have been variously described but not rigorously tested for effectiveness. One exception is a study of a Vietnamese intervention in Santa Clara County (Lai, McPhee, Jenkins, et al., 2000) that found reasonable participation rates and high quit rates.

Pederson, Ahluwalia, Harris, (2000) reviewed cessation programs and self-quitting for African Americans in 56 studies from 1988-98. The study, which examined 56 studies, concluded that church-based cessation programs may provide an appropriate location for interventions but did not demonstrate unequivocal effectiveness. Community-based interventions showed no differences between African Americans and whites. Although clinic-based programs for AA smokers did not demonstrate effectiveness in this review, a double-blind, placebo-controlled, randomized trial at an inner-city hospital outpatient program conducted by Ahluwalia, McNagny, Clark, et al., (1998) showed 17.1% 6-month quit rates with the nicotine patch as compared to 11.7% with the placebo patch. More recently, Ahluwalia, Harris, Catley, et al., (2002) examined the effects of bupropion versus placebo along with 8 motivational counseling sessions by AA counselors, in a randomized double-blind, placebo controlled trial in 600 African American adult smokers treated at a community-based health care center over a 7 week period. The intervention group experienced a significantly greater mean reduction in depression symptoms at week 6 compared to the placebo group, and the intervention group also gained significantly less weight.

Fisher, Auslander, Munro et al., (1998) examined a community intervention in low-income AA neighborhoods in St. Louis that involved cessation classes, a billboard campaign and door-to-door distribution of self-help materials. The program reduced prevalence from 34% to 27% in the intervention neighborhoods as compared to a 1% reduction (from 34% to 33%) in control neighborhoods in Kansas City. Schorling, Roach, Siegel, et al., (1997) studied a church-based intervention in Virginia – consisting of individual counseling and self-help materials within the context of community activities – implemented in one rural community demonstrated changes in smokers' stages of change compared to a control county (Schorling, et al., 1997). Another stages-of-change intervention, developed and tested in Harlem by the Harlem Health Connection (involving a culturally-tailored cessation guide, a cessation video featuring AA historical figures and telephone support) did not reveal a significant difference in quit rates compared to a control group that received non-tobacco specific health education materials. An intervention by Goldberg to train medical students found changes in stages of change of outpatient smokers compared to control groups, but not in quit rates (Goldberg, Hoffman, Farinha, et al., 1994).

One study with great salience for tobacco use by elders of color found that quitting tobacco extends life regardless of age of quitting. This study by Taylor et al (2002) analyses data compiled on 676,306 women and 508,351 men participating in Cancer Prevention II, a prospective study begun in 1982. Taylor et al., found that tobacco users who quit at age 65 gain 2.0 years of life expectancy among men and 3.7 years among women. Despite the gains in life extension and quality of life from smoking cessation at any age, elders may be less likely to perceive the benefits of quitting or the continued harm of smoking, according to a RAND evidence review and meta-analysis, 'Interventions to Promote Smoking Cessation in the Medicare Population'. The RAND study identified 488 articles (248 of which satisfied screening criteria), of which 149 related to patient education, 118 to individual counseling, 104 self-help, and 76 involving patient financial incentives. This study concluded that individual, telephone and group counseling as well as pharmacotherapy are effective in promoting smoking cessation.

Multi-Component and Disease Self-Management Interventions

A growing literature reports on interventions that promote disease self-management by targeting multiple behaviors. We found impressive evidence for the effectiveness of elder chronic disease self-management programs (Lorig, Sobel, Stewart, et al., 1999; Leveille, 1998). Lorig and her colleagues examined the effects of a nurse-supervised self-management program for 952 adults with chronic disease during a six-month randomized controlled trial at community-based sites such as churches, senior centers, community centers, libraries, and health care facilities. They found that treatment subjects demonstrated significant improvement in exercise minutes per week as well as fewer hospitalizations and days in the hospital so that health care expenditure savings approximated $750 per participant, more than 10 times the cost of the intervention (Lorig et al., 1999). Leveille et al provided evidence that a one year senior center based randomized, controlled, chronic disease self-management and physical activity program which collaborated with primary care providers for 201 chronically ill older adults, significantly improved physical activity levels. The study also concluded that the intervention reduced hospital days in the intervention group (increased number of hospitalized participants by 69% in controls and decreased by 38% in intervention group), thus yielding a savings of at least $400 per participant per year. The intervention consisted of a targeted health management plan developed by the participants and a geriatric nurse practitioner focusing on risk factors along with physical activity (either senior center or home based) and chronic illness programs, three follow-up visits, and 9 phone contacts by the nurse. These studies were done in predominantly white, relatively educated communities and it is unclear how these models may need to be adapted to other populations and communities.

Findings from a meta-analysis of randomized and non-randomized controlled trials evaluating patient education and counseling for preventive health behaviors including 39 studies on smoking/alcohol, 17 studies on nutrition/weight control, and 18 studies on other topics in patients without diagnosed disease, made a strong case for systematic delivery of these interventions by health care providers (Mullen, Simons-Morton, Ramirez, et al., 1997). Using behavioral techniques specifically self-monitoring and using several communication channels such as media plus personal communication produced larger effects for the smoking/alcohol and nutrition/weight groups.

Another randomized controlled 6-month pilot study of disability prevention and health promotion of 100 elders was also identified (Wallace, Buchner, Grothaus, et al., 1998). This study conducted at a senior center serving predominantly White elders, included a health promotion program with supervised exercise three times a week for 6 months, nutrition counseling, smoking and alcohol cessation interventions as needed, and telephone follow-up by a nurse at 2, 4 and 16 weeks to review subjects' progress. Improved SF-36 scores and disability days demonstrated the feasibility and efficacy of providing a health-promotion program in a community senior center where physical activity improved, thus impacting health and functional status. Involvement with a health provider and social activation at the senior center could have contributed towards the improved outcomes.

Gold and colleagues examined the effectiveness of a telephone-based health promotion program targeting 1741 high risk, ready-to-change adults using a quasi-experimental design with pre/post between-group comparisons of lifestyle related health risks (Gold, Anderson, Serxner, 2000). Programs were offered in cholesterol control, eating habits, exercise and activities, stress management, tobacco use, weight control, and back care, and conducted by a health educator providing 3-5 telephone counseling contacts designed to produce change over a one-year period. Participants were 1.6 to 3.5 times as likely as non-participants to reduce targeted risk in six of seven risk areas. Overall, participants significantly reduced their number of risks whereas non-participants significantly increased their risks. In this study, subjects were not randomized to either control or treatment group. Wilcox et al conducted a quantitative literature review that examined the magnitude of the effects of 32 studies on dietary and physical activity interventions delivered in health care settings in reducing cardiovascular risk factors (Wilcox, Parra-Medina, Thompson-Robinson, 2001). Intervention effects were modest but statistically significant for physical activity, body mass index, dietary fat, blood pressure, and total and low-density cholesterol.

Cost-Effectiveness Studies in Medicare Populations

Several initiatives have explored health promotion interventions for the Medicare population. Two reports discuss a demonstration health-promotion program implemented in a staff-model HMO designed to test cost-effectiveness and outcomes of the program at 24 and 48 months for 2558 Medicare beneficiaries (Patrick, Grembowski, Durham, et al., 1999). Researchers offered intervention participants a health-risk assessment, health promotion visit, disease prevention visit, and follow-up classes compared to usual care for control group participants. At 24 and 48 months, the treatment group participated in significantly more exercise and consumed less dietary fat. But the intervention did not yield lower cost per quality-adjusted life years and total cost of care did not significantly differ between the two groups, except for the capitation amount of $186 per treatment-group enrollee per year.

Another demonstration study determined whether adding a benefit for yearly preventive visits for 2 years and optional counseling visits to their primary care provider to 4,195 older Medicare beneficiaries affected costs, comparing Medicare claims data for the two years in which preventive visits occurred (Burton, Paglia, German, et al, 1995). They reported no significant differences in charges between the intervention and control groups with a modest health benefit seen in the intervention group. German, et al., (1995) reporting results on this same demonstration noted that 63% of beneficiaries in the intervention group made a preventive clinical visit and approximately 50% made a counseling visit. The results of this study showed that those in the intervention group had a greater health benefit as measured by mortality. The death rate in the intervention group was 8.3% compared to 11.1% in the control intervention group.

Health Risk Appraisals and Motivational Interviewing

The RAND Evidence Report on Health Risk Appraisals (HRA) and Medicare provided evidence-based recommendations regarding the use of HRA in health promotion programs for elders (Shekelle, 2002). Out of a total of 267 journal articles, unpublished reports, and conference presentations, 27 were controlled trials and data indicated that the more intensive interventions, which included follow-up and feedback following HRA, are the most effective. This data agreed with the Leveille study in which follow-up telephone contact was essential after establishing the initial health promotion program (Leveille, 1998). However, out of the 27 controlled trials, 7 studies were reported to have 85% or more white persons, 18 gave no data regarding race/ethnicity, one study with mean age 39-43 years had >50% white persons, and another study had >84% white. The study concluded that these interventions were most likely to be effective when feedback on health risks is combined with follow-up interventions and materials, but programs that use HRA alone or with a single follow-up contact do not appear to hold promise.

Health risk appraisals that follow-through with programs using tailored print communications (TPCs) created especially for an individual based upon knowledge about that individual were particularly effective in conveying risk information that was comprehensible to the individual. These materials provide individually relevant and appropriate information. For example, Rimer and Glassman (1999) described the uses and effectiveness of TPC for several areas of cancer risk communication such as dietary change, smoking cessation, mammography use, hormone replacement therapy, and genetic susceptibility to cancer. Following health risk appraisals, the use of individualized learning plans and motivational interviewing has also been proven to increase the motivation of individuals who need to change health behaviors.

Miller and Moyers (2002) described theoretical assumptions of motivational interviewing, controversies surrounding denial and resistance, and combinations of motivational interviewing with other treatments. Motivational Interviewing is a technique that has potential for successful application in effecting behavior change. Since it is by definition customized to the individual, it should be an effective method amongst underserved populations as well. Dunn and colleagues conducted a systematic review of 29 randomized trials of motivational interventions for four behavioral domains: substance abuse, smoking, HIV risk and diet/exercise (Dunn et al, 2001). Out of the 29 studies, 60% yielded at least one significant behavior change effect. Substantial evidence existed that motivational interviewing techniques are effective for substance abuse when used by clinicians who are non-specialists in substance abuse treatment, but data were inadequate to judge the effect of motivational interviewing for the other domains. There was no significant association between length of follow-up time and magnitude of effect size.

Stein and colleagues tested motivational interviewing for reducing alcohol use on 187 needle exchange clients through a randomized clinical trial (Stein, Charuvastra, Maksad et al, 2002). The brief motivational interview consisted of two 1-hour therapist sessions following assessments visits, one month apart, and focused on alcohol use and HIV risk-taking. Drinking days were significantly reduced in both groups, but comparisons on dichotomous outcomes showed that those in the motivational interview group were over two times more likely than controls to report reductions of 7 days or more. Heavier drinkers appeared more suited for this intervention, but further research is needed on optimal intensity of treatments and which components of motivational interview are most effective.

A further study reported preliminary and modest support of a motivational interview strategy used for 269 resistant pregnant smokers (Stotts, Diclementa, Dollan-Mullen, 2002). In this prospective, randomized, controlled trial, all participants received brief counseling plus a self-help booklet at their first pre-natal visit and seven booklets mailed weekly, while the intervention groups received a stage of change-based personalized feedback letter and two telephone counseling calls using motivational interviewing strategies. All participants reported smoking in the past 28 days at 28 weeks. An implementation analysis suggested that 43% of women in the intervention group were classified as not smoking compared to 34% of the control group and at 6 weeks postpartum, 27% of the experimental group reported being abstinent or light smokers, versus 14.6% of the controls.

Discussion and Conclusions

We are of the firm conviction that the next paradigm shift needed to improve overall health status will emerge from extensive education about, awareness of, and adherence to health-promoting lifestyles and behaviors. Yet healthcare financing and delivery systems as well as healthcare practitioners are largely focused on diagnosis and treatment of acute disease. Noteworthy barriers to adopting and adhering to recommended health promoting behavior patterns have been erected. Not only are interventions such as those directed towards the need for physical activity, good nutrition, and avoiding substance abuse (including tobacco) under-utilized; they are rarely, if ever, targeted towards older adults and especially older adults of color, because of three popular concepts: 1) The benefits of prevention activities diminish rapidly in the face of 'normal aging'; 2) Prevention is not as effective once chronic disease processes have begun; and 3) Older adults are less responsive to health education and promotion activities.

These concepts may be even more insidious in the case of underserved R/E populations, but recent research in gerontology, geriatrics, and chronic disease management suggests that all three concepts may be somewhat remediable (Rowe, 1999; Vita, Terru, Hubert, 1998; Russell, Carson, Taylor, 1998; Ornish, Scherwitz, Billings et al., 1998). In order to do so, recognition of a failure by public policy, health care provider organizations, and practitioners needs to be a starting place for major re-thinking of how our society cares for elders. The disconnect between current understanding of cancer prevention and health promotion and current practice in care for older adults can be addressed through efforts directed to: 1) Reducing barriers erected by patients; 2) Reducing barriers created by providers; 3) Reducing barriers connected to program design or financing of care.

Reducing Patient Barriers

Gaps exist in educating older adults regarding primary prevention. They are bombarded on a daily basis with conflicting information on behavioral changes and their relationships to cancer or other health outcomes. Yet they receive little support from health professionals and others in sorting through this information, distinguishing credible and actionable recommendations from commercial claims, or finding sources of support for appropriate lifestyle modification. In response to this confusing environment and the failure of the health care system to provide consistent and clear recommendations and support, elders may develop a sense that continuing existing behaviors is the best response. At the same time, many of the proposed options for adopting healthy behaviors that have received the greatest attention and support are presented in culturally insensitive ways or seem to require extraordinary efforts. Elders may find such activities too time-consuming, report that they cause discomfort, or say that the benefits are not immediately tangible. Moreover, older adults may develop an attitude of hopelessness regarding growing older, and become seemingly resigned to the immutability of lifelong habits that are harmful to health. They may accept functional limitations as an inevitable consequence of aging and think it is too late to gain advantages from incorporating healthful practices into their daily routine.

Reducing Provider Barriers

An emerging body of evidence has demonstrated that physicians and other health practitioners are not being as effective as they might be in intervening with elders and particularly R/E minority elders around cancer prevention and health promotion issues. Although these practitioners are not the only, or necessarily the best sources of motivation and support for behavior modifications, their lack of adequate involvement in supporting healthy lifestyles has emerged as a significant barrier.

Most providers are trained to treat disease. There is inadequate training and sensitivity to the need for preventive services, and inconsistency in how preventive services are prescribed. Physicians acknowledge both the importance of delivering preventive services to their patients and their responsibility, but few consider themselves successful at highlighting prevention and many do not even try (Wechsler, Levine, Idelson, et al., 1996). Training about prevention is not always thoroughly incorporated into clinical syllabi and does not emphasize the importance of such practices in the treatment of individuals throughout the lifespan.

Both established practitioners and trainees have been reluctant to focus on behavioral risk reduction interventions because of ongoing uncertainties in current understanding of the roles of behavior in carcinogenesis and other disease processes. As indicated in our review more and more studies seek to elucidate the multi-factorial nature of carcinogenesis. For example, understanding the gradual process of the transition from adenomatous polyp to adenocarcinoma allows one to examine and modify lifestyle (reducing red meat, alcohol and tobacco, increasing physical activity, using chemoprevention) (Alberts, 2002). Similarly, since oxidative damage is increasingly recognized as an important factor in the pathogenesis of numerous diseases including cancer and cardiovascular disorders, studies are being done to learn more about the constellation affecting antioxidant capacity. For example, non-smoking, regular activity and a nutrient-rich diet are positively associated with increased antioxidant capacity, while smoking, psychological stress, alcohol consumption, low fruit and low fish consumption were shown to be negatively associated with antioxidant capacity (Lesgards, Durand, Lasarre, et al., 2002). The authors conclude that 'the evaluation of the total human resistance against free-radical aggression, taking into account nutritional habits, lifestyle, and environmental factors, maybe useful in preventive medicine as a precocious diagnosis to identify healthy subjects' (who are at risk for cancer).

It is expected that answers to the relationship between lifestyle factors, environmental exposures, and the risk of cancer, mortality, and survival will require the conduct of large-scale, prospective cohort studies such as the Cancer Prevention Study II sponsored by the American Cancer Society, (Calle, Rodriguez, Jacobs, et al., 2002). This study investigates for dietary, hormonal, genetic, physical activity, medication use and other factors and association with cancer risk. Meanwhile, large gaps exist in our understanding of these causes of cancer. For example, the association between fat intake and prostate or breast cancer remains inconclusive (Moyad, 2002). Recommendations to modify behavior need not wait, however, until the results of these prospective studies.

While it is imperative that those charged with managing older patients (such as geriatricians and geriatric nurse practitioners) understand the ongoing benefits of prevention at any age, and even as disease advances, such understanding is equally important for practitioners trained in other specialties or serving other age populations. In particular, community-based social and supportive service and lifestyle enrichment practitioners serving elders and other older adults may play pivotal roles in supporting health promoting choices and activities. As the aging patient population grows larger, many practitioners will likely encounter older adults in their professional careers, and unless practitioners are aware of the potential, they may miss opportunities to advocate and practice prevention for older adults. Similarly, as the demographics change, and our elderly become more racially and ethnically diverse, providers will need to be more sensitive to, and capable of, delivering culturally competent care.

Current programs for delivering health care preferentially reimburse for acute care services, rather than for prevention and health promotion. Other than a few underutilized clinical preventive and screening procedures, this is especially true for older adults. Furthermore, once chronic conditions become apparent, we fail to make use of continuing prevention efforts to slow progression and improve the functioning of older adults. This places an inordinate burden on the health care system.

Reducing Programmatic Barriers

Serious health insurance barriers also exist. For those without insurance, the problem is compounded by the fact that there is often no usual source of care and that even basic screening services are not available. Even when some preventive services are covered, as through Medicare, their rate of use is erratic (Wennberg,

1999). Particularly for elders living alone, loss of mobility as one gets older, social isolation, and poverty hamper access to prevention services even if they are available in the community.

Unless these features of most delivery systems are altered, it is unlikely that several proven prevention interventions will actually become widespread. Different mechanisms for promoting their use therefore need to be encouraged. Likewise, until delivery systems allocate sufficient time for meaningful communication between health care providers and their older patients, lack of knowledge and awareness, misunderstandings, and 'lack of compliance' will certainly persist. The literature shows that the best preventive care for older adults is composed of a combination of ambulatory services including patient education, life-style counseling, and clinical oversight through routine check-ups and timely screening (Waltzer, 1998), both able to be done in an efficient and cost-effective way despite resource constraints. Although the literature on behavior change for elders in underserved R/E groups is sparse, several scholars have suggested that there might be few differences between white elders and elders from non-white groups in their responses to these interventions. Major conclusions from systematic reviews of behavioral interventions from studies addressing general (primarily White) populations shows that there is evidence for effective programs that target specific behavioral changes. However, it has proven difficult to engage and maintain engagement of white older adults and R/E diverse adult populations in these programs.

References

Agurs-Collins, T., Kumanyika, S., Ten Have, T. et al. (1997). A randomized controlled trial of weight reduction and exercise for diabetes management in older African-American subjects. *Diabetes Care*, 20(10): 1503-1511.

Ahluwalia, J.S., McNagny, S.E. and Clark, S. (1998). Smoking cessation among inner-city African-Americans using the nicotine transdermal patch. *Journal of General Internal Medicine*, 13(1): 1-8.

Ahluwalia, J.S., Harris, K.J., Catley, D., Okuyemi, K.S. and Mayo, M.S. (2002). Sustained-release bupropion for smoking cessation in African Americans: A randomized controlled trial. *Journal of the American Medical Association*, 288(4): 468-474.

AHRQ. (2000). *Efficacy of Interventions To Modify Dietary Behavior Related to Cancer Risk* (Evidence Report/Technology Assessment: Number 25 AHRQ Publication No. 01-E028). Rockville, MD: Agency for Healthcare Research and Quality.

Alberts, D.S. (2002). Reducing the risk of colorectal cancer by intervening in the process of carcinogenesis: A status report. *Cancer Journal*, 8(3): 208-21.

Ard, J., Rosati, R. and Oddone, E. (2000). Culturally-sensitive weight loss program produces significant reduction in weight, blood pressure, and cholesterol in eight weeks. *Journal of the National Medical Association*, 92(11): 515-523.

Astrup, A., Gurnwald, G. and Melanson, E. (2000). The role of low-fat diets in body weight control: A meta-analysis of ad libitum dietary intervention studies. *International Journal of Obesity*, 24:1545-1552.

Au, G.K. (2000). Evaluation of the benefits and risks of hormone replacement therapy. *Hong Kong Medical Journal*, 6(4): 381-389.

Baskin, M., Resnicow, K. and Campbell, M.K. (2001). Conducting health interventions in Black churches: A model for building effective partnerships. *Ethnic Disparities*, 11: 823-833.

Bowen, D. and Bereford, S. (2002). Dietary interventions to prevent disease. *Annual Review of Public Health*, 23: 255-286.

Burton, L., Paglia, M.J., German, P.S. et al. (1995). The effect among older persons of a general preventive visit on three health behaviors: Smoking, excessive alcohol drinking, and sedentary lifestyle. *Preventive Medicine*, 24(5): 492-497.

Burton, L., Shapiro, S. and German, P. (1999). Determinants of physical activity initiation and maintenance among community-dwelling older persons. *Preventive Medicine*, 29(5): 422-430.

Calle, E.E., Rodriguez, C., Jacobs, E.J. et al. (2002). The American Cancer Society Cancer Prevention Study II Nutrition Cohort: Rationale, study design, and baseline characteristics. *Cancer*, 94(9): 2490-2501.

Carlos Poston II, W., Haddock, K., Olvera, N.E. et al. (2001). Evaluation of a culturally appropriate intervention to increase physical activity. *American Journal of Health Behavior*, 25(4): 396-406.

CDC – U.S. Centers for Disease Control and Prevention, National Center for Chronic Disease Prevention and Health Promotion, and Office on Smoking and Health. (1999). *Best Practices for Comprehensive Tobacco Control Programs – August 1999 (Reprinted, with corrections)*. Atlanta G.A.: U.S. Department of Health and Human Services.

Christensen, S. and Shinogle, J. (1997). Effects of supplemental coverage on use of services by Medicare enrollees. *Health Care Financing Review*, 19(1): 5-17.

Clark, D.O., Stump, T.E. and Damush, T.M. (2003). Outcomes of an exercise program for older women recruited through primary care. *Journal of Aging and Health*, 15(3): 567-585.

Clarke, G. and Whittemore, A.S. (2000). Prostate cancer risk in relation to anthropometry and physical activity: The National Health and Nutrition Examination Survey I Epidemiological Follow-Up Study. *Cancer Epidemiology, Biomarkers and Prevention*, 9(9): 875-881.

Coates, R.J., Bowen, D.J., Kristal, A.R. et al. (1999). The Women's Health Trial Feasibility Study in Minority Populations: Changes in dietary intakes. *American Journal of Epidemiology*, 149(12): 1104-1112.

Conn, V.S., Minor, M.A., Burks, K.J. et al. (2003). Integrative review of physical activity intervention research with aging adults. *Journal of the American Geriatrics Society*, 51(8): 1159-1168

Damush, T., Stump, T., Saportio, A. et al. (2001). Predictors of older primary care patients' participations in a submaximal exercise test and a supervised, low-impact exercise class. *Preventive Medicine*, 33: 485-494.

Djuric, Z., Lababidi, S., Heilbrun, L. et al. (2002). Effect of low-fat and/or low-energy diets on anthropometric measure in participants of the Women's Diet Study. *Journal of the American College of Nutrition*, 21(1): 38-46.

Dunn, C., Deroo, L. and Rivara, F.P. (2001). The use of brief interventions adapted from motivational interviewing across behavioral domains: a systematic review. *Addiction*, 96(12): 1725-1742.

Eakin, E.G., Glasgow, R.E. and Riley, K.M. (2000). Review of primary care-based physical activity intervention studies: effectiveness and implications for practice and future research. *The Journal of Family Practice*, 49(2): 158-168.

Eakin, E. (2001). Promoting physical activity among middle-aged and older adults in health care settings. *Journal of Aging and Physical Activity*, 9: S29-S37.

Ettner, S.L. (1999). The relationship between continuity of care and the health behaviors of patients: does having a usual physician make a difference? *Medical Care*, 37(6): 547-555.

Fiore, M.C., Bailey, W.C., Cohen, S.J. et al. (2000). *Treating Tobacco Use and Dependence*. Rockville MD: Public Health Service.

Fisher, E.B., Auslander, W.F., Munro, J.F. et al. (1998). Neighbors for a smoke free north side: Evaluation of a community organization approach to promoting smoking cessation among African Americans. *American Journal of Public Health*, 88(11): 1658-1663.

Frank, E., Winkleby, M.A., Altman, D.G. et al. (1991). Predictors of physicians' smoking cessation advice. *Journal of the American Medical Association*, 266(22): 3139-3144.

Gentry, D., Longo, D.R., Housemann, R.A. et al. (1999). Prevalence and correlates of physician advice for prevention: impact of type of insurance and regular source of care. *Journal of Health Care Finance*, 26(1): 78-97.

German, P., Burton, L. and Shapiro, S. (1995). Extended coverage for preventive services for the elderly: Response and results in a demonstration population. *American Journal of Public Health*, 85(3): 379-386.

Glass, J., Miller, W., Szymanski, L. et al. (2002). Physiological responses to weight-loss intervention in inactive obese African-American and Caucasian Women. *The Journal of Sports Medicine and Physical Fitness*, 42(1): 56-64.

Gold, D., Anderson, D.R. and Serxner, S.A. (2000). Impact of a telephone-based intervention on the reduction of health risks. *American Journal of Health Promotion*, 15(2): 97-106.

Goldberg, D.N., Hoffman, A.M., Farinha, M.F. et al. (1994). Physician delivery of smoking-cessation advice based on the stages-of-change model. *American Journal of Preventive Medicine*, 10(5): 267-274.

Goldstein, M.G., Niaura, R., Willey-Lessne, C. et al. (1997). Physicians counseling smokers: A population-based survey of patients' perceptions of health care provider-delivered smoking cessation interventions. *Archives of Internal Medicine*, 157(12): 1313-1319.

Gregg, E. and Narayan, K.M.V. (1998). Culturally appropriate lifestyle interventions in minority populations. *Diabetes Care*, 21(5): 875.

Janes, G.R., Blackman, D.K., Bolen, J.C. et al. (1999). Surveillance for use of preventive health care services by older adults, 1995-1997. *Morbidity and Mortality Weekly Report*, 48(SS-8): 51-88.

Keyserling, T., Ammerman, A. and Davis, C. (1997). A randomized controlled trial of a physician-directed treatment program for low-income patients with high blood cholesterol: The Southeast Cholesterol Project. *Archives of Family Medicine*, 6(2): 135-145.

King, A., Rejeskim, J. and Buchner, D.M. (1998). Physical activity interventions targeting older adults. *American Journal of Preventive Medicine*, 15(4): 316-333.

King, A.C. (2001). Interventions to promote physical activity by older adults. *Journal of Gerontology: Biological Sciences and Medical Sciences*, 562(2): 36-46.

Kochevar, A., Smith, K.L. and Bernard, M.A. (2001). Effects of a community-based intervention to increase activity in American Indian elders. *Journal of the Oklahoma State Medical Association*, 94(10): 1-6.

Kumanyika, S., Espeland, M. and Bahnson, J. (2002). Ethnic comparison of weight loss in the trial of nonpharmacologic interventions in the elderly. *Obesity Research*, 10(2): 96-106.

Lai, K.Q., McPhee, S.J., Jenkins, N.H. et al. (2000). Applying the Quit and Win contest model in the Vietnamese community in Santa Clara County. *Tobacco Control*, 9(2) 56-59.

Lesgards, J.F., Durand, P., Lassarre, M. et al. (2002). Assessment of lifestyle effects on the overall antioxidant capacity of healthy subjects. *Environmental Health Perspective*, 110(5): 479-486.

Leveille, S.G., Wagner, E.H., Davis, C. et al. (1998). Preventing disability and managing chronic illness in frail older adults: A randomized trial of a community based partnership with primary care. *Journal of the American Geriatrics Society*, 46(10): 1191-1198.

Lorig, K., Sobel, D.S., Stewart, A.L. et al. (1999). Evidence suggesting that a chronic disease self-management program can improve health status while reducing hospitalization. *Medical Care*, 37(1): 5-14.

Mallin, R. (2002). Smoking cessation: integration of behavioral and drug therapies. *American Family Physician*, 65(6): 1107-1114.

Marcus, A., Morra, M. and Rimer, B. (1998). A feasibility test of a brief educational intervention to increase fruit and vegetable consumption among callers to the Cancer Information Service. *Preventive Medicine*, 27: 250-261.

Marin, G. and Perez-Stable, E. (1995). Effectiveness of disseminating culturally appropriate smoking cessation information: Programa Latino Para Dejar de Fumar. *Journal of the National Cancer Institute Monographs*, 18: 155-163.

McKeown, T. (1979). *The Role of Medicine: Dream, Mirage, or Nemesis?* Princeton University Press: Princeton, NJ.

McMahon, F., Fujioka, K., Singh, B. et al (2000). Efficacy and safety of sibutramine in obese White and African American patients with hypertension: A 1-year, double-blind, placebo-controlled, multi-center trial. *Archives of Internal Medicine*, 160(14): 2185-2191.

Miller, J.H. and Moyers, T. (2002). Motivational interviewing in substance abuse: applications for occupational medicine. *Occupational Medicine*, 17(1): 51-65.

Miller, W.C., Koceja, D.M. and Hamilton, E.J. (1997). A meta-analysis of the past 25 years of weight loss research using diet, exercise or diet plus exercise intervention. *International Journal of Obesity*, 21(10): 941-947.

Moyad, M.A. (2002). Dietary fat reduction to reduce prostate cancer risk: controlled enthusiasm, learning a lesson from breast or other cancers, and the big picture. *Urology*, 59(4 Suppl 1): 51-62.

Moyers, T.B. and Rollnick, S. (2002). A motivational interviewing perspective on resistance in psychotherapy. *Journal of Clinical Psychology*, 58(2): 185-93.

Mullen, P.D., Simons-Morton, D.G., Ramirez, G. et al. (1997). A meta-analysis of trials evaluating patient education and counseling for three groups of preventive health behaviors. *Patient Educational Counseling*, 32(3): 157-173.

Narayan Venkat, K., Hoskin, M., Kozak, A.M. et al. (1998). Randomized clinical trial of lifestyle interventions in Pima Indians: A pilot study. *Diabetic Medicine*, 15(1): 66-72.

Ornish, D., Scherwitz, L.W., Billings, J.H. et al. (1998). Intensive life type changes for reversal of coronary heart disease. *Journal of the American Medical Association*, 280; 2001-2007.

Parra-Medina, D., D'antonio, A., Smith, S.M. et al. (2004). Successful recruitment and retention strategies for a randomized weight management trial for people with diabetes living in rural, medically underserved counties of South Carolina: the POWER study. *Journal of the American Dietetic Association*, 104(1): 70-75.

Patrick, D., Grembowski, D., Durham, M. et al. (1999). Cost and outcomes of Medicare preventive reimbursement for HMO preventive services. *Health Care Financing Review*, 20(4): 25-43.

Pederson, L., Ahluwalia, J., Harris, K. et al. (2000). Smoking cessation among African-Americans: What we know and do not know about intervention and self-quitting. *Preventive Medicine*, 31(1): 23-38.

Perez-Stable, E.J., Marin, B.V. and Marin, G. (1993). A comprehensive smoking cessation program for the San Francisco Bay Area Latino community: Programa Latino Para Dejar de Fumar. *American Journal of Health Promotion*, 7(6): 430-442, 475.

Petrella, R. and Lattanzio, C.N. (2002). Does counseling help patients get active? Systematic review of the literature. *Canadian Family Physician*, 18: 23-32.

Resnicow, K., Jackson, A. and Wang, T. (2001). A motivational interviewing intervention to increase fruit and vegetable intake through Black churches: Results of the Eat for Life Trial. *American Journal of Public Health*, 91(10): 1686-1693.

Rimer, B.K. and Glassman, B. (1999). Is there a use for tailored print communications in cancer risk communication? *Journal of the National Cancer Institute Monograph*, 25: 140-148.

Rowe, J.W. (1999). Geriatrics, prevention, and the remodeling of Medicare. *New England Journal of Medicine*, 340(9): 720-721.

Royo-Bordonada, M.A., Martin-Moreno, J.M., Guallar, E. et al. (1997). Alcohol intake and risk of breast cancer: the euramic study. *Neoplasma*, 44(3): 150-156.

Russell, L.B., Carson, J.L., Taylor, W.C. et al. (1998). Modeling all cause mortality: Projections of the impact of smoking cessation based on the NHEFS. NHANES I Epidemiologic Follow-up Study. *American Journal of Public Health*, 88(4): 630-636.

Schorling, J.B., Roach, J., Siegel, M. et al. (1997). A trial of church-based smoking cessation interventions for rural African Americans. *Preventive Medicine*, 26(1): 92-101.

Shekelle, P. (2002). *Health Risk Appraisals and Medicare*. Southern California Evidence-Based Practice Center.

Shi, L. (1999). Experience of primary care by racial and ethnic groups in the United States. *Medical Care*, 37(10): 1068-1077.

Smith, D., Heckemeyer, C., Kratt, P. et al. (1997). Motivational interviewing to improve adherence to a behavioral weight-control program for older obese women with NIDDM: A Pilot Study. *Diabetes Care*, 20(1): 52-54.

Song, R., Lee, E.O., Lam, P. et al. (2003). Effects of tai chi exercise on pain, balance, muscle strength, and perceived difficulties in physical functioning in older women with osteoarthritis: a randomized clinical trial. *The Journal of Rheumatology*, 30(9): 2039-2044.

Stein, M.D., Charuvastra, A., Maksad, J. et al. (2002). A randomized trial of a brief alcohol intervention for needle exchangers (BRAINE). *Addiction*, 97(6): 691-700.

Stewart, A.L., Verboncoeur, C.J., McLellan, B.Y. et al. (2001). 2nd Physical activity outcomes of CHAMPS II: A physical activity promotion program for older adults. *The Journals of Gerontology: Series A, Biological Sciences and Medical Sciences*, 56(8): M465-70.

Stewart, J.H.I. (2001). Lung carcinoma in African Americans. *Cancer*, 91(12): 2476-2482.

Stotts, A.L., Diclemente, C.C. and Dolan-Mullen, P. (2002). One-to-one: A motivational intervention for resistant pregnant smokers. *Addictive Behavior*, 27(2): 275-292.

Taira, D., Safran, D.G., Seto, T.B. et al. (1997). The relationship between patient income and physician discussion of health risk behaviors. *Journal of the American Medical Association*, 278(17): 1412-1417.

Lee, P.R. and Estes, C.L. (eds) (1994). *The Nation's Health*. Fourth Edition, Boston, MA: Jones and Bartlett Publishers.

Tilley, B., Glanz, K. and Kristal, A. (1999). Nutrition intervention for high-risk auto workers: Results of the Next Step Trial. *Preventive Medicine*, 28: 284-292.

U.S. National Center for Chronic Disease Prevention and Health Promotion, U.S. Department of Health and Human Services, Public Health Service, Surgeon General, and Satcher, D. (1998). *Tobacco Use Among U.S. Racial/Ethnic Minority Groups – African Americans, American Indians and Alaskan Natives, Asian Americans and Pacific Islanders, and Hispanics: A Report of the Surgeon General*. Atlanta, GA. Department of Health and Human Services.

van der Bij, A., Laurant, M.G.H. and Wensing, M. (2002). Effectiveness of physical activity interventions for older adults. *American Journal of Preventive Medicine*, 22(2): 120-133.

Vita, A.J., Terry, R.B., Hubert, H.B., et al. (1998). Aging, health risks, and cumulative disability. *New England Journal of Medicine*, 338(15): 1035-1041.

Von Korff, M. Gruman, J., Schaefer, J. et al. (1997). Collaborative management of chronic illness. *Annals of Internal Medicine*, 127(12): 1097-1002.

Walcott-McQuigg, J.A., Chen, S.P., Davis, K. et al. (2002). Weight loss and weight loss maintenance in African-American women. *Journal of the National Medical Association*, 94(8): 686.

Wallace, J., Buchner, D.M., Grothaus, L. et al. (1998). Implementation and effectiveness of a community-based health promotion program for older adults. *Journal of Gerontology: Medical Science*, 53A(4): M301-M306.

Waltzer, K.B. (1998). Simple, sensible preventive measures for managed care settings. *Geriatrics*, 53(10): 65-68, 75-77.

Warnecke, R.B., Flay, B.R., Kviz, F.J. et al. (1991). Characteristics of participants in a televised smoking cessation intervention. *Preventive Medicine*, 20(3): 389-403.

Wee, C.C., McCarthy, E.P., Davis, R.B. et al. (1999). Physician counseling about exercise. *Journal of the American Medical Association*, 282(15): 1583-1588.

Wennberg, J.E. (1999). Understanding geographic variations in health care delivery. *New England Journal of Medicine*, 340(1): 52-53.

Wechsler, H., Levine, S., Idelson, R.K. et al. (1996). The physician's role in health promotion revisited: A survey of primary care practitioners. *New England Journal of Medicine*, 334(15): 996-998.

Wilcox, S., Parra-Medina, D., Thompson-Robinson, M. et al. (2001). Nutrition and physical activity interventions to reduce cardiovascular disease risk in health care setting: A quantitative review with a focus on women. *Nutrition Reviews*, 59(7): 197-214.

Yanek, L., Becker, D. and Moy, T. (2001). Project Joy: Faith based cardiovascular health promotion for African American women. *Public Health Reports*, 116(1): S68.

Young, D.G.J., Charleston, J., Felix-Aaron, K. et al. (2001). Motivations for exercise and weight loss among African-American women: Focus group results and their contributions towards program development. *Ethnic and Health*, 6(3/4): 227-245.

Zaza, S., Aguero, L.K.W-D., Briss, P.A. et al. (2000). Data collection instrument and procedure for systematic reviews. In *The Guide to Community Preventive Services*. *American Journal of Preventive Medicine*, 18(1S): 44-74.

Chapter 5

Racial/Ethnic Disparities in Breast Cancer

Introduction

This chapter considers opportunities for reducing racial/ethnic (R/E) disparities in breast carcinoma (breast cancer) outcomes among elders. Although men also develop breast cancer, the numbers are too few for R/E comparisons and so this chapter focuses exclusively on women. It describes R/E differences in breast cancer incidence, prevalence, survival, and mortality as well as the roles of screening, detection, treatment and aftercare in these outcomes. Also examined are studies of the effectiveness of culturally tailored interventions.

The R/E disparity in breast cancer outcomes exemplifies the wealth/health paradox. Paradoxically, health may suffer in a wealthy nation that produces highly advanced medical care. The relationship between health and wealth at the national level is shaped in part by equitable access to advanced preventative and curative technologies. The United States (US) has worse health outcomes than would be expected given its relative wealth (Jameson, Bobadilla, Hetcht et al., 1993) because of disparities by race/ethnicity and other socio-economic factors. The evidence presented in this chapter shows that for elders the R/E differences in breast outcomes cannot be attributed primarily to individual factors, such as risk behaviors, biology, and attitudes towards the disease. Rather, socio-economic and other group differences in capacity to access emerging technology seem to account for this pattern.

Since the first breast cancer treatment was introduced in 1902 in the form of radical mastectomy, there have been important developments in breast cancer management. The introduction of mammography in 1973 and new treatment modalities, such as combination chemotherapy, local radiation therapy, newer chemotherapy and hormonal therapy, since then, have increased survival odds. Similarly, breast-conserving surgery has improved the cosmetic aspects of treatment for this cancer. On the policy and advocacy fronts, since 1988 breast cancer has received an unprecedented attention in terms of national programs. For example, in 1990, Congress enacted the Breast and Cervical Cancer Mortality Prevention Act, which authorized the Centers for Disease Control and Prevention (CDC) to set up the National Breast and Cervical Cancer Demonstration Program (NBCDP). Since 1991, the NBCCP has provided free mammograms and referrals to low-income women including elders (CDC, 2001); and Medicare coverage was introduced. There have also been many private sector programs to increase awareness and to facilitate access to screening since the early 1990s. Consequently, between 1980 and 1992 there was a 200 fold increase in mammography use among women 40 years and older and between 1991-1992 mortality began to decline (Newcomb and Lantz, 1993). Although mortality rates have now stabilized, the increase in mammography use has been paralleled by a noticeable decline of about 18%. Elders from R/E minorities have benefited least from these technological and program advancements: disparities in early detection and mortality have persisted and the gap is widening.

Methods

We conducted electronic searches of Medline and the NCI CancerLit from 1985 to 2004, supplemented by backward citation searches using Social Science Citation Index/Web of Science for selected papers. All searches used the following key words to locate reports on cancer among persons of color, 'minority elderly, race, elders of color, elders, minority, older adults, adults, African American, Blacks, Hispanic, Latino, Spanish surname, American Indians, Native Americans, Alaskan Native, Hawaiian Native, Pacific Islanders, and Asian American.' As in other chapters, we have found it necessary to use the R/E group label 'Asian and Pacific Islander' because most published research has not yet adopted the Census 2000 classification. Although the US Census and other sources now differentiate 'Asian' and 'Native Hawaiian and other Pacific Islanders (NHOPI),' most of the national level data reported for breast cancer do not make this distinction, combing all Asian and Pacific Islanders (API). Much of this literature also uses the terms 'Black' and 'non-white' despite ongoing concerns about operational definitions. We use the R/E classifications adopted by primary data sources. Additional key words included 'prevalence, incidence, mortality, survival, screening, diagnosis, treatment, surgery, chemotherapy, radiotherapy, radiation, quality of life, relapse, monitoring, culture, intervention, RCT, community health worker, case management, quality improvement.' Other sources of information were the RAND reports on Health Aging prepared for CMS and the reviews supporting the AHRQ Task Force on Clinical Preventive Services guidelines, Cochrane group reviews, other review papers.

Racial/Ethnic Differences in Prevalence and Mortality

Breast cancer is a major public health problem in the United States. Based on 1993 estimates: 1 in 8 women will develop breast cancer and 1 in 28 will die from it over a lifetime (estimated up to age 85 years, (Feuer, Wun, Boring et al., 1993)). Case fatality is also quite high. In recent years, 1 in 5 cases of invasive breast cancer die of this disease. For example, the 2004, the American Cancer Society estimates 215,990 female breast cancer cases and 40, 110 deaths (Ahmedin, Tiwari, Murray, and Ghafoor et al., 2004).

Breast cancer incidence Breast cancer is equally important for each of the five R/E groups considered in this review (white, African-American (AA),

Hispanics/Latinos, American Indian/Alaska Natives (AI/AN) and API). It is a leading cause of cancer morbidity for women in all groups. It is also the leading cause of cancer mortality for Latinas and the second leading cause for white, AA, AI/AN, and API women (Howe, Wingo, Thun et al., 2001).

The incidence rate is highest for white and lowest for AI/AN women. There is however, a wide racial/ethnic variation: 141.7, 119.9, 96.8 and 89.6, 54.2/100, 000 population, (Year 2000 standard population) for white, AA, API, Hispanic, and AI/AN women, respectively (Ries, Eisner, Kosary et al., 2004). There is a possible underestimation of some of these rates although the relative ranking is likely to remain the same. For example, using data from the National Breast Cancer Early Detection Program (NBCCEDP), May, Lee, Richardson et al., (2000), found less variation in breast cancer detection rates among R/E groups. They used 1991-1998 mammography and diagnostic data for 573,751 women who received breast cancer screening through the NBCCEDP. In Table 5.1, using incidence data collected within the same period, we compare each minority group to the white group on incidence and detection rates using rate ratios. Table 5.1 shows that incidence rate ratios (IRR) for Hispanic, API and AI/AN are lower than the detection rate ratios (DRR) with the exception of AA where the IRR are close to the DRR. This suggests an underestimation of the incidence rates for API, Hispanics and AI/AN and that differences in screening rates might be partly responsible for the wider variation in population-based incidence rates.

Table 5.1   Breast cancer incidence, detection rates and rate ratios by racial/ethnic group: 1991-1998

Race	White*	AA	API	Hispanic.	AI/AN
Incidence Rate[1]	137	120.7	93.4	82.6	59.4
Incidence Rate Ratio	1	0.88	0.68	0.60	0.43
Detection Rate[2]	7.7	6.4	6.2	4.9	4.9
Detect Rate Ratio	1	0.83	0.81	0.64	0.64

*White women are the comparison group for ratios and constitute the denominator [1]Rates are per 100, 000 population, year 2000 standard; [2]Rates are per 1,000 mammograms:

Source: Ries et al., 2002.SEER CSR, 1973-1999, data for 1992-1998; May et al., 2000, data for 1991-1998.

Because breast cancer risk increases with age, older women have a higher incidence than younger women. According to National Cancer Institute's Surveillance, Epidemiology and End Results (SEER) data for 1997-2001(Ries et al 2004), invasive breast cancer is five times higher in women 65 years of age and older than in younger women.

Breast cancer mortality Like incidence, mortality varies by age and R/E. For the period 1997-2001 mortality estimates for white, AA, API, AI/AN, and for Hispanic women varied widely: 27.0, 35.4, 12.6.4, 13.6, 17.3 per 100,000 population (Year 2000 standard) respectively (Ries et al 2004). Older women, however, had a disproportionate share of the breast cancer mortality. The odds of dying from breast cancer were 8 times greater for women 65 years and older than for younger women. This risk was greatest for older black women, especially women 65-84 years of age who, despite having lower incidence, are more likely to die from this cancer than their white peers. This can be better appreciated by examining the trends in relative mortality rates between white and Black women, covering the period 1979-1996 and the age group 65-79, which are presented in Figure 5.1.

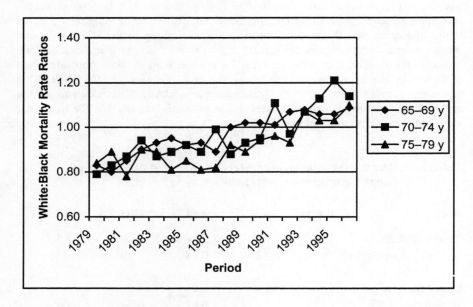

Figure 5.1 Trends in black/white mortality rate ratios* among older women by age group: 1979-1996

Source: Marbella and Layde, 2001.
* 1=no difference, less than 1=mortality is less for Black women, greater than 1=mortality is higher for Black women.

As shown in Figure 5.1, through the 1980s, breast cancer mortality was lower for older Black women (65 years and over) than for older white women. A shift in relative mortality rate is seen starting 1989. Therefore, for the entire period under consideration (1979-1996) there was a relative increase in breast cancer mortality for Black women compared to white women of the same age: about 26 percentage points for the age groups 65-69, 75-79, 80-84 (80 to 84 is not shown here) and 35 percentage points for the age group 70-74 (Marbella and Layde, 2001). Notably, the 1980s saw major improvements in availability and efficacy of breast screening and treatment of regional disease in general (Chu, Tarone, Kessler et al., 1996; Delgado, Lin, and Coffey, 1995, Frost, Tollestrup, Hunt et al., 1996). These data, therefore, suggest the role of health care access in the observed R/E disparities in breast cancer mortality i.e. as the efficacy of treatment improved, positive outcomes for whites compared to that for Blacks also increased; exceeding that for Blacks. For the other R/E groups no comparable analyses were found to assess such shifts in mortality rate. But as seen under survival, similar R/E shifts did occur in early detection and survival, over this same period, particularly for Hispanic and AI/AN women (Frost et al., 1996). This is further explored under survival differences.

Stage and Race/ethnic survival differences One major contributor to age and R/E disparities in breast cancer mortality is a later stage at diagnosis. Many studies report a more advanced stage of breast cancer at diagnosis in R/E subgroups. The race-stage association for this cancer, however, seems complex. There are age and R/E variations.

Table 5.2   Stage-specific prevalence of breast cancer among women by race and ethnicity: 1996-2000*

	White (%)	AA (%)	Hispanic (%)	AI/AN (%)	API (%)
Localized	66	55	57	56	65
Regional	29	36	35	36	30
Distant	5	9	7	8	5
Unstaged	8.5	9.0	NA	NA	NA

*Source: Ries et al., 2004, SEER statistical review, 1975-2000; NA=not available.

Considering all age groups as shown in Table 5.2, national estimates of the stage-specific prevalence of breast cancer for the period 1996-2001 shows that AA, Hispanic/Latino and AI/AN are less likely to be diagnosed at localized stage and are more likely to be diagnosed at regional stage. A more advanced stage for older AA than white women is also supported by a number of analytic studies (McCarthy, Burns, Coughlin et al., 1998; Jones, Kasi, Curnen et al., 1995; Bibb, 2001; Reeves, Newcomb, Remington et al., 1996; Wu, Andrews, Correa et al., 2001; Jacobellis and Cutter, 2002; Joslyn and West, 2000).

A more heterogeneous picture is seen in Hispanics and API than in AI/AN and AA women. Although studies typically show that Hispanic women are more likely have advanced stage than white women, age-specific analyses are needed to assess how age moderates this effect. Two large analytic studies (Li, Marlone and Daling, 2003, Hardeen and White, 2001) involving a substantial number of elders 60 years and over (31-56% and 59% respectively) found Hispanics to have advanced stage and larger tumors than were white women. Li et al., (2003), using SEER data on a sample of 124,934 women diagnosed with primary invasive breast cancer between 1992 and 1998, found Hispanics were 50% more at stage II, 90% more at stage III, and 80% more at stage IV. One study, however, using a sample from San Diego, California showed the Hispanic/white difference in stage to be significant only for younger women but not older women. The sample comprised all incident cases (10,161) from in the county that were identified through the California Tumor Registry (Bentley, Delfino, Taylor et al., 1998). This may or may not apply to other settings.

An intergenerational difference has also been shown. Hedeen and White (2001), using data from 4 SEER regions and a sample of 28,826 women diagnosed between 1992 and 1995, found first generation immigrants (born outside the US) to have larger tumors than second generation (born in the US); although no ethnic difference in stage was seen. It is not clear from this study if intergenerational differences are related to age; the age interaction was not tested. For AI/AN women, two studies (Sugarman, Dennis and White 1994; Frost et al., 1996) conducted earlier show that they present at similar stage as the white women. The larger studies mentioned earlier (Li et al., 2003; Hardeen and White, 2001) found no racial difference in being diagnosed at stage II compared to stage I, but found that American Indians were 70% more likely to be diagnosed at stage III than were white women and twice as likely to be at stage IV.

The difference in stage at diagnosis observed among AI/AN and Hispanics for the period 1992-1998 represents a second historical shift in stage at diagnosis, compared to white women. During 1973-82 Hispanics and AI/AN were less likely to be diagnosed at local stage but during 1983-1992, breast cancer stage became comparable for all three groups (Frost et al., 1996).

Within the pan-ethnic API group, Chinese, Filipinos and NHOPI are more likely to have late stage than white women (Meng et al., 1997). Japanese women, however, tend to have less advanced stage than either white women or other API women (Natarajan, Nemoto and Mettlin, 1988).

Impact of stage on survival   Survival rates vary by stage with better survival experienced at localized (stages 0 and I) than at advanced stage (stages II and over). As shown in Table 5.4, based on SEER estimates for 1995-2000 (Ries et al 2004), regional stage reduces survival for women 50 years and older by 20 percentage points (97.3 vs. 77.7); while distant metastasis reduces it by 78 percentage points (97.3 vs. 19.6). For most women of color, particularly AA women, the influence of stage on survival is greater than for white women. Although survival rates for both AA and white women decline with increasing stage of the disease, Black women experience less survival at every stage of the disease (Ries et al., 2001) with the greatest differential being for regional disease (Ries et al., 2004). For example, for the period 1995-2000, at regional disease, AA women 50 years and older experienced 13% less survival than white women compared to 6.4% and 11.2% at local and distant metastasis. During this period survival rates for Black women 50 years and older were 92.6, 69.1, and 12.9 compared to 99.0, 81.6 and 24.1 among white women for localized, regional and distance metastasis respectively. As we will indicate in greater detail below, these stage-specific 5-year survival differentials between Black and white women are primarily explained by differences in appropriateness of cancer treatment and management of co-morbid chronic conditions (Shavers and Brown 2002, Mancino, Rubio, Henry-Tillman et al., 2001*)*. This frustrates early detection efforts.

The impact of stage on 5-year survival in general (McCarthy et al., 2000) and on R/E disparities suggested by the national data is supported by analytic studies (Yood Johnson, Blount, et al., 1999; Meng et al., 1997; El-Tamer, Homel and Wait 1999). For example, El-Tamer et al (1999) used registry data from two institutions collected for the period 1982-1995 on a sample of 1,745 patients, (1,297 AA and 448 white women) to evaluate whether race was a prognostic factor in breast cancer survival after taking into account other factors which included, age, income, stage, histologic findings, type of operation, and treating institution. AA patients with breast cancer were 1.27 times more likely to die than were white women. Only stage, age, and whether the patient had a therapeutic surgical treatment significantly contributed to survival.

Table 5.3   Influence of stage on breast cancer survival rates for white and black women >= 50 years: 1995-2000

	All	**White**	**AA**	**AA difference**
In Situ	100	100	100	0
Localized	97.5	99.0	92.6	-6.4
Regional	80.4	81.6	69.1	-12.5
Distant	25.5	24.1	12.9	11.2
Unstaged	54.9	52.1	46.2	4.9

Source: Ries et al., 2004. SEER Cancer Statistics Review, 1975-2001.

Stage-specific differences have also been described for Hispanics, American Indians, and some API subgroups. A historical review shows that between 1983-1992, relative survival improved for white women at all stages, and for AI/AN women with local disease. Despite earlier stages at diagnosis, Hispanic females showed less improvement in overall or stage-specific survival than white females; similar survival during 1973-1982; but significantly worse survival during 1983-1992. AI/AN women experienced poorer survival than whites during both time periods (Frost et al., (1996). These findings re-affirm the role of both screening and treatment access in breast racial/ethnic disparities in breast cancer outcomes.

Factors Explaining Racial/Ethnic Differences in Breast Cancer Stage

Role of screening mammography A few studies have explicitly analyzed the role of mammography in breast cancer stage at diagnosis. These studies show that lack of mammography use significantly contributes to R/E differences in stage (McCarthy et al., 1998, Jones et al., 1995; Bibb et al., 2001; Reeves et al., 1996; Wu et al., 1999; Jacobellis and Cutter, 2002). These papers suggest that lack of routine regular screening may result in about 5-13 percentage points excess late stage diagnosis, in either AA or white sample (Jones et al., 1995; McCarthy et al., 1998; Jacobellis and Cutter, 2002). McCarthy et al. (1998) examined the association between mammography and stage among women age 67 and older from three states, finding that mammography use can attenuate the race-stage disparity. Mammography use explained about 30% of the stage difference between AA and white women. They also found that the Black-white difference in cancer stage occurred only among non-users of mammography. In another study, Jacobellis and Cutter (1998) used a 1990-1998 mammography database (N=5,182) of Denver, Colorado women to examine each R/E cohort's incident cancer cases (N=1,902) and tumor stage distribution given similar patterns of routine screening use. They found that regardless of R/E, women participating in routine screenings had earlier-stage disease by 5 to 13 percentage points.

The foregoing studies demonstrate that lack of mammography use contributes about 5-30-percentage points difference in stage. The studies also suggest that mammography is not the only factor. Other factors hypothesized to influence stage of breast cancer at time of diagnosis include obesity and biologic factors such as tumor characteristics (Reeves et al., 1996; Moorman, Jones, Millikan et al., 2001), structural context variables, (Mandelbaltt and Kanetsky, 1995), and socio-cultural factors (Lannin, Mathews, Mitchell et al., 1998). Although tumor characteristics have been associated with faster growth; given that R/E differences in tumor characteristics tend to diminish with age; therefore, we conclude that the role of tumor characteristics in explaining R/E differences in stage at the time of diagnosis is small among older women (65 and older) and smaller than may be true for younger women. Studies are required to examine a possible interaction of the other factors with screening mammography, lack of follow-up after an abnormal screen or interval detected lesions and delay in diagnostic workup. More age-specific analysis of impact of mammography on stage is also needed.

Breast Cancer Screening for Early Detection

Although primary prevention of breast cancer is desirable, its utility is limited. Less than 50% of breast cancer cases are attributable to well established risk factors. In addition, many of the established risk factors are not easily modifiable

(NCI, 1998) while hormonal therapy is in clinical trial stage. Screening for breast cancer and detecting it at early more treatable stages, therefore, is the only means now widely available for preventing deaths from this disease. There is consensus among professional organizations regarding annual or biennial mammography screening for the age group 50-69 (NGC 2002; NCI 2002; Smith Cokkinides, von Eschenbach et al., 2002) although organizational recommendations for other age groups differ. For example, the NCI continues to recommend that 'women in their 40s, and women aged 50 and older should be screened every one to two years; while women who are at higher than average risk of breast cancer should seek expert medical advice about whether they should begin screening before age 40 and the frequency of screening' (NGC, 2002; NCI, 2002). The American Cancer Society (ACS) recommends yearly mammography for all women 40 years of age and older and for women under the age of 40 if they have additional risk factors. The ACS has no upper age limit (NGC 2002; Smith et al, 2002). For women 70 years and older, there is currently no consensus mainly because the data are lacking to recommend or withhold recommendation. The American Geriatric society, recommends 'annual or at least biennial mammography until age 75 and biennially or at least every three years thereafter with no upper age limit for women with an estimated life expectancy of four or more years'(AGS, 2000). Medicare coverage for mammography began in 1991 subject to co-payment and deductible; while in 1998 expanded (authorized by the 1997 Balanced Budget Act) from biennial to annual and co-payment and deductible were waived.

Because mammography is not perfect (about 10-20% of breast cancer will not be detected by mammography), professional organizations also recommend complementary screening modalities. The ACS, for example, recommends monthly breast self-exam and clinical breast examination every three years. 'Newer but more expensive imaging technologies, such as digital mammography, magnetic resonance imaging (MRI), radio nuclei imaging and high resolution ultra-sonography are also available, but are still in clinical trial and have not proven to be more superior than mammography for routine monitoring' (Muss, 2000).

The recommendation to adopt mammography as a mass-screening tool is based partly on evidence of its efficacy taking into consideration its safety. The evidence comes from meta-analyses of randomized controlled studies which indicate that screening mammography is substantially efficacious in preventing breast cancer deaths, by about 17%, in women 40-49 years of age and 25-30% in women aged 50-69 years (NCI, 1998; Shapiro 1997; Miller, 1992; Alexander 1997; Kerlikowske Grady, Rubin, et al., 1995). Despite the controversy regarding the efficacy of mammography (Gotzsche and Olson 2000) there is still consensus among professional organizations that mammography saves lives (NGC, 2002; NCI, 2002; Smith, 2002). The consideration for mass screening is based on (1) high prevalence for the pre-clinical stage, (2) treatment for pre-clinical phase more effective than for clinical stage and (3) serious consequences of the disease if left untreated (NCI, 2002)

It should be noted, nonetheless, that mammography screening has never been tested in R/E minorities or for persons older than age 70. There are however many reasons to believe that elders of color can benefit from mammography, including that: risk of breast cancer increases with age; elders tend to have more favorable tumor characteristics (Diab, Elledge and Clark, 2000; Furberg, Millikan, Dressler, et al., 2001; Porter, El-Bastawissi, Mandelson et al., 1999) and tumor characteristics are comparable for different racial/ethnic groups (Diab et al, 2000; Furberg et al., 2001).

Mammography Screening and Racial/Ethnic Differences

There are significant R/E and age disparities in breast cancer screening that reduce the effectiveness of early detection efforts. Over the past two decades, the proportion of women who report lifetime use of mammography (ever using) and recent mammography (use in the past 2 years) has been increasing for all ages and R/E groups (Blackman, Bennett and Miller 1999). But older Black women are less likely to have repeat mammograms or to adhere to recommended screening intervals (Lee and Vogel, 1995; Hawley, Earp, O'Malley et al., 2000; Hegarty et al., 2000). Elder Latina and AI/AN women have the lowest mammography screening rates, both lifetime and recent.

Mammography ever and use past 2 years Although in general mammography use has been increasing, older women of color are less likely to have ever had a mammogram and to have repeat screens (Parker, Sabogal and Gebretsadik, 1999; Burns McCarthy; Freund et al., 1996a/1996b, Coleman and O'Sullivan, 2001; (CDC 1995; Hegarty et al., 2000). Burns et al., (1996b) found age-related R/E disparities among elders. They used Medicare billing data data, to examine mammography use among women age 65 or older residing in one of 10 states that had part B coverage up to December 31, 1990. They found mammography use to be lower for AA than for white women age 65 - 74 (14% vs 21%) and 75 - 84 (9% vs 12%).

Interactions between R/E and region in mammography screening rates have been noted. These seem to have persisted even after the BCCDP. For example elder Black women in eastern Massachusetts were 9 times as likely to report mammography screening than their peers in eastern Long Island (Coleman and O'Sullivan, 2001). Both ethnicity and region differences in screening have also been noted among Latinas. Ramirez, Saurez, Laufman et al., (2000) in a study involving 8 locations across the US and focused on four distinct Hispanic populations: Central American, Cuban, Mexican-American and Puerto-Rican. The sample consisted 2,383 women age 40 and older. They found that Mexican Americans in Houston, Brownsville and Laredo were the least likely to be screened.

Persistent racial/ethnic disparities despite increasing uptake Medicare reimbursement for mammography and the NBCCP projects (CDC, 1994: Kelaher and Stellman 2000) have increased overall prevalence of first time breast cancer screening, but have had little impact on reducing R/E disparities in screening adherence (Preston, Scinto, Ni et al., 1997; Kelaher. and Stellman, 2000: CDC, 1997; Hegarty et al., 2000) among older women. Studies done after 1990 demonstrate persistent racial/ethnic differences in mammography use. For example, Coleman and O'Sullivan (2001) used a sample of 13,545 women, aged 65-74, from Medicare records to examine trends in mammography use. They found that mammography use increased for white but not for Black women. Similarly, Preston et al (2001) used Medicare Part B mammography claims and small area analysis methodology to identify mammography in Connecticut. They found that mammography use rates among Black women 65 years and older were significantly lower than for their white peers.

Disparities in repeat use and adherence to recommended schedules The increasing prevalence of lifetime and recent mammography says little about age and R/E differences in repeat mammography use or adherence to schedule. Epidemiologic studies designed to answer these questions indicate significant R/E differences in repeat mammography and adherence to schedule among both Black and other women of color. For example, Gilliland, Rosenberg, Hunt et al., (2000) examined patterns of mammography use among Hispanic, AI/AN, and white women in New Mexico for the period 1994-1997. They found generally low prevalence of routine screening rates in this population: only 50% of the women aged 50-74 years and less than one third of women aged 75 and older were screened annually. Routine screening annually or biennially was especially low among Hispanics and American Indians. For example, the proportion of Hispanics 50-74 years of age who had annual routine screening was about 20% compared 30% among non-Hispanic white women.

Earlier studies found similar patterns. Bastani Kaplan, Maxwell et al., (1995) examined initial and repeat mammography screening in a low-income multi-ethnic population in Los Angeles. After review of medical records they found that only 21% received a mammogram in the prior 12 months. Approximately 5% of the total sample received a repeat mammogram in the 21-month period over which they were tracked. Song and Fletcher s (1998) evaluated breast cancer re-screening rates among low-income women and examined factors associated with re-screening for women enrolled in Breast and Cervical Health Program (BCHP) in King County, Washington. They found that overall, percentages of women who re-screened at 15 and 27 months for women aged 50-69 was 25.7% and 45.0%, respectively.

Follow-up after abnormal screening and race/ethnic patterns

After an abnormal mammogram, multiple procedures are conducted to reach a diagnostic resolution. These may include additional screening, needle or excision biopsy, histological examination to confirm the cancer diagnosis and additional tests to identify pathologic characteristics (e.g. nuclear grade) and other tumor markers that have prognostic or treatment significance such as progesterone receptor and estrogen receptor (ER/PR) status. Timely and complete diagnostic work-up is important because the choice of treatment for breast cancer depends primarily on the clinical and tumor characteristics (particularly stage, hormonal receptor status) and co-morbidity. Clinical factors and tumor status determine primary treatment choice, while positive ER/PR determines the decision to use tamoxifen for systemic treatment. Women who have incomplete diagnostic work-up are therefore likely to have inappropriate treatment and delayed diagnostic resolution is likely to delay treatment onset.

Although there have been very few studies on this subject, they suggest that women of color are less likely to have timely confirmation of diagnosis and diagnostic work-up (Kerlikowske, 1996). Chang, Kerlikowske, Napoles-Springer et al., (1996), used a retrospective review of records from a North Carolina van and a sample of 317 women aged 33-85 who were reported to have abnormal screen to determine whether patient race was associated with timeliness of follow-up. They found that non-white women had significantly longer time from the date of index abnormal screen to final disposal (median=19 days for non-white vs. median 12 days for white women) and longer time between index abnormal screen and first diagnostic test (median 12 days for non-white vs. 7 days for white). Kerner, Yerdidia, Padgett et al., (2003) conducted a study in New York using a sample of 184 Black women who in 1992 had abnormal mammograms. They found that within 3 months, 39% Black women were without a diagnostic resolution and 28% did not have a resolution within 6 months. These rates of non-completion are lower than rates reported else where for the general population of about 1-31% (69-99% completion) and 1-11% (89-99% completion with computer tracking) after 8-12 weeks (Kerlikowske, 1996). In a Colorado study involving a multi-racial sample of 167,232 (white, AA, Hispanic, Asian, AI/AN and other) for 1990-1997, Strzelczyk and Dignan (2002) found AA, Hispanic, AI/AN, Asians and other were less likely to adhere to follow-up recommendation. They found significant interaction between race and age, education, health insurance and family history of breast cancer.

Explaining Racial/Ethnic Disparities in Mammography Screening

An extensive epidemiological literature has explored factors that may account for R/E disparities in mammography, emphasizing provider and individual factors.

Practitioner factors   Two practitioner factors are reported to influence R/E disparities: practitioner characteristics and practitioner recommendation. Burns, Freund, Ash et al (1995), used administrative data for 791 women aged 50 years and older. They found that 73% of women had received repeat mammography. Practitioner features associated with repeat use were gender, practicing in the women's health group rather than the general internal medicine service, and being a fellow or an attending physician. Practitioner recommendations also influence R/E disparities in mammography according to several studies.

For older women, provider recommendation is a more important predictor of mammography use than other cues to action such as mass media (Danigelis, Worden 1996; Taylor Thompson, Montano et al., 1998). Although practitioner recommendations and enthusiasm are among the strongest predictors of mammography use, older Black women are less likely than their white peers to receive referrals for screening mammography (Potosky, Breen, Graubard et al., 1998). Similarly, O'Malley, Earp and Harris, (1997), found less Black (25%) than white women (52%) reported physician recommendation. They also estimated that physician recommendations might account for 60 to 75% of the initial racial differences in mammography use. Fox and Roetzheim (1994) found racial differences in physician recommendation as well as enthusiasm of recommendation. Non-white women were significantly less likely than were white women to report physician recommendation.

Individual factors Individual differences in economic, cultural and logistical barriers have also been linked to R/E disparities. Economic factors associated with mammography, included income, having supplemental health insurance to Medicare. These factors have been associated with provider recommendation (Coleman et al., 2001), recent use (Ramirez et al., 2000; Maxwell Bastani and Warda, 1998) and ever having a mammogram (Ramirez et al, 2000).

Having no supplemental insurance is major source of R/E disparities. Kelaher and Stellman (2000), compared mammography use between Medicare-eligible and ineligible women in the years before 1990 and 1993 (after the 1991 policy change to provide mammography to Medicare Part B holders). Using NHIS data they showed that disparities had persisted despite increase in use. Having additional health insurance was the only significant predictor of having a usual source of care among the Medicare population. Dolan, Reifler, McDermott et al (1995) showed that older women of color, although more likely to accept recommendations for repeat screening than older white women, were less likely to adhere to recommendations, especially those who had Medicare but no co-insurance. The sample comprised 343 women 50 years and older who had received recommendation for screening. They found that acceptance of the recommendation differed by race: more AA women (89%) than white women (82%) accepted recommendation. In multivariate analysis, only age remained independently predictive of acceptance. However, among women who accepted the recommendation, adherence significantly differed by race, with more white (70%) than non-white women (59%) actually participating in repeat screening. In logistic regression insurance type and health care provider training but not race remained independently predictive of adherence.

Regarding cultural factors, various analytic approaches and single measures have been used to determine the impact of cultural factors on mammography use, including: (1) the health belief model; (2) acculturation scales; (3) knowledge scales and (4) level of education. Not all health beliefs or acculturation constructs have been associated with mammography use. Cultural variables that have been associated with mammography use include high school education, English speaking (Solis Marks, Garcia et al., 1990; Woloshin, Schwartz, Katz et al., 1997; Ramirez et al., 2000; Suarez, Roche, Nichols et al., 1997), some health beliefs such as low risk perception (Tang, Solomon and McCracken, 2000; Austin, Ahmad, McNally et al., 2002), perceived benefit of screening, modesty (Maxwell et al., 1998) and knowledge (Sung, Blumenthal, Coates et al., 1997).

Evidence for the role of health beliefs in determining R/E disparities in mammography use has been inconsistent. Although a number of studies show that health beliefs and attitudes differ by R/E, these measures do not consistently predict use and their inclusion in multivariate models of use does not consistently reduce or eliminate the independent effects of R/E (Laws and Mayo 1998). Health beliefs more consistently associated with mammography use include concern about cost (Stein, Fox and Murata 1991) and low perceived need (Tang et al, 2000). In contrast to health beliefs, knowledge including that about cancer screening guidelines and cancer prevention (Sung et al, 1997) has been consistently associated with screening behavior.

Only a few studies were found that analyzed the role of logistical barriers in mammography use. In a study conducted prior to broad Medicare coverage for mammography, Kiefe, McKay, Halevy et al., (1994) used a randomized controlled trial to evaluate the effectiveness of initiatives to remove financial barriers to mammography for low-income older women. The sample (N=119) had a mean age 71, with 77% black and 52% reported prior mammogram. They found that 'for women without the voucher, the main reason for not obtaining a mammogram was financial; the main reason for women with the voucher was transportation.' In another study, Maxwell et al., (1998) found transportation to be a significant barrier to mammography use for a sample of Korean Americans. In contrast, Solis et al., (1990) using data from the HHANES, found that for diverse Hispanic adults (ages 20-74), facility type and travel time produced no consistent impacts on mammography use. Lack of age stratification and the heterogeneity within Hispanic groups might account for this inconsistency. Rural residency is another factor that seem to affect R/E disparities in breast cancer screening among the elderly (Cummings Whetstone, Earp et al., 2002).

Barriers to Diagnosis Confirmation and Completion

Women of color not only face barriers to screening, but also to timely confirmation of diagnosis and diagnostic work up. As noted earlier, two studies were found that explicitly examined factors that influenced R/E disparities to diagnostic work-up (Caplan, Helzlsouer, Shapiro, et al., 1996; Rojas Mandelblatt, Cagney, et al., 1996). Caplan et al., (1996) examined provider and health care system barriers associated with delay in diagnostic work-up among 367 breast cancer cases that were part of the NCI's Black-white survival study. They found that 45% of the delay was due to provider and health care system, through difficulties in scheduling or physician inaction, 25% was due to patient factors and 17% due to both patient and provider factors. Rojas et al., (1996) performed a cross-sectional survey of three cancer screening clinics and found high rates of non-compliance (50%) with follow-up after abnormal screening. Overall, non-compliers were less likely to report being told to follow-up (65% vs. 100) and more likely to report barriers to follow-up such as cost of lost wages, medical care system barriers or fears than compliers, 61% vs. 9%

Interventions to Reduce Racial/Ethnic Disparities in Mammography Use

There is currently great interest in determining interventions to increase mammography screening. This area has also been subject to intensive reviews and meta-analyses (Legg et al, 2000; Mandelblatt, and Kanetsky, 1995; Mandelblatt and Yabroff, 1999; Wagner, 1998; Yabroff and Mandelblatt, 1999; Shekelle, Stone, Mangolione et al., 2001). Interventions to increase mammography use range from simple low cost computer generated reminders to interventions that involve human intermediaries. Both simple and more complex interventions seem effective in increasing uptake and adherence to screening, although few studies have examined whether these effects are sustainable over time. Interventions directed at the practitioner, such as reminders to providers, audit, and feedback, organizational change, such as information systems to enhance follow up or scheduling changes and those directed at the client such as mailed reminders using automated reminder systems, telephone counseling, or customized reminders, or lay health workers, seem to be equally effective. But provider directed interventions seem optimal especially when at least two strategies are used, according to these reviews. For example, according to Mandelblatt and Yabroff (1999) behavioral interventions for providers increased mammography screening rates from usual care of 65 percent by 13.2 percentage points, and by 6.8% compared to active controls. Similarly, behavioral interventions aimed at the individual client increased mammography screening by 13.2% compared with usual care, and by 13.0% for multiple strategies and 5.6% and for single intervention. The setting of the intervention also seems to matter. For example, according to Mandelblatt and Kanetsky (1995) in academic medical settings, physician reminders and audit with feedback each increased use of mammography and clinical breast examination by approximately 5% to 20%, while in community settings, the effect of physician education were slightly less ranging from 6% to 14%.

Although these interventions have been found effective in the general population, their ability to increase screening among R/E groups who are Medicare beneficiaries as well as the costs of these strategies, are unknown, according to all of these reviews. Different strategies may be required for populations such as the rural and low-income women and low education women. These women experience additional socio-cultural barriers beyond health insurance and provider barriers. These include generally low perceived risk for breast cancer, lack of knowledge or appreciation for prevention as medical care approach and fear of discovering breast cancer, (Gregg and Curry 1994; Suarez, Roche, Nichols et al., 1997; Austin Ahmad, McNally et al., 2002). These women also face geographical access barriers such as lack of transportation (Lannin et al., 1998; Maxwell et al., 1998) and opportunity costs.

Further, none of the prior meta-analyses focused on the set of breast cancer initiatives that explore the use of explicitly culturally adapted intervention strategies to improve adherence by older women of color to screening guidelines. To fill this gap, our review focuses on interventions that are culturally tailored to women of color. Culturally tailored studies were defined as ones using any of the following interventions: (1) Language appropriate education materials or role model media education; (2) use of lay health workers chosen from the respondents' community and either of the same ethnicity as the participant or with deep roots in the community and competence in its language as the participant; and (3) use of social networks such as church or other culturally significant community based organizations. Articles were searched from various sources, including Medline. Publications were also sought from prior reviews and the CDC database. Key words for this search included 'interventions and breast cancer screening, patient support and breast cancer screening, breast cancer screening and lay health worker, breast cancer screening and lay health advisor, breast cancer screening and volunteers, breast cancer screening and lay educators, breast cancer screening and lay advisor, breast cancer screening and community interventions.' The database was also searched using leading author names to identify prior studies on same subject by these authors. Additional article sources were recommendations by expert consultants and review of bibliographies in prior reviews.

Promising culturally tailored interventions   Twenty-eight reports met inclusion criteria, but some of these were multiple papers on a single intervention, while other studies did not meet minimal methodological standards. To be included, studies needed to report on an experimental or quasi-experimental project. Acceptable control strategies were: (1) Pre-test and post-test (paired control) design with independent concurrent control at each point in time; or (2) independent concurrent controls. In addition, non-randomized studies had to have both baseline and follow-up data to be included. Twelve programs, yielding 17 comparisons between intervention and comparison groups, met these criteria and were included in the meta-analysis.

Measures of adherence were mammography rate changes among women who had some prior use and mammography uptake measures were mammography changes among women who had some prior use. We used the absolute rate difference as the Effect Size measure. We used comprehensive meta-analysis software developed by Biostat, Inc., to compute fixed effects point and variance measures. This software uses a two-by-two table of measures of actual events to calculate effect sizes. For both the control and the intervention group, the change in number of screened women was calculated by subtracting the follow-up number from the baseline number. Thus, the effect measure included in the meta-analysis reflects a so-called difference-in-differences approach. Because we wanted to identify moderator effects, we report the Mantel-Hanszel fixed effects estimates without adjustment for program heterogeneity.

Characteristics of the studies   The twelve studies and seventeen intervention arms contributed a total sample of 7,376 participants. The target populations included AI/ANs, Hispanic/Latinas, Native Hawaiians and AAs. The ages of the populations were typically 40 and over but all included elders. Eleven studies, contributing fourteen intervention arms, used the outreach method to recruit participants. Only two studies, with three intervention arms, used inreach or both inreach and outreach recruitment strategies. While seven programs used individualized interventions (i.e. Community Health Worker (CHW) as educator or lay advisor providing education, counseling or screening referrals to individual patients) ten programs used group approaches. Seven intervention arms focused on screening uptake, while ten focused on screening adherence as their outcomes. Appendix 5.1 provides a summary of these projects and their findings.

Meta-analysis findings Table 5.6 provides a summary of the meta-analysis. The meta-analysis showed that as a group, these programs achieved small but significant impacts on screening rates – a rate difference (RD) of about 10% (RD=0.078; 95% CI =0. 062, 0.103); Z=9.46, p<0.001). Nonetheless, the program findings were remarkably heterogeneous (Q=146.15, p<0.000). That is, these programs did not produce consistent findings, but rather there were differences in their designs and populations that influenced outcomes.

To determine the proportion of heterogeneity attributable to program features and not chance, we calculated I^2 a new index developed by the Cochrane group calculated as $100\%x(Q-df)/Q$ where Q is the Cochrane's heterogeneity statistic and df are the degrees of freedom (Higgins Thompson, Deeks et al., 2003). The I^2 has several advantages over Q statistic, including intuitive interpretation. The I^2 showed that 89% of the heterogeneity was due to program factors rather than chance (I^2=89). Heterogeneity within programs was found in two studies: Earp, Eng and O'Malley (2002) and Gotay, Banner, Matsunaga, Hedlund et al., (2000). The Earp et al., (2002) study produced positive impact for low income but not for high income, the Gotay et al., (2000) show no program effect for adherence but positive impact for uptake and similarly and the Margolis et al., (1998) showed positive impact for uptake but not adherence.

Moderator effects Because of the small number of final interventions included, only three control variables were tested: (1) Outreach vs. Inreach recruitment strategy, (2) Individualized vs. Group communication and (3) Screening Uptake vs. Adherence. We found two significant moderator effects – individual vs. group strategies and Outreach vs. Inreach. Programs that utilized individualized strategies produced smaller effects, about 5% percentage points higher than the control groups (RD=0.051; 95% CI=0.022, 0.080; Z=3.49, p=0.005), while rates for group strategies were 10% higher compared to the control groups (RD=0.101 CI=0.083, 0.119) a significant difference, (Z=10.81, p<0.000). Programs that emphasized screening uptake produced similar effects as those that used adherence as an out come (average rate difference about 8% points higher for treatment than control groups (RD=0.079; 95% CI=0.059, 0.099; Z=7.69, p<0.000 for adherence and RD=0.078; 95% CI=0.050, 0.105; Z=5.58, p<0.000) for uptake.)

Stability of the estimates and publication bias To determine stability of effect size estimates, we calculated Fail-Safe-N (FSN). FSN is defined as the number of unpublished null studies that would render the effect size statistically insignificant and was first described by Rosenthal (1979) as a file drawer problem meaning that there are likely to be unpublished studies lying in file cabinets because publication is usually based on statistical significance findings. We calculated FSN using

Rosenthal's file drawer approach as described by Begg (1994) as: $k_0 > -(\Sigma Z_i)^2/(Z_{1\alpha/2})^2$ where: $(\Sigma Z_i)^2$ is the square of the sum of Z values associated with the effect size, $(Z_{1\alpha/2})^2$ is the square of the critical Z value at p=0.05 in two tails and k is the number of programs involved and k_0 is the number of unpublished null studies that would be required to render the estimated effect size non-significant. The FSN calculations showed overall 6 additional studies that found no effect of these interventions would be needed to render our estimates statistically insignificant. In stratified analyses the estimate for Group Interventions were the most stable (FSN=20) followed by those for Outreach Interventions (FSN=9.2). It is unlikely that so many unpublished studies exist. We also examined a funnel plot to determine if there was any publication bias and found no evidence of publication bias.

Table 5.4   Meta-analysis of mammography screening interventions for older women of color

Citation	Recruitment	Strategy	Effect	-0.25	0.00	0.25
Bird, 1998	Outreach	Group	.220			
Bird, 1998	Outreach	Group	.111			
Duan, 2000	Outreach	Individual	.073			
Duan, 2000	Outreach	Individual	.025			
Earp, 2002	Outreach	Group	-.057			
Earp, 2002	Outreach	Group	.108			
Erwin, 1999	Outreach	Group	.090			
Gotay, 2000	Outreach	Group	.003			
Gotay, 2000	Outreach	Group	-.002			
Margolis, 1998	Both	Individual	.096			
Margolis, 1998	Both	Individual	-.027			
Navarro, 1998	Outreach	Group	.070			
Paskett, 1999	Outreach	Group	.151			
Slater, 1998	Outreach	Group	.063			
Sung, 1997	Outreach	Individual	.091			
Webber, 1997	Both	Individual	.132			
Zhu, 2002	Outreach	Individual	.000			
Fixed Combined (17)			**.078**			
				Negative		Positive

Effect: Absolute rate difference; Both: Inreach or both inreach and outreach

We conclude that these findings provide some confidence that culturally tailored strategies for improving breast cancer screening can be effective, although the overall impacts on mammography use were modest. We found strong evidence for studies that used Group Intervention and Outreach Strategies and fairly strong evidence for both Uptake and Adherence outcomes. More primary studies involving two strategies, (in-reach and individualized interventions) are required to determine the stability of the estimates for these two approaches. Further, we were unable to test the impact of population attributes such as age R/E because there were relatively few studies; and reporting did not support sub-group analyses.

Breast Cancer Treatment and Racial/Ethnic Differences

Treatment Consensus and Treatment Efficacy

Treatment for breast cancer is a multi-step and multimodal in nature. Treatment options for primary breast cancer include surgery, adjuvant radiation therapy and adjuvant systemic therapy with tamoxifen or chemotherapy. Treatment recommendations are generally based on breast cancer stage. Further refinement is based on tumor characteristics such as lymph node status, estrogen receptor or progesterone receptor (ER/PR) status, and menopausal status. There are also ongoing evaluations of optimal treatment options for systemic therapy especially for treatment of advanced stage breast cancer. Stage I, II, IIIA, and operable IIIC breast cancer are treated with curative intent. Local-regional treatment includes (1) Breast-conserving therapy (lumpectomy, breast irradiation, and surgical staging of the axilla) or (2) Modified radical mastectomy (removal of the entire breast with level I-II axillary dissection) with or without breast reconstruction. In some cases, sentinel lymph node biopsy is performed with these patients but this is currently is under clinical evaluation. However, surgical staging of the axilla should also be performed. Primary treatment is followed by adjuvant therapy in form of radiation therapy or systemic therapy. Radiation therapy is aimed at reducing local recurrences while systemic therapy is aimed at reducing the risk of distance metastasis and contra lateral breast cancer. Administration of adjuvant radiation therapy depends on number of axillary nodes involved. For patients with 1-3 positive nodes the role of regional radiation (infra/supraclavicular nodes, internal mammary nodes, axillary nodes and chest wall) is unclear. Regional radiation is advised for patients with more than 4 nodes or extra nodal involvement. Adjuvant systemic therapy is administrated according to lymph node status, ER/PR status and menopausal status. Patients with lymph node negative are sub-classified in a 3-tier risk groups proposed by an International Consensus Panel: (Low risk=Tumor size   cm; ER/PR$^+$ Tumor grade 1; Intermediate risk=Tumor size , 1-2 cm; ER/PR$^+$; Tumor grade 1-2; High risk=Tumor size, >2 cm; ER/PR $^{(-)}$; Tumor grade 2-3). With the exception of patients with negative ER/PR tumor receptor status, the preferred systemic therapy for postmenopausal women in general is tamoxifen. Women receive either tamoxifen alone or tamoxifen with chemotherapy. The only choice available for women with ER/PR negative tumors is chemotherapy. Treatment with chemotherapy is for about 6 months; longer duration treatment has no additional benefit (NCI/PDQ, 2004).

Patients with inoperable stage IIIB or IIIC or inflammatory breast cancer should also be treated with curative intent, although the evidence of benefit is much more limited. Treatment for stage IV and distant metastasis is palliative, usually involving hormone therapy and or chemotherapy with or without trastuzumab (Herceptin). Radiation therapy and/or surgery may be indicated for patients with limited symptomatic metastases (NCI/PDQ, 2004).

Treatment efficacy   Survival for BCS plus radiation is equivalent to that for mastectomy according to randomized prospective trials. Radiation therapy after breast conserving surgery consists of postoperative external-beam radiation to the entire breast with daily doses extending over a 5-week period. Older women are just as likely to benefit from BCS as their younger counterparts in terms of survival and disease free status (Solin, Schultz and Fowble, 1995). If radiation therapy is omitted after breast conserving surgery, then BCS ceases to be equivalent to mastectomy and is associated with higher local recurrence rates, (NCI-PDQ, 2004; Fisher, Anderson, Bryant et al., 2002; Veronesi, Salvadori, Luini, et al., 1995;; Clark, McCulloch, Levine et al., 1992) hence the emphasis on radiation adjuvant therapy.

The reduction of risk recurrence for those treated with chemotherapy is similar with or without tamoxifen (NCI/PDQ, 2004). In general patients with ER-positive breast cancer are likely to benefit from tamoxifen. In addition benefits from tamoxifen seem to accrue with prolonged use (Fisher, Dignam, Bryant, et al., (2001). In one review, 10-year proportional reductions in recurrence and mortality associated with 5 years of use were 47% and 26%, respectively (EBCTCG, 1998, NCI-PDQ, 2004). However, Tamoxifen is efficacious irrespective of lymph node status (positive or negative) or menopausal status. Addition of chemotherapy to tamoxifen in postmenopausal women with ER-positive disease results in a significant but small survival advantage (NCI-PDQ, 2004). A disadvantage of tamoxifen is its association with certain side effects such as development of endometrial cancer and deep vein thrombosis. Unlike tamoxifen, chemotherapy is efficacious regardless of ER/PR status, menopausal status, although impact varies by patient age. For women 50 to 69 years, combination chemotherapy improved 10-year survival by 2% compared to 7% for younger women for those with node-negative disease and by 3% compared to 11% for younger women for those with node-positive disease (EBCTCG, 1998; NCI/PDQ, 2004).

Racial/Ethnic Disparities in Breast Cancer Treatment

Although poorer breast cancer survival among women of color is mainly attributed to stage at the time of diagnosis, the R/E disparity in survival is not fully explained by stage (Eley, Hill, Chen, et al., 1994; Simon and Severson 1997). Alternative explanation include (1) differences in treatment efficacy or and (2) differences in treatment effectiveness. Shavers and Brown (2002) reviewed R/E group differences in treatment and survival. Although the study was not focused on Medicare beneficiaries, it served as a basis for this review. We sought additional and more recent articles, especially articles that examined treatment patterns for breast cancer for the period before and after 1990. Although the literature neither supports clear conclusions on temporal trends in treatment and treatment outcome disparities by R/E or compelling accounts for the specific determinants of these disparities, several conclusions can be drawn.

Equal treatments yield equal outcomes Evidence in support of treatment disparity as a contributory factor to R/E survival differences is demonstrated by examining both randomized controlled trials (efficacy studies) in which patients have equal disease and equal treatment and observational studies of prognostic factors in which patients are either equally treated or have equal disease. The strongest indirect evidence that perhaps disparities in treatment could be responsible for the residual disparity in survival comes from randomized controlled trials of treatment efficacy by race. For example, the National Surgical Adjuvant Breast and Bowel Project (NSABP) compared AA and white women on impact of treatment on survival. There was no AA/white difference in survival in this 'equal disease/equal treatment trial'. This study demonstrated that when R/E groups have similar stage and disease characteristics and are equally treated, there is little or no racial in breast cancer treatment or survival (Dignam 2000/2001; Dignam et al., 1997). There are no equivalent studies comparing white women to Hispanics, Asians/Pacific Islanders, and American Indian/Alaskan Natives.

Tumor characteristics and efficacy Tumor characteristic play an important role in the choice of breast cancer treatment strategies. It has been hypothesized that differences in molecular tumor characteristics (which are associated with faster breast cancer growth and lymph node metastasis) could be responsible for stage-specific differences in survival. It has also been suggested that R/E disparities in molecular tumor characters may influence treatment outcomes (Shavers and Brown, 2002). Although poorer survival has been associated with more aggressive breast tumor characteristics (such as high nuclear grade, p53 gene alteration, and HER-2/neu expression, negative estrogen and progesterone receptors), especially among younger women, R/E differences in these factors are not consistent and contribute little to survival disparities among the elderly. R/E differences in unfavorable tumor characteristics among the elderly are small (Furberg, Millikan, Dressler, et al., 2001) because these features tend to diminish with age (Diab, Elledge, and Clark, 2000). For example, Furberg et al (2001) found that younger AA and white women differed only with respect to ER/PR status, while older AA and white women differed only with respect to stage at diagnosis. In addition, although observational studies report disparities in survival, randomized controlled trials show little or no difference in breast cancer survival by R/E group (Dignam Redmond, Fisher et al., 1997; Roach Cirrincione, Budman et al., 1997; Dignam et al., 2001). This suggests a R/E difference in treatment efficacy is not the major factor accounting for residual disparity in breast cancer survival after accounting for difference in stage at diagnosis and treatment quality.

Treatment Effectiveness and Racial/Ethnic Differences

Four studies we reviewed demonstrated that disparities in treatment are the major contributing factor to survival differences (Bain, Greenberg, and Whitaker 1986; Bradley, Given, and Roberts, 2002, Mancino et al., 2001, McWhorter and Mayer 1987). All these studies found that (1) disparities occurred in primary treatment and were associated with poorer survival among AA women; (2) AA women were less likely to have surgery or other breast cancer directed treatment and (3) when AA women did receive treatment, they were likely to be treated less optimally.

Breast conserving therapy versus mastectomy   In 1990 the National Institutes of Health Consensus Panel recommended breast conserving surgery (BCS) with radiation therapy (RT) for stage I and II cancer as a preferable method of primary treatment rather than mastectomy because survival outcomes for these two treatment modalities are equivalent and in addition BCS provides better quality of life (QOL) because it preserves breast tissue. Appropriate BCS now includes complete tumor resection, axillary lymph node dissection (LND) and RT to the local area. Appropriate mastectomy is also accompanied by axillary LND and breast reconstruction. Although breast reconstruction is not essential to survival, it improves quality of life.

The evidence shows that up to 1990, women of color who had invasive breast cancer were less likely to receive minimal expected therapy (Breen, Wesley, Merrill et al., 1999, Diehr, Yergan, Chu, et al., 1989; Farrow, Hunt, and Samet, 1992; Michalski and Nattinger, 1997; McWhorter et al., 1987; Muss, Hunter, Wesley et al., 1992). There was, however, no R/E difference in the use of BCS among women who had ductal carcinoma-in-situ (Adams-Cameron, Gilliland, Hunt, et al., 1999). In contrast, after 1990, use of BCS increased even among women of color especially AA women (Bradley Given and Roberts, 2002; Morris, Cohen, Schlag et al., 2000; Polednak 2002). Variations by R/E in use still persist (Gilligan, Kneusel, Hoffmann et al., 2002; Polednak, 1997; Polednak, 2002; Legorreta, Liu, and Parker, 2000). There is consistent evidence of R/E disparities in the receipt of BCS particularly for AI/AN, Hispanic, and API women, who are less likely to receive BCS (Legorreta et al., 2000; Morris et al., 2000; Shavers and Brown 2002). Elderly AA women are still less likely to receive BCS (Morris et al., 2000). A more recent study involving 11 SEER registries and 124,934 of women (with 31-56% elders 60 years and older) diagnosed between 1992 and 1998, show that Black women were 40% more likely to receive inappropriate care. AI/AN were just as likely to receive appropriate care as white women. There was, however, a heterogeneous picture for Asians and Hispanics, where rates of appropriate care varied by sub-group. For example, Mexicans and Puerto Ricans, but not Cubans and other Hispanics, were more likely to receive inappropriate treatment than white women (Li, Malone and Daling, 2003).

Four factors have been found to contribute to disparities in primary surgical treatment: Provider organization characteristics, patient characteristics, and systems of care and geographical location of treatment or patient residence. Primary surgical treatment disparities are more common in smaller facilities. Patient age, insurance status, SES, urban/rural residence, census tract education level, and census tract income level are consistent correlates of primary surgical treatment disparities (Michalski et al., 1997; Morris et al., 2000; Velanovich, Yood, Bawle et al., 1999; Bradley et al., 2002; Diehr et al., 1989; Muss et al., 1992).

Omission of radiation therapy after breast conserving surgery   Because BCS requires a separate incision for LND and requires local RT, it has a greater potential to be administered inappropriately (radiation therapy or lymph node dissection might be omitted). Although the use of BCS has been increasing for women of color since 1990, the proportion of women receiving appropriate therapy has also declined. For example, according to Nattinger, Hoffmann, Kneusel et al., (2000), the proportion of women receiving appropriate care fell from 88% in 1983-1989 to 78% by 1995. Reviewers have concluded that all women of color and the elderly are less likely to receive RT after BCS (Ballard-Barbash, Potosky, Harlan et al., 1996; Shavers and Brown 2002). The differential is greater for women aged 65 and older.

Omission of systemic adjuvant therapy Statistically significant benefits have been observed with systemic adjuvant therapy (Aapro, 2001). However, omission of systemic adjuvant therapy, tamoxifen or chemotherapy, following BCS or mastectomy, is another potential source of treatment disparity. Much of the difference in survival between AA and white women is attributed to greater proportions of AA never becoming disease free. The likelihood is greater for women in later stage than for those in early stage. For example, Mancino et al., (2001) performed a retrospective review of 1,345 women who were entered during 1990-1998 in a local tumor registry with invasive breast cancer ranging from stages I-IV. This data revealed no difference in *survival* between Black and white women who had presented with either Stage I or Stage II breast cancer. They however, found significant differences between Blacks and whites that had presented with either stage III or IV. They also found a significantly lower percentage of Black women who became disease free after initial therapy compared to white women particularly in the stage III and IV sample. This difference in ability to achieve disease free status is not explained by differences in stage, but by failure to complete systemic adjuvant therapy. By contrast, efficacy studies in which conditions of treatment are controlled show that women of color who have access to adjuvant therapy have similar disease free rates as white women (Dignam 2001).

Two of the studies reviewed suggest that transportation and distance to treatment sites are potential barriers to completion of systemic adjuvant therapy among women of color and the elderly. For example, Guidry, Aday, Zhang et al., (1997) compared distance and mode of transportation to radiation therapy and chemotherapy and perceptions of transportation as a barrier to care among 593 breast cancer patients from multiple R/E groups receiving treatment from a Texas consortium. Women of color reported barriers such as distance, access to automobile and availability of someone to drive them to the treatment center. In a follow-up analysis, Guidry (1998) found significant insurance barriers to completion of adjuvant therapy for Hispanic and Black women (Guidry et al, 1998).

Omission of Breast reconstruction One study was found that addressed the issue of R/E disparities in breast reconstruction surgery after mastectomy. Polednak (1999) used Connecticut cancer registry data to examine among 10, 756 cases (diagnosed with breast cancer between 1988-1995) trends and predictors of breast reconstruction after mastectomy. Women of color and the elderly were less likely to have breast reconstruction after mastectomy. They found breast reconstruction surgery to be negatively associated with Black race, age and poverty (Polednak 1999).

As a group, these studies examined provided evidence for racial/ethnic disparity in treatment as a contributory factor to survival differences both before and after 1990. These studies suggest that the primary factors contributing to survival differences are regional and systemic failure, i.e. failure to eliminate breast cancer cells that spread to the regional and distant sites. Studies also show that women of color are more likely to receive inappropriate treatment (incomplete) than are their counterparts. Limitations to identifying racial/ethnic disparities in treatment include, limited number of studies that are based exclusively on more recent data (post 1990), and the fact that some studies combine data from different periods (for example, combining the 1980s and 1990s) despite the major shift in breast treatment modalities over time.

Interventions to Reduce Race/Ethnic Disparities in Cancer Treatment

Interventions aimed either at the individual level or at reducing R/E disparities in cancer treatment were sought from the Medline database using endnote software. Consultants and other review papers were other potential sources for these. There are currently no intervention studies in these areas that we could identify. The few observational studies on barriers to treatment by R/E women of color suggest interventions aimed at reduction in out-of-pocket expenses related to treatment, help with navigating the care system and education regarding treatment options and reducing transportation barriers might be useful in reducing non-clinical barriers to radiation therapy and systemic adjuvant therapy.

Summary and Conclusions

Although breast cancer incidence is higher among white women, traditionally excluded R/E group women have a more advanced stage at diagnosis and experience disproportionate rates of mortality. Both underlying risk and access to mammography appear to play a role in increasing breast cancer incidence; however, the pattern of increase with more early stage tumors suggests a clear role of screening. There is evidence that R/E differences in stage at the time of diagnosis account for a significant share of mortality and survival disparities. Nonetheless, there are also stage-specific racial differences in survival that cannot be explained by clinical factors.

Some decline in breast cancer mortality has been reported. It appears that screening and treatment have contributed to reduced mortality rates. White women have benefited more from this than women of color. Higher mortality for AA women in recent years represents a major shift (from lower to higher), which began almost a decade after the introduction of mammography and accelerated during the decade of improved local and systemic therapy (1990s). Although tumor characteristics may influence R/E differences breast cancer stage and treatment efficacy, we found little evidence for this among elders. The observed R/E differences are unlikely to be due to inherent differences in tumor characteristics.

Differences in breast cancer tumor characteristics tend to diminish with age and few available studies showed comparable tumor characteristics. The exception may be Japanese Americans. The overall survival advantage of Japanese-American, suggests more favorable tumor characteristics with a possible environmental role as suggested by one study of breast cancer and green tea among Japanese patients (Nakawachi, Suemasu, Suga et al., 1998) but more conclusive studies of this possibility are needed.

There is consensus regarding recommendations for use of screening methods on timing of screening for breast cancer. Breast cancer screening rates are below the recommended levels for all Medicare beneficiaries, but notably lower for underserved R/E minorities. Different R/E groups seem to be at different stages in a screening-re-screen and follow-up continuum and many in these groups face additional barriers to breast cancer screening compared to white women. Although many factors account for R/E disparities in breast cancer screening, SES, health insurance, practical access barriers (such as transportation) and inconsistent attention by practitioners play major roles.

There are reports of culturally tailored interventions to increase screening that typically involve use of community health workers to conduct educational programs using culturally and linguistically adapted materials. Some programs used multiple strategies that included assistance in overcoming barriers to access. Our meta-analysis of these studies shows that overall breast cancer screening interventions aimed at women of color and employing community health workers and other cultural tailoring components produce modest significant impacts on screening rates, but they are extremely heterogeneous in their effects. Group educational approaches rather than individualized produced had stronger findings.

Final diagnosis and staging of breast cancer requires a multi-step process involving multiple tests, procedures, and professional consultations. There is evidence that AA women are less likely to receive complete diagnostic work-ups and valid clinical staging. The reasons for these are not clear from this review, due to a dearth of studies exploring this issue.

There is compelling evidence for R/E disparities in breast cancer treatment. Members of traditionally excluded R/E groups are less likely to receive appropriate care and are less likely to receive systemic adjuvant therapy after breast conserving surgery and were less likely to undergo breast reconstruction. The strength of available evidence varies across these measures of use. At the individual patient level, non-clinical factors were associated with disparity in primary breast cancer treatment choice: insurance status, SES, geographical location of residence, and neighborhood-level measures of SES. Women also reported barriers such as distance, access to automobile and availability of someone to drive them to the treatment center. There is increasingly strong evidence that R/E survival differences within stage at diagnosis are primarily explained by disparities in primary treatments and completion systemic adjuvant treatments.

This chapter reveals R/E disparities at every stage of the breast cancer management continuum. These findings suggest that interventions aimed at both reducing R/E disparities in breast cancer detection and treatment have the potential to influence overall differences in outcomes. The available research shows that both differences in stage at diagnosis and differences in treatment influence breast cancer and health outcomes. Improving screening participation and adherence for R/E elders are clearly worthwhile goals in light of these findings. Although the evidence could be stronger, it appears that culturally tailored screening interventions that focus group education and counseling approaches had greater potential to influence R/E differences than individualized approaches. Unlike prior efforts, new demonstrations might focus on programming that specifically targets screening adherence, follow-up after abnormal screening and removal of practical access barriers such as transportation as an additional strategy. Interventions that increase the likelihood that patients and practitioners follow-up on suspicious screening findings and perform complete diagnostic work-ups can reduce R/E differentials. No less important than complete diagnosis is timely completion of all recommended primary and adjuvant treatments. These findings underscore the potential to improve breast cancer survivorship by ensuring that patient and practitioners complete the process. Although demonstrations and evaluations of breast cancer treatment management services were not identified in the literature, this review highlights treatment management as a potential area for important and cost-effective reductions in cancer care disparities. A treatment management intervention that draws upon a community health worker serving as a patient navigator holds the potential to increase the share of elders of color who receive the current standard of care.

References

Aapro, M.S. (2001). Adjuvant therapy of primary breast cancer: a review of key findings from the 7th International Conference, St. Gallen, February 2001. *Oncologist*, 6(4): 376-385.

Ahmedin, J., Tiwari, R.C., Murray, T. et al. (2004). Cancer Statistics 2004. *CA, Cancer Journal of Clinicians*, 54:8-29. Available online at: http://CAonline.AmCancerSoc.org.

ACS – American Cancer Society. (2001). *Cancer Facts and Figures 2001*. Atlanta, GA: American Cancer Society.

AGS Clinical Practice Committee. Journal of the American Geriatrics Society, 48:842-8442000; http://www.ameriacangeriatrics.org/products/positionpapers/brstcncr.shtml.

Alexander, F.E. (1997). The Edinburgh randomized trial of breast cancer screening. *Journal of the National Cancer Institute, Monograph*, 22: 31-35.

Austin, L.T., Ahmad, F., McNally, M.J. et al. (2002). Breast and cervical cancer screening in Hispanic women: a literature review using the health belief model. *Womens Health Issues*, 12(3): 122-128.

Bain, R.P., Greenberg, R.S. and Whitaker, J.P. (1986). Racial differences in survival of women with breast cancer. *Journal of Chronic Diseases*, 39(8): 631-642.

Ballard-Barbash, R., Potosky, A.L., Harlan, L.C. et al. (1996). Factors associated with surgical and radiation therapy for early stage breast cancer in older women. *Journal of the National Cancer Institute*, 88(11): 716-726.

Bastani, R., Kaplan, C.P., Maxwell, A.E. et al. (1995). Initial and repeat mammography screening in a low-income multi-ethnic population in Los Angeles. *Cancer Epidemiology, Biomarkers, and Prevention*, 4(2): 161-167.

Begg, C.B. (1994) Publication bias. In Cooper H and Hedges LV (eds). (1994). The Handbook of Research Synthesis (pp 399-437). New York Russell Sage Foundation.

Bentley, J.R., Delfino, R.J., Taylor, T.H. et al. (1998). Differences in breast cancer stage at diagnosis between non-Hispanic White and Hispanic populations, San Diego County 1988-1993. *Breast Cancer Research Treatment*, 50(1): 1-9.

Bibb, S.C. (2001). The relationship between access and stage at diagnosis of breast cancer in African American and Caucasian women. *Oncology Nurses Forum*, 28(4): 711-719.

Bird, J.A., McPhee, S.J., Ha, N.T. et al. (1998). Opening pathways to cancer screening for Vietnamese-American women: lay health workers hold a key. *Preventative Medicine*, 27(6):821-829.

Blackman, D.K., Bennett, E.M. and Miller, D.S. (1999). Trends in self-reported use of mammograms (1989-1997) and Papanicolaou tests (1991-1997) – Behavioral Risk Factor Surveillance System. *Morbidity and Mortality Weekly Report*, 48(6): 1-22.

Bradley, C.J., Given, C.W. and Roberts, C. (2000). Disparities in Cancer Diagnosis and Survival. *Cancer*, 91(1): 178-188.

Breen, N., Wesley, M.N., Merrill, R.M. et al. (1999). The relationship of socio-economic status and access to minimum expected therapy among female breast cancer patients in the National Cancer Institute Black-White Cancer Survival Study. *Ethnic Diseases*, 9(1): 111-125.

Burns, R.B., McCarthy, E.P., Freund, K.M. et al. (1996a). Black women receive less mammography even with similar use of primary care. *Annals of Internal Medicine*, 125(3): 173-182.

Burns, R.B., McCarthy, E.P., Freund, K.M. et al. (1996b). Variability in mammography use among older women. *Journal of the American Geriatric Society*, 44(8): 922-926.

Caplan, L.S., Helzlsouer, K.J., Shapiro, S. et al. (1996). Reasons for delay in breast cancer diagnosis. *Preventive Medicine*, 25(2): 218-224.

CDC (1994). Results from the National Breast and Cervical Cancer Early Detection Program, October 31, 1991 – September 30, 1993. *Morbidity and Mortality Weekly Report*, 43(29), 530-534.

CDC (1997). Use of Clinical Preventive Services by Medicare Beneficiaries Aged greater than or equal to 65 Years – United States, 1995. *Morbidity and Mortality Weekly Report*, 46(48): 1138-1143.

CDC (2001). National breast cancer and Early Detection Program, Authorizing and Related Legislation: http//www.cdc.gov/cancer/nbccedp/law.htm.

Chang, S.W., Kerlikowske, K., Napoles-Springer, A. et al. (1996) Racial differences in timeliness of follow-up after abnormal mammography. *Cancer*, 78(7) 1395-1340.

Chu, K.C., Tarone, R.E., Kessler, L.G. et al. (1996). Recent trends in U.S. breast cancer incidence, survival, and mortality rates. *Journal of the National Cancer Institute*, 88(21), 1571-1579.

Clark, R.M., McCulloch, P.B., Levine, M.N. et al. (1992). Randomized clinical trial to assess the effectiveness of breast irradiation following lumpectomy and axillary dissection for node-negative breast cancer. *Journal of the National Cancer Institute*, 84(9): 683-689.

Coleman, E.A. and O'Sullivan, P. (2001). Racial differences in breast cancer screening among women from 65 to 74 years of age: Trends from 1987-1993 and barriers to screening. *Journal of Women and Aging*, 13(3): 23-39.

Cummings, D.M., Whetstone, L.M., Earp, J.A. et al. (2002). Disparities in mammography screening in rural areas: analysis of county differences in North Carolina. *Journal of Rural Health*, 18(1): 77-83.

Danigelis, N.L., Worden, J.K. and Mickey, R.M. (1996). The importance of age as a context for understanding African-American women's mammography screening behavior. *American Journal of Preventive Medicine,* 12(5): 358-366.

Delgado, D.D., Lin, W.Y. and Coffey, M. (1995). The role of Hispanic race/ethnicity and poverty in breast cancer survival. *Puerto Rico Health Sciences Journal,* 14(2): 103-116.

Deutsch, M. and Flickinger, J.C. (2001). Shoulder and arm problems after radiotherapy for primary breast cancer. *American Journal of Clinical Oncology,* 24(2): 172-176.

Diab, S.G., Elledge, R.M. and Clark, G.M. (2000). Tumor characteristics and clinical outcome of elderly women with breast cancer. *Journal of the National Cancer Institute,* 92(7): 550-556.

Diehr, P., Yergan, J., Chu, J. et al. (1989). Treatment modality and quality differences for Black and White breast-cancer patients treated in community hospitals. *Medical Care,* 27(10): 942-958.

Dignan, M., Michielutte, R., Blinson, K. et al. (1996). Effectiveness of health education to increase screening for cervical cancer among eastern-band Cherokee Indian women in North Carolina. *Journal of the National Cancer Institute,* 88(22):1670-1676.

Dignam, J.J., Redmond, C.K., Fisher, B. et al. (1997). Prognosis among African-American women and White women with lymph node negative breast carcinoma: findings from two randomized clinical trials of the National Surgical Adjuvant Breast and Bowel Project. *Cancer,* 80(1): 80-90.

Dignam, J.J. (2000). Differences in breast cancer prognosis among African-American and Caucasian women. *CA Cancer Journal of Clinicians,* 50(1), 50-64.

Dignam, J.J. (2001). Efficacy of systemic adjuvant therapy for breast cancer in African-American and Caucasian women. *Journal of the National Cancer Institute Monograph,* 30: 36-43.

Dolan, N.C., Reifler, D.R., McDermott, M.M. et al. (1995). Adherence to screening mammography recommendations in a university general medicine clinic. *Journal of General Internal Medicine,* 10(6): 299-306.

Duan, N, Fox, S.A., Derose, K.P. et al. (2000). Maintaining mammography adherence through telephone counseling in a church-based trial. *American Journal of Public Health,* 90(9):1468-1471.

Earp, J.A., Eng, E., O'Malley, M.S. et al. (2002). Increasing use of mammography among older, rural African American women: results from a community trial. *American Journal of Public Health,* 92(4): 646-654.

EBCTCG (Early Breast Cancer Trialists' Collaborative Group). (1998). Tamoxifen for early breast cancer: an overview of the randomised trials. *Lancet,* 351(9114): 1451-1467.

EBCTCG (Early Breast Cancer Trialists' Collaborative Group). (1998). Polychemotherapy for early breast cancer: an overview of the randomised trials. *Lancet,* 352(9132): 930-942.

El-Tamer, M.B., Homel, P., and Wait, R.B. (1999). Is race a poor prognostic factor in breast cancer? *Journal of the American College of Surgeons,* 189(1): 41-45.

Eley, J.W., Hill, H.A., Chen, V.W. et al. (1994). Racial differences in survival from breast cancer. Results of the National Cancer Institute Black/White Cancer Survival Study. *Journal of the American Medical Association,* 272(12): 947-954.

Erwin, D.O., Spatz, T.S., Stotts, R.C. et al. (1999). Increasing mammography practice by African American women. *Cancer Practices,* 7(2):78-85.

Farrow, D.C., Hunt, W.C. and Samet, J.M. (1992). Geographic variation in the treatment of localized breast cancer. *New England Journal of Medicine,* 326(17): 1097-1101.

Fisher, B., Anderson, S., Bryant, J. et al. (2002) Twenty-year follow-up of a randomized trial comparing total mastectomy, lumpectomy, and lumpectomy plus irradiation for treatment of invasive breast cancer. *New England Journal of Medicine,* 347(16): 1233-1241.

Fisher, B., Dignam, J., Bryant, J. et al. (2001). Five versus more than five years of tamoxifen for lymph node-negative breast cancer: Updated findings from the National Surgical Adjuvant Breast and Bowel Project B-14 randomized trial. *Journal of the National Cancer Institute*, 93 (9): 684-690.

Fox, S.A. and Roetzheim, R.G. (1994). Screening mammography and older Hispanic women. Current status and issues. *Cancer*, 74(7 Suppl): 2028-2033.

Frost, F., Tollestrup, K., Hunt, W.C. et al. (1996). Breast cancer survival among New Mexico Hispanic, American Indian, and non-Hispanic White women (1973-1992). *Cancer Epidemiology, Biomarkers and Prevention*, 5(11): 861-866.

Feuer, E.J., Wun, L.M., Boring, C.C. et al. (1993). The lifetime risk of developing breast cancer. *Journal of the National Cancer Institute*, 85(11): 892-897.

Furberg, H., Millikan, R., Dressler, L. et al. (2001). Tumor characteristics in African American and White women. *Breast Cancer Research Treatment*, 68(1): 33-43.

Gilligan, A.M., Kneusel, R.T., Hoffmann, R.G. et al. (2002). Persistent differences in sociodemographic determinants of breast conserving treatment despite overall increased adoption. *Medical Care*, 40(3): 181-189.

Gilliland, F.D., Rosenberg, R.D. and Hunt, W.C. (2000). Patterns of mammography use among Hispanic, American Indian, and non-Hispanic White Women in New Mexico, 1994-1997. *American Journal of Epidemiology*, 152(5): 432-437.

Gotay, C.C., Banner, R.O., Matsunaga, D.S. et al. (2000). Impact of a culturally appropriate intervention on breast and cervical screening among native Hawaiian women. *Preventive Medicine*, 31(5): 529-537.

Gregg, E.W., Kriska, A.M., Narayan, K.M. et al. (1996). Relationship of locus of control to physical activity among people with and without diabetes. *Diabetes Care*, 19(10): 1118-1121.

Gotzsche, P.C. and Olsen, O. (2000). Is screening for breast cancer with mammography justifiable? *Lancet*, 355(9198): 129-34.

Guidry, J.J., Aday, L.A., Zhang, D. et al. (1997). Transportation as a barrier to cancer treatment. *Cancer Practice*, 5(6): 361-366.

Guidry, J.J., Aday, L.A., Zhang, D. et al. (1998). Cost considerations as potential barriers to cancer treatment. *Cancer Practice*, 6(3): 182-187.

Hardy, R.E., Ahmed, N.U., Hargreaves, M.K. et al. (2000). Difficulty in reaching low-income women for screening mammography. *Journal of Health Care for the Poor and Underserved*, 11(1): 45-57.

Hawley, S.T., Earp, J.A., O'Malley, M. et al. (2000). The role of physician recommendation in women's mammography use: is it a 2-stage process? *Medical Care*, 38: 392-403.

Hegarty, V., Burchett, B.M., Gold, D.T. et al. (2000). Racial differences in use of cancer prevention services among older Americans. *Journal of the American Geriatric Society*, 48(7): 735-740.

Higgins, J.P., Thompson, S.G., Deeks, J.J. et al. (2003). Measuring inconsistency in meta-analyses. *British Medical Journal*, 327(7414): 557-560.

Howe, H., Wingo, P.A., Thun, M.J. et al. (2001). Annual report to the nation on the status of cancer (1973 through 1998), featuring cancers with recent increasing trends. *Journal of the National Cancer Institute*, 93(11): 824-842.

Hunter, C., Stemmermann, G., Jackson, J.S. et al. (1997). Aggressiveness of colon cancer in Blacks and Whites. National Cancer Institute Black/White Cancer Survival Study Group. *Cancer Epidemiology Biomarkers, and Prevention*, 6(12): 1087-1093.

Jacobellis, J. and Cutter, G. (2002). Mammography screening and differences in stage of disease by race/ethnicity. *American Journal of Public Health*, 92(7): 1144-1150.

Jameson, D.T., Bobadilla, J., Hetcht, R. et al. (1993) World Development Report, 1993. Investing in Health Oxford University Press, 200 Maddison Avenue, New York.

http://www-wds.worldbank.org/servlet/WDSContentServer/WDSP/IB/1993/06/01/
000009265_ 3970716142319/Rendered/PDF/multi0page.pdf.

Jones, B.A., Kasl, S.V., Curnen, M.G. et al. (1995). Can mammography screening explain the race difference in stage at diagnosis of breast cancer? *Cancer*, 75(8): 2103-2113.

Joslyn, S.A. and West, M.M. (2000). Racial differences in breast carcinoma survival. *Cancer*, 88(1): 114-123.

Kelaher, M. and Stellman, J.M. (2000). The impact of Medicare funding on the use of mammography among older women: implications for improving access to screening. *Preventative Medicine*, 31(6): 658-664.

Kerlikowske, K., Grady, D., Rubin, S.M. et al. (1995). Efficacy of screening mammography. A meta-analysis. *Journal of the American Medical Association*, 273(2): 149-154.

Kerlikowske, K. (1996). Timeliness of follow-up after abnormal screening mammography. Breast Cancer Res Treat. 40(1): 53-64

Kerner, J.F., Yedidia, M., Padgett, D. et al (2003). Realization of breast cancer screening: clinical follow-up after abnormal screening among Black women. *Preventative Medicine*, 37(2): 92-101.

Lannin, D.R., Mathews, H.F., Mitchell, J. et al. (1998). Influence of socioeconomic and cultural factors on racial differences in late-stage presentation of breast cancer. *Journal of the American Medical Association*, 279(22): 1801-1807.

Larson, D., Weinstein, M., Goldberg, I. et al. (1986). Edema of the arm as a function of the extent of axillary surgery in patients with stage I-II carcinoma of the breast treated with primary radiotherapy. *International Journal of Radiation, Oncology, and Biology for Physics*, 12 (9): 1575-1582.

Laws, M.B. and Mayo, S.J. (1998). The Latina Breast Cancer Control Study, year one: factors predicting screening mammography utilization by urban Latina women in Massachusetts. *Journal of Community Health*, 23(4): 251-267.

Lee, J.R. and Vogel, V.G. (1995). Who uses screening mammography regularly? *Cancer Epidemiology, Biomarkers, and Prevention*, 4(8): 901-906.

Legg, J.S. (2000). Provider efforts to increase mammography screening. *Radiology Technology*, 71(5), 435-440.

Legorreta, A.P., Liu, X. and Parker, R.G. (2000). Examining the use of breast-conserving treatment for women with breast cancer in a managed care environment. *American Journal of Clinical Oncology*, 23(5): 438-441.

Li, C.I., Malone, K.E. and Daling, J.R. (2003). Differences in breast cancer stage, treatment and survival by race and ethnicity. *Archives of Internal Medicine*, 163: 49-56.

Link, B.G., Northridge, M.E., Phelan, J.C. et al. (1998). Social epidemiology and the fundamental cause concept: On the structuring of effective cancer screens by socioeconomic status. *Milbank Quarterly*, 76(3): 375-402, 304-375.

Mancino, A.T., Rubio, I.T., Henry-Tillman, R. et al. (2001). Racial differences in breast cancer survival: the effect of residual disease. *Journal of Surgical Research*, 100(2): 161-165.

Mandelblatt, J., Andrews, H., Kao, R. et al. (1995). Impact of access and social context on breast cancer stage at diagnosis. *Journal of Health Care for the Poor Underserved*, 6(3): 342-351.

Mandelblatt, J.S. and Yabroff, K.R. (1999). Effectiveness of interventions designed to increase mammography use: A meta-analysis of provider-targeted strategies. *Cancer Epidemiology, Biomarkers and Prevention*, 8(9): 759-767.

Marbella, A.M. and Layde, P.M. (2001). Racial trends in age-specific breast cancer mortality rates in US women. *American Journal of Public Health*, 91(1): 118-121.

Margolis, K.L., Lurie, N., McGovern, P.G. et al. (1998). Increasing breast and cervical cancer screening in low-income women. *Journal of General Internal Medicine*, 13(8): 515-521.

Maxwell, A.E., Bastani, R. and Warda, U.S. (1998). Mammography utilization and related attitudes among Korean-American women. *Women's Health*, 27(3): 89-107.

May, D.S., Lee, N.C., Richardson, L.C. et al. (2000). Mammography and breast cancer detection by race and Hispanic ethnicity: Results from a national program (United States). *Cancer Causes Control*, 11(8): 697-705.

McCarthy, E.P., Burns, R.B., Coughlin, S.S. et al. (1998). Mammography use helps to explain differences in breast cancer stage at diagnosis between older Black and White women. *Annals of Internal Medicine*, 128(9): 729-736.

McWhorter, W.P. and Mayer, W.J. (1987). Black/White differences in type of initial breast cancer treatment and implications for survival. *American Journal of Public Health*, 77(12): 1515-1517.

Meng, L., Maskarinec, G. and Lee, J. (1997). Ethnicity and conditional breast cancer survival in Hawaii. *Journal of Clinical Epidemiology*, 50(11): 1289-1296.

Michalski, T.A. and Nattinger, A.B. (1997). The influence of race and socioeconomic status on use of breast-conserving surgery for Medicare beneficiaries. *Cancer*, 79: 314-319.

Moorman, P., Jones, B., Millikan, R. et al. (2001). Race, anthropometric factors, and stage at diagnosis of breast cancer. *American Journal of Epidemiology*, 153(3): 284-291.

Morris, C.R., Cohen, R., Schlag, R. et al. (2000). Increasing trends in the use of breast-conserving surgery in California. *American Journal of Public Health*, 90(2): 281-284.

Muss, H.B. (2000). Breast Cancer and Differential Diagnosis of Benign Nodules. In: Goldman L G and Bennett J.C. Cecil (eds). *Text Book of Medicine 21st Edition*. WB Saunders Company: Phildelphia, PA.

Nakawachi, K., Suemasu, K., Suga, K.T. et al. (1998). Influence of drinking tea on breast cancer malignancy among Japanese patients. *Japan Journal of Cancer Research*, 89: 254-261.

Natarajan, N., Nemoto, D., Nemoto, T. et al. (1988). Breast cancer survival among Orientals and Whites living in the United States. *Journal of Surgical Oncology*, 39(3): 206-209.

Nattinger, A.B. (2000). Care for breast cancer: the adoption of newer clinical paradigms. *Medical Care*, 38(7): 693-695.

Navarro, A.M., Senn, K.L., McNicholas, L.J. et al. (1998). Por La Vida model intervention enhances use of cancer screening tests among Latinas. *American Journal of Preventative Medicine*, 15(1):32-41.

NCI (1998). *Screening for Breast Cancer*, [electronic document]. National Cancer Institute. Available: http:/www.cancer.gov. Last update 11/98.

NCI (2002). NCI Statement on Mammography Screening. http://www.cancer.gove/new center/mammstatement31jan02.

NCI/PDQ (2004). Breast cancer (PDQ) treatment. http://www.cancer/gov/cancertopics/ pdq/treat-ment/breast/healthprofessional/page7#section_165.

Newcomb, P.A. and Lantz, P.M. (1993). Recent trends in breast cancer incidence, mortality, and mammography. *Breast Cancer Research Treatment*, 28(2): 97-106.

NGC National Guideline Clearinghouse. (2001). Guideline synthesis: Screening for breast cancer. In: *National Guideline Clearinghouse (NGC) [website]. Rockville (MD): 2001 Jun 12. [cited 7/18/2002. Available: http://www.guideline.gov.*

O'Malley, M.S., Earp, J.A. and Harris, R.P. (1997). Race and mammography use in two North Carolina counties. *American Journal of Public Health*, 87(5): 782-786.

Parker, J.D., Sabogal, F. and Gebretsadik, T. (1999). Relationship between earlier and later mammography screening – California Medicare, 1992 through 1994. *Western Journal of Medicine*, 170(1): 25-27.

Paskett, E.D., Tatum, C.M., D'Agostino, R. et al. (1999). Community-based interventions to improve breast and cervical cancer screening: results of the Forsyth County Cancer

Screening (FoCaS) Project. *Cancer Epidemiological Biomarkers and Prevention,* 8(5):, 453-459.

Pearlman, D.N., Rakowski, W., Ehrich, B. et al. (1996). Breast cancer screening practices among Black, Hispanic, and White women: reassessing differences. *American Journal of Preventive Medicine,* 12(5): 327-337.

Polednak, A.P. (1997). Predictors of breast-conserving surgery in Connecticut, 1990-1992. *Annals of Surgical Oncology,* 4(3): 259-263.

Polednak, A.P. (1999). Post-mastectomy breast reconstruction in Connecticut: Trends and predictors. *Plastic Reconstructive Surgery,* 104(3): 669-673.

Polednak, A.P. (2002). Trends in, and predictors of, breast-conserving surgery and radiotherapy for breast cancer in Connecticut, 1988-1997. *International Journal of Radiation Oncology Biology and Physics,* 53(1): 157-163.

Porter, P.L., El-Bastawissi, A.Y., Mandelson, M.T. et al. (1999). Breast tumor characteristics as predictors of mammographic detection: comparison of interval- and screen-detected cancers. *Journal of the National Cancer Institute,* 91(23): 2020-2028.

Preston, J.A., Scinto, J.D. and Ni, W. (1997). Mammography under utilization among older women in Connecticut. *Journal of the American Geriatric Society,* 45(11): 1310-1314.

Ramirez, A.G., Villarreal, R., McAlister, A. et al. (1999). Advancing the role of participatory communication in the diffusion of cancer screening among Hispanics. *Journal of Health Communication,* 4(1):31-36.

Ramirez, A.G., Suarez, L., Laufman, L. et al. (2000). Hispanic women's breast and cervical cancer knowledge, attitudes, and screening behaviors. *American Journal of Health Promotion,* 14(5): 292-300.

Reeves, M.J., Newcomb, P.A., Remington, P.L. et al. (1996). Body mass and breast cancer. Relationship between method of detection and stage of disease. *Cancer,* 77(2): 301-307.

Ries, L., Eisner, M.P., Kosary, C.L. et al. (eds). (2002). *SEER Cancer Statistics Review, 1973-1999.* Bethesda, MD: National Cancer Institute.

Ries, L.A.G., Eisner, M.P., Kosary, C.L. et al. (eds). (2003). *SEER Cancer Statistics Review, 1975-2001,* National Cancer Institute. Bethesda, MD, http://seer.cancer.gov/csr/1975_2001/, 2004.

Roach III, M., Cirrincione, C., Budman, D. et al. (1997). Race and survival from breast cancer: based on Cancer and Leukemia Group B trial 8541. *Cancer Journal Scientific American,* 3(2): 107-112.

Rojas, M.J., Cagney. K., Kerner, J. et al. (1996). Barriers to follow-up of abnormal screening mammograms among low-income minority women. Cancer Control Center of Harlem. *Ethnic Health,* 1(3): 221-228.

Rosenthal, R. (1979). The 'file drawer problem' and tolerance for null studies. *Psychological Bulletin,* 86: 638-641P.

Shapiro, S. (1997). Periodic screening for breast cancer: the HIP Randomized Controlled Trial. Health Insurance Plan. *Journal of the National Cancer Institute, Monograph,* (22): 27-30.

Shavers, V.L. and Brown, M.L. (2002). Racial and ethnic disparities in the receipt of cancer treatment. *Journal of the National Cancer Institute,* 94(5): 334-357.

Simon, M.S. and Severson, R.K. (1997). Racial differences in breast cancer survival: The interaction of socioeconomic status and tumor biology. *American Journal of Obstetrics and Gynecology,* 176(6): S233-239.

Slater, J.S., Ha, C.N., Malone, M.E. et al. (1998). A randomized community trial to increase mammography utilization among low-income women living in public housing. *Preventative Medicine,* 27(6):862-870.

Smith, R.A., Cokkinides, V., Eschenbach, A.C. et al. (2002). American Cancer Society guidelines for arly detection of cancer. *CA, Cancer Journal for Clinicians,* 52(8): 8-23.

Solin, L.J., Schultz, D.J. and Fowble, B.L. (1995). Ten-year results of the treatment of early-stage breast carcinoma in elderly women using breast-conserving surgery and definitive breast irradiation. *International Journal of Radiation, Oncology, Biology, and Physics,* 33 (1): 45-51.

Song, L. and Fletcher, R. (1998). Breast cancer re-screening in low-income women. *American Journal of Preventive Medicine,* 15(2): 128-133.

Swedborg, I. and Wallgren, A. (1981) The effect of pre- and post-mastectomy radiotherapy on the degree of edema, shoulder-joint mobility, and gripping force. *Cancer,* 47(5): 877-881.

Suarez, L., Roche, R.A., Pulley, L.V. et al. (1997). Why a peer intervention program for Mexican-American women failed to modify the secular trend in cancer screening. *American Journal of Preventive Medicine,* 13(6): 411-417.

Sugarman, J.R., Dennis, L.K. and White, E. (1994). Cancer survival among American Indians in western Washington State (United States). *Cancer Causes Control,* 5(5): 440-448.

Sung, J.F., Blumenthal, D.S. and Coates R.J. (1997). Knowledge, beliefs, attitudes and cancer among inner city African Americans. *Journal of the National Medical Association,* 89(6): 405-411.

Tang, T.S., Solomon, L.J. and McCracken, L.M. (2000). Cultural barriers to mammography, clinical breast exam, and breast self-exam among Chinese-American women 60 and older. *Preventative Medicine,* 31(5): 575-583.

Taylor, V.M., Thompson, B., and Montano, D.E. et al. (1998). Mammography use among women attending an inner-city clinic. *Journal of Cancer Education,* 13(2): 96-101.

Veronesi, U., Salvadori, B., Luini, A., et al. (1995). Breast conservation is a safe method in patients with small cancer of the breast. Long-term results of three randomized trials on 1,973 patients. *European Journal of Cancer,* 31A(10): 1574-1579.

Velanovich, V., Yood, M.U., Bawle, U. et al. (1999). Racial differences in the presentation and surgical management of breast cancer. *Surgery,* 125(4): 375-379.

Woloshin, S., Schwartz, L.M., Katz, S.J. et al. (1997). Is language a barrier to the use of preventive services? *Journal of General Internal Medicine,* 12(8): 472-477.

Wagner, T.H. (1998). The effectiveness of mailed patient reminders on mammography screening: a meta-analysis. *American Journal Preventive Medicine,* 14(1): 64-70.

Weber, B.E. and Reilly, B.M. (1997). Enhancing mammography use in the inner city. A randomized trial of intensive case management. *Archives of Internal Medicine,* 157(20): 2345-2349.

Wu, X.C., Andrews, P.A., Correa, C.N. et al. (2001). Breast cancer: incidence, mortality, and early detection in Louisiana, 1988-1997. *Journal of the Louisiana State Medical Society,* 153(4): 198-209.

Wu, Y., Khan, H., Chillar, R. et al. (1999). Prognostic value of plasma HER-2/neu in African American and Hispanic women with breast cancer. *International Journal of Oncology,* 14(6): 1021-1037.

Yabroff, K.R. and Gordis, L. (2003). Does stage at diagnosis influence the relationship between socioeconomic status and breast cancer incidence case fatality and mortality? *Social Sciences Medicine,* 57(12): 2265-2279.

Yabroff, K.R. and Mandelblatt, J.S. (1999). Interventions targeted toward patients to increase mammography use. *Cancer Epidemiology, Biomarkers and Prevention,* 8(9): 749-757.

Yood, M.U., Johnson, C.C., Blount, A. et al. (1999). Race and differences in breast cancer survival in a managed care population. *Journal of the National Cancer Institute.* 91(17): 1487-1491.

Zhu, K., Hunter, S., Bernard, L.J. et al. (2002). An Intervention Study on Screening for Breast Cancer among Single African-American Women Aged 65 and Older. *Preventative Medicine,* 34(5):536-545.

Appendix 5.1 Culturally tailored mammography screening interventions

Author	Disparity	Design	Setting	Age
Bird (1998)	Adherence	CPT	Community based	40+
Bird (1998)	Uptake	CPT	Community based	40+
Duan (2000)	Adherence [A2]	RCT	Sample of churches [B2]	50+
Duan (2000)	Adherence [A2]	RCT	Sample of churches [B2]	50+
Earp (2002)	Adherence	CPT	Population based [A3]	50+
Earp(2002)	Adherence	CPT	Population based [A3]	50+
Erwin (1999)	Uptake	CCBT	Sample of churches [A4]	40+
Gotay (2000)	Uptake	CPT	Population based [A5]	40+
Gotay (2000)	Adherence	CPT	Population based [A5]	40+
Margolis (1998)	Adherence	CCT	In reach [A6]	40+
Margolis (1998)	Adherence	CCT	In reach [A6]	40+
Navarro (1998)	Adherence	RCT [A7]	Community based	40+ [B7]
Paskett (1999)	Adherence	CPT	Outreach [A8]	40+
Slater (1998)	Adherence	RCT	Outreach [A9]	50+
Weber (1997)	Adherence	RCT	Primary care sites	52+
Sung (1997)	Adherence	RCT	Community based	18+
Zhu (2002)	Adherence	RCT	10 housing sites	65+

Mammography Intervention Studies Notes

CHW:Community Health Worker; CCT: Controlled clinical trial; RCT: Randomized clinical trial; CCBT: Controlled community based trial; RD: Rate absolute rate difference; BLN: Baseline sample; CGBL Rate: Control group baseline sample; MD: Medical doctor; NP: Nurse practitioner.

[A1]. Small group education session by lay health workers, plus education material distribution, promotional events.

Target Group	Intervention	BLN	CG BL Rate	RD
Vietnamese Americans	CHW, education materials, events [A1]	705	32	22
Vietnamese Americans	CHW, education materials, events [A1]	705	43	11
Latina, AA	Telephone counseling [C2]	522	na	7.5
Latina, AA	Telephone counseling [C2]	291	na	2.6
AA	Volunteer CHW [B3]	514	49[C4]	11
AA	Volunteer CHW [B3]	204	73	-6
AA	CHW, Witness Team [B4]	310	60.4[C4]	9.1
NHOPI	Volunteer CHW, Kokua groups [B5]	287	75	0[c5]
NHOPI	Volunteer CHW, Kokua groups [B5]	228	60	0[C5]
Native American	CHW invite and NP [B6]	835[C6]	na	9.6
Native American	CHW invite and NP [B6]	719[C6]	na	-2.7
Latina	Por La Vida Model [C7]	361	24.6	7
AA	Multiple out-reach tools. CHW [B8]	248	30	15
White, AA	CHW-, Friend-to-Friend [B9]	427	53.5	6.3
AA, Asian, Latina	MD letter and CHW follow-up [A10}	376	16	17
AA	CHW in-home education [A11]	321	34.3	4.8
AA	CHW in-home education[A12]	323	47[B12]	0

[A2]. Rates are the 1-year non-adherence rates. Rates were broken into maintenance (M) for those adherent at baseline and conversion (C) for those who became adherent during the study. Rates were not reported for the entire control or experimental groups as a whole. Only those who completed the study were included in the final analysis. 1113 subjects began the study. [B2.] 30 churches randomized to telephone counseling and control: 8 mostly Latino churches, 12 mostly Black churches, and 10 mostly white churches in southern CA were included in the study. Churches were blocked on dominant race/ethnicity, size, and resources. [C2]. The intervention was telephone counseling annually over two years.

[A3]. Population based probabilistic sampling in NC, 37% non-white, 5 intervention counties. [B3]. 170 volunteer lay health advisors prompted awareness of mammography in the community.

[A4]. Two intervention counties with 11 churches, 2 control counties, 48% of members were African American. [B4]. Seven local AA women were witness role models and spoke to church member groups about their experiences, highlighting the need for early detection and resources for free/reduced cost mammograms. Program also provided vouchers for free mammograms. About 32 vouchers were distributed within a 6-month f/u, women made their own appointments and transportation. There was no federal funding or systematic screening program. [C4]. Baseline samples were not explicitly provided. We calculated baseline samples from given proportions provided under baseline characteristics. Intervention group was 75% of 216 minus 2 who were not Black; for the control group- 69% of 217.

[A5]. Study used random digit telephone sampling. Kokua neighborhood was intervention community with neighborhood control communities identified through census tracts. [B5]. Kokua groups were composed of community women gathered by friends or colleagues. Female lay health advisors led the groups. The definition of Kokua is: Help without being requested and without expectation of payment. [C5]. There was no difference in these unadjusted estimates between the intervention and control communities, although the authors using nonhierarchical linear regression found the Kokua group to be significant predictor of mammography use as compared to the control.

[A6]. Senior aides recruited American Indian women from non-primary care clinics. Female low-income lay health advisors were paid by a federal job-retraining program. A study coordinator supervised lay aides. [B6] Lay health advisors assessed participants' breast cancer screening status and offered appointments with a female NP at a women's cancer screening clinic. Each clinic visit was linked to a mammography on the same day. [C6]. Sample sizes for each group were calculated from baseline data in table 2 of the article.

[A7]. Study recruited Consejeras (CHWs) through social networks. Randomization was by Consejera. [B7]. Age range in text is 18-72 because study also looked at pap test. [C7]. The Por La Vida model involved 36 lay health 'natural' helpers conducting educational sessions with an average of 14 members. Natural helpers are described as people who have a reputation in the community for good judgment, sound advice discretion, and caring. [A8]. Education brochures to address identified barriers: e.g. where to get a mammogram. [B8]. Multifaceted education and promotional intervention such as free party in the community that included educational classes and information booths, prizes, cholesterol and diabetes screening.

[A9]: ACS and a high-rise resident volunteer planned Community involvement [B9]. The Friend to Friend (FTF) Project involved education, limited provider and patient reminders, limited free mammograms, screening promotion, scheduling assistance small group discussions, health professional talks, opportunities to request assistance in obtaining a mammogram, and provider reminder. Recruitment involved FTF parties, fliers, posters and presentations at resident council meetings, educational newsletters sent to building residents, personal invitations. Women who attended FTF parties were encouraged to invite those who did not.

[A10]. Physician intervention was a letter on practice letterhead reminding the woman she was due for a mammogram. CHE group received the same letter, but then a follow-up letter written in English and Spanish, telephone calls, other reminders, home visits, and assistance facing barriers.

[A11]. Lay health workers visited from a community-based women's health organization.

[A12]. Baseline rates were calculated by subtracting the pre-post difference from the posttest rate

Chapter 6

Race/Ethnicity and
Cervical Cancer

Introduction

In this chapter we explore opportunities for reducing racial/ethnic (R/E) disparities in uterine cervix carcinoma (cervical cancer) morbidity and mortality. As for breast cancer, we focus on the burden of the disease (incidence, mortality and survival) utilization of services (screening and follow-up, and treatment) and on interventions to reduce disparities in screening, and treatment. A major theme here is that cervical cancer appears more readily controlled than breast cancer, and thus differential incidence and mortality by R/E group appears even more unnecessary. Unlike breast cancer, the cervical cancer major risk factors, such as infection with Human Papilloma virus (HPV), are exogenous. Further, there is more clear evidence that the pre-cancerous phase of cervical lesions may progress to become cancerous in a multi-step process involving a long lead-time. As a result, there are ample opportunities for effective interventions to abort the disease.

Although the incidence of invasive cervical cancer has significantly declined over the last four decades, it remains an important public policy issue. The introduction of Papanicolaou (Pap) test has made it possible to prevent pre-cancerous and pre-invasive lesions of the more common type of cervical cancer, squamous cell carcinoma (SCCA), from progressing to the invasive type and for health practitioners to intervene at more treatable localized stages. Like breast cancer, however, women in traditionally underserved racial/ethnic (R/E) groups have benefited least from these developments. For example, between 1997 and 2001, elderly African American (AA) women were more likely to develop invasive cervical cancer and 3 times more likely to die from it than were white women of the same age group (18.9/100,000 for AA women vs. 6.5/100,000 for white women (Ries, Eisner, Kosary et al., 2004). This is mainly because elder R/E minority women suffer a triple jeopardy in relation to cervical cancer–longer life time exposure to risk factors, lower rates of screening and follow-up, and inability to receive timely effective treatment.

Invasive cervical cancer remains substantially higher among R/E minority elders largely due to ineffective screening. For example, although the incidence varies widely by R/E, detection rates are less variable. Bernard, Lee, Piper, et al., (2001) using a large national multiethnic sample of women, found the R/E variation in the prevalence of abnormal screens to be much smaller and ironically, white women, had the highest rates of high risk screens. This suggests that the observed wide difference in cervical cancer incidence is due to differences in effectiveness of screening and follow-up rather than due to large differences in underlying risk and that this may account for better survival observed among white women. Many factors including inadequate health insurance, lack of recommendation by providers, practical access barriers and possible provider-patient miscommunication account for racial differences in screening. Culturally tailored interventions that include community health workers, as cultural brokers are therefore promising as interventions to reduce R/E disparities in screening.

Stage-at-diagnosis of cervical cancer plays a big role in R/E survival differences but does not fully explain the R/E differences in survival, suggesting the role of other factors. The role of histology remains inconclusive. Although adenocarcinoma (ADCA) is associated with worse prognosis at advanced stages, and over the past 25 years has been increasing, particularly among older AA women (Wang; Sherman, Hildesheim et al, 2003, its clinical significance has not been established mostly due to smaller proportions of this cell type. None of the studies however have tested the interaction between histology and R/E in stage-specific survival.

More important is the role of treatment effectiveness and perhaps co-morbidity; and hence the need for multilevel/multidisciplinary approaches. As demonstrated by studies of 'equal disease, equal treatment' and efficacy studies, there is no reason to believe that there is a R/E difference in the efficacy of cervical cancer treatment. There is, however, a clear difference in treatment, particularly choice of treatment for local and regional disease, inability to adhere to treatment protocol, and lower rates of timely treatment completion. For example, more use of radiotherapy than hysterectomy has been reported for AA than white women. This coupled by the failure to adhere to radiotherapy treatment (RT) may account for some difference in treatment effectiveness. Further, although the role of treatment in improving survival is limited at advanced stages of cervical cancer, elder women in underserved R/E groups could further benefit from better treatment of the regional disease. More recent data shows a narrowed gap in stage-specific survival differences, suggesting some improvement in treatment effectiveness, although mortality differences still persist.

Identification and Selection of Reports for Systematic Reviews

We conducted electronic searches of Medline and the NCI CancerLit from 1985 to 2003, supplemented by backward citation searches using Social Science Citation Index/Web of Science for selected papers. Cervical cancer keywords i.e. uterine cervix carcinoma or cervical cancer, were combined with other key words in each search. All searches used the following key words to locate reports on cancer among women from R/E minority groups: minority elderly, race, elders of color, elders, minority, older adults, adults, African-American, Black, Hispanic, Latino, Spanish surname, American Indian, Native American, Alaskan Native, Hawaiian Native, Pacific Islanders, and Asian American. Additional key words included: prevalence, incidence, mortality, survival, screening, diagnosis, treatment, surgery, chemotherapy, radiotherapy, radiation, quality of life, relapse, monitoring, culture, intervention, RCT, community health worker, case management, quality improvement. Other sources of information were the review of intervention to increase use of Medicare services prepared for CMS by RAND (Shekelle, Stone, and Manglione et al., 2001) and the reviews supporting the AHRQ Task Force on Clinical Preventive Services guidelines. As in other chapters, we use the R/E categories adopted in primary sources even when these were not consistent within current census classifications.

Cervical Cancer Prevalence and Mortality: Race/Ethnic Differences

Cervical cancer is 100% preventable if caught and treated at the pre-cancerous or pre-invasive stage. Improvements in SES coupled with increased access to Pap screening have shifted the incidence of cervical cancer from mostly invasive to most pre-invasive types known as cervical intra-epithelial lesion (SIL), cervical intra-epithelial neoplasia 2 (CIN 2) and cervical intra-epithelial neoplasia[3] (CIN3). In 2002 for example an estimated 1,250,000 women were diagnosed with SIL, CIN 2 and CIN3 compared to 13,000 who were diagnosed with invasive cervical cancer. Between 1975 and 2001 the incidence of invasive cervical cancer declined by 49% (14.8 in 1975 to 7.6 per 100,000 in 2001) (Ries et al, 2004). Cervical cancer, however, remains an important public policy issue because of its high fatality rate. One in three women diagnosed with cervical cancer dies. In 2004, for example 10,500 invasive cervical cancer cases and 3,900 deaths are estimated (ACS, 2004).

Incidence and Racial Ethnic Patterns

Like breast cancer, older women have higher cervical cancer incidence and mortality rates than younger women. Between 1997 to 2001, invasive cervical cancer incidence rates for women aged 65 years and over were 2 times higher than incidence rates for younger women (13.2 vs. 7.7 per 100,000); and older women were 3 times more likely to die from cervical cancer than were younger women (7.6 vs. 2.2 per 100,000 women at risk) (Ries et al., 2004). Unlike breast cancer, however, cervical cancer is more common in minority R/E groups ((Hispanics, African-American (AA), Asians/Pacific Islanders (API), American Indians/Alaska Natives (AI/AN) in that order)) than in whites. Of the top 15 cancers (considering both genders), it is overall 10th most common. But it is 4th for Hispanics, 6th for AA, 7th for API and AI/AN and 9th for white women (Ries, Eisner, Kosary et al., 2001). Its incidence rate varies similarly: 16.2, 11.8, 9.5 and 6.0 per 100,000 for Hispanics, AA, API, AI/AN respectively (see Table 6.1). In contrast with breast cancer R/E minorities with cervical cancer tend to be older than their white counterparts, perhaps representing missed opportunities to prevent this disease.

Although the past two decades has seen a decline in the incidence of invasive SCCA for all women, the rates for underserved R/E groups have remained above average. There has also been an increase in the less common cell type, ADCA. This has been reported for older AA and for younger women in all groups. There has been no similar trend among elder White women. The reasons for rising incidence of ADCA are not clear. A cohort effect implying different, underlying risk factors for women born since the sexual revolution has been suggested (Wang; Sherman, Hildesheim et al., 2003. The higher rate of incidence of ADCA among older AA women has been attributed to both possible differences in risk factors and less effective screening. There are also notable intra-ethnic variations in cervical cancer incidence. Among API for example, its incidence rate for the period 1988 to1992, varied widely: 21.1 for Chinese, 28.2 for Filipino, 55.2 for Koreans, 181.6 for Vietnamese and 9.5 per 100,000 for Japanese American women (Miller et al., 1996).

Table 6.1 Cervical cancer incidence by race/ethnicity: SEER sites, 1997-2001

Race/Ethnicity	Incidence [I] 1997-2001	EAPC1992-2001 (%)[1]
All Races	9.3	-2.6*
Hispanic	16.2	-3.3*
White non-Hispanic	7.3	-2.5*
African American	11.8	-3.1*
Asian/Pacific Islander	9.5	-4.7*
AI/Alaskan Natives	6.0	-7.7

[1]The EAPC is the estimated annual percentage change over the time interval.
*The EAPC is significantly different from Zero (p<05)

Source: Ries, et al (2004). http://seer.cancer.gov/csr/1975_2001/, 2004.

Mortality, Survival and Racial/Ethnic Patterns

The trend in cervical cancer mortality for the period 1975-2001 shows a gradual but substantial decline of about 47% (from 5.5 per 100,000 for 1975/76 to 2.9 per 100,000 for 1997/01) similar to the rate of decline in invasive cervical cancer incidence (about 43%). (See Table 6.1) Mortality, however, remains relatively higher for underserved R/E groups and for elderly women than for younger white women. From 1997-2001, for example, cervical cancer mortality rates were 5.6 for Blacks, 3.6 for Hispanics, 2.8 for AN/AI and .8 for API women compared to 2.5 per 100,000 for white women. Similarly women 65 years and older had 3.5 greater odds of dying from cervical cancer compared to younger women. AA women 65 years and older had 5.0 times greater odds of dying from cervical cancer than younger AA women (compared to 3 times the rate for older White women relative to younger white women). (See Table 6.1).

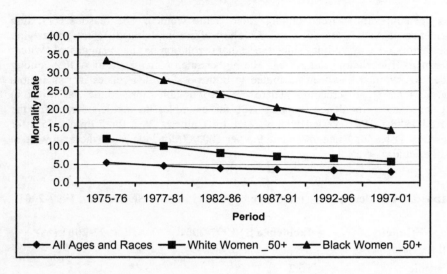

Figure 6.1 Trend in invasive cervical cancer mortality: overall and among black and white women 50 years of age and over; 1975-2001

Source: Ries et al. (2004). Mortality rate is per 100,000 women at risk.

In contrast to mortality, the trend in cervical cancer survival is disappointing. From 1974–2000, for example there was overall no significant improvement in cervical cancer five-year survival rates (69.2% in 1974 to 72% in 2000). Slight improvement in survival during this period is seen only among white women (from 69.9% in 1974 to 74% in 2000). This data suggests that the decline in mortality is attributed mostly to early detection efforts rather than to improvements in treatment efficacy. This is better demonstrated in the next section by analyzing stage-specific survival rates. This new data (adjusted to 2000 standard population) also suggests a narrowing gap in survival between older white women and older black women since 1989 (see Figure 6.2) suggesting that early detection efforts have started paying off.

Stage, Survival and Race/Ethnic Differences

A number of researchers have noted that AA and other underserved R/E group women generally have less favorable cervical cancer survival than white women and that stage at diagnosis plays a major role. It is not clear, however, whether this is true for cervical cancer and if the R/E disparity in survival is fully explained by differences in stage of disease at diagnosis.

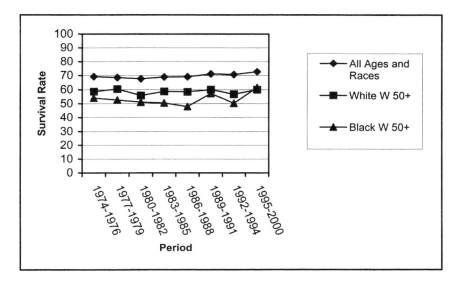

Figure 6.2 Trends in cervical cancer survival for all ages/races, older black and white women: 1975-2001

Source: Ries et al. (2004). Rates are 5-year survival rates per 100 cases.

As for breast cancer, cervical cancer five-year survival declines with increasing stage for both white and non-white older women but stage specific racial differences in survival are also common. Ragland, Selvin and Merrill (1991) used SEER data for the period 1974-1985 to examine R/E patterns of stage at diagnosis for seven selected sites including cervical cancer. They did not find a consistent pattern in the association between stage and race among cervical cancer patients. They found racial differences at some stages but not all.

SEER data for the period 1973-1999 (Ries et al., 2004) shows that at localized stage, older AA and white women experienced nearly equal survival (89% and 86%, respectively). But that for regional (stage IIB and III) and distant metastasis (stage IV), older AA women had significantly worse survival) and this was also true for distant metastasis (11.5 for older white and 3% for older AA women). More recent data suggests that the survival gap between white women and Black women 50 years of age and over has narrowed. As shown in table 6.3 stage-specific survival rates are comparable with a trend toward better survival at every stage for AA women. The narrowed gap in stage-specific survival suggests improvement in treatment effectiveness for Black women. The data for this period also shows comparable five-year survival between Black and white women 65 years of age and over. Stage-specific comparisons, however, are not available for this age group and the relative contributions of early detection and improved treatment cannot be delineated for this age group. Black/white stage-specific differences in survival, however, persist for younger women. The data for the period 1996-2000 also shows that R/E differences in stage at diagnosis have persisted. AA and API women are still less likely to be diagnosed at localized stage than were White women (ACS, 2004) and were more likely to be diagnosed at regional and distant metastasis stage. Hispanic women seem to have comparable stage at diagnosis to white women according to this new data. No stage-specific survival data are available for this group in this dataset.

For AI/AN women, Sugarman, Dennis and White (1994) compared stage-specific survival for AAN (n=551) and whites (n=110,899) diagnosed from 1974-1989 from the Seattle-Puget Sound Cancer Registry. They found that AI/AN women experienced worse survival despite having similar stage distribution. This poor survival persisted after adjustment for differences in cancer stage at diagnosis, lack of cancer treatment, age, and residence in a non-urban county. Interestingly the authors observed that the survival experience among AI/AN women incorrectly classified as white cancer in the registry records was more favorable than those correctly classified as American Indians in the cancer registry. The significance of this finding is not clear from this study in terms of impact on population estimates. Further, more recent studies on relative stage-specific survival of AI/AN are required.

Table 6.2   Cervical cancer survival by stage, age and race: 1995-2000

	W< 50	AA< 50.	W50 +	AA50 +.
Localized	95.7	85.6	85.9	90.5
Regional	58.6	51.9	47.9	48.1
Distant	25.9	11.	11.9	12.3
Unstaged	76.7	54.8	47.5	52.6
All Stages	82.4	69.	60.0	61.5

Source: Ries et al, 2004. AA=African-American W=White.

Among the API women, the stage-survival association is heterogeneous for subgroups. Lin, Clarke, Preen et al., (2002) used data from SEER to compare the distributions of stage at diagnosis and computed 5-year cause specific survival probabilities, overall and by stage of disease, for cancer patients whose diagnosis was in 1988-1994 and who were observed through 1997. They found significant variations in the association between stage and survival among the Asian American subpopulations. The Chinese, experienced worse survival than did white women. They also had worse survival than the Filipino and the Japanese. The survival experience of the Chinese was worse than that of white women even for early stage cervical carcinoma (Lin, Clarke, Preen, Glaser et al., (2002). The Japanese in contrast experienced better survival than white women did.

A possible role of histology in stage-specific survival difference Some age and R/E differences in the incidence of ADCA have been reported and some histology types have features with poor prognostic potential (Lopez, Kudelka, Edwards, et al., 1997). Could these or other histological differences help explain the stage-specific survival patterns? Some histology types have poor prognostic features such as being difficult to detect at pre-invasive stage (ADCA), having a high risk for lymph node metastasis (e.g. adenosquamous carcinoma); poor response to surgery and radiation (e.g. glassy cell carcinoma), or potential for neuroendocrine differentiation and very poor prognosis (e.g. small cell carcinoma). ADCA is less likely to be detected by pap screening and is associated with more aggressive behavior such as lymph node involvement, early metastasis and higher recurrence rates (Lopez, et al., 1997). Although ADCA has been associated with higher mortality at advanced stages, its clinical significance in terms of influencing mortality differences has not been established. The association between histology of cervical cancer and stage-specific survival has been reported for stage IB and stage IIB and not all stages.

A number of earlier studies examined the association between histology and stage-specific survival. These studies have been small and they show an inconsistent association of histology type to stage-specific survival, suggesting that this phenomenon may apply to some subpopulations but not all. In a more recent large population study (n= 21,434 for SCCA and 4,650 for ADCA) conducted over a 24-year period, (1973-1996), Smith, Tiffany, Qualls and Charles (2000) found a statistically significant difference in survival in favor of squamous cell carcinoma, the difference in survival was, however small. Because none of the studies directly addressed the interaction between histology and R/E group in survival, the role of histology differences in cervical cancer survival disparities cannot be ruled out. Primary studies should specifically examine impact of histology differences on stage-specific survival differences for elder R/E minorities.

Cervical Cancer Screening and Race/Ethnicity Differences

There is currently no effective primary prevention for cervical cancer. Two possible primary intervention methods are immuno-prevention (vaccination) against Human Papilloma Virus (HPV) and modification of sexual behavior. The potential for immuno-prevention has been recognized and there are currently studies developing vaccines for certain types of HPV, which would make this possible, (NCI Cancer facts 2001). Modification of sexual behavior is often advised, though its effectiveness and relevance to Medicare populations are unclear. There is also some evidence to show that incorporating a focus on sexual behavior under cervical cancer preventive policy would stigmatize the disease and thus potentially reduce participation in screening and treatment. For example in one study among Hispanic women, Hubbell, Chavez, Mishra, et al., (1996), found that women who associated cervical cancer with sexual conduct were less likely to report ever having had a Pap smear. This review therefore focuses on Pap screening and follow-up after abnormal screening.

Cervical cancer is one cancer that best meets the criteria for disease screening (Cole and Morrison, 1978; NCI 2001). It is characterized by a long lead time with pre-cancerous lesions progressing through a succession of identifiable stages from least severe to most severe (termed as atypical squamous cell carcinoma of undetermined significance (ASCUS) through low grade intraepithelial lesion (LSIL) or Cervical intraepithelial neoplasia (CIN 1), to high grade squamous intraepithelial lesion (HSIL) or cervical intraepithelial neoplasia 2-3 (CIN 2-3) – prior to invasive disease (Smith, Mettlin, Davis, et al., 2000; NCI Cancer facts, 2001). If detected in the pre-clinical phase there are options to treat the pre-cancerous lesions and cure is almost 100% (Smith, et al., 2000). Although there have been no formal randomized trials to test the efficacy of Pap smear in preventing mortality, the test is widely accepted as an effective screening tool and its effectiveness is supported by several observational studies. Introduced in 1940 by Dr. George Papanicolaou, the Pap smear is now recognized as a major contributor to reduced cervical cancer incidence and mortality. There is broad consensus among professional organizations regarding screening policy. For example, the American Cancer Society recommends that women who are sexually active or those who are 18 years and over be screened with Pap smear test annually. After 3 or more consecutive satisfactory screenings with normal findings, the Pap test may be done less frequently (ACS, 2002, Smith, et al., 2000). To increase screening by elders, Medicare introduced coverage for cervical cancer screening in 1998.

Older Women and Potential Benefits of Pap Screening

Current scientific data shows the need for repeat screening in order to benefit from a Pap test. Assuming life expectancy of 84 years, the lead-time and prevalence of pre-cancerous phase of cervical cancer lesions suggest that older women would benefit from at least two screenings and necessary follow-up for abnormal screens. The pre-cancerous lesions form a continuum of progressively increasing abnormal changes and patterns; and timing of persistence, regression, and progression to invasive cervical cancer vary. For example, the average time for progression of CIN 3 to invasive cancer is 10 to 15 years, but there is a small subset of rapidly progressive cervical cancers, which are diagnosed within 3 years of a confirmed negative Pap test (NCI-PDQ 2002b). Repeat screening at least every 3 years is necessary, however, because of the high possibility of false negatives and due to this subset of rapidly progressing cervical cancer. Like other screening tests, Pap test is not perfect. It is highly liable to technical and interpretive errors with both false positive and false negatives being common. The Pap test has a high sensitivity and specificity for pre-cancerous lesions. Its reliability however depends on the technique used to obtain the cytological specimen and the adequacy of its review by the cytologist. Pap test failure rate in diagnosing invasive cancer can be as high as 50% (NCI-PDQ, 2002b). This necessitates repeat screening. Studies also suggest an unmet need for follow up of abnormal screenings for R/E minorities.

Although the incidence rate for cervical cancer varies widely, the R/E variation in abnormal Pap smear and high-risk rates is smaller. Bernard, Lee, Piper, et al., (2001) used the National Breast and Cervical Cancer Early Detection

Program data collected for 1991-1998 to describe Pap screening and biopsy results by R/E group. They examined the percentage of abnormalities detected by Pap tests and the rate of biopsy-diagnosed high-grade pre-cancerous or cancerous lesions by R/E group. The sample included 628,085 women of which about 50% were R/E minorities. They found that AI/AN women had the highest proportion of abnormal Pap tests for first program screens (4.4%), followed by AA (3.2%), White (3.0%), Hispanic (2.7%), and API (1.9%) women. They also found that AI/AN women were more likely than others to report never having had a prior Pap test. With regard to high-risk lesions, white women had the highest biopsy detection rate of high-grade lesions for first program screens (9.9 per 1000 Pap tests). They also found that AA women with a high-grade Pap test were less likely to get complete diagnostic testing or preventive treatment of pre-cancerous conditions. These findings suggest that access to screening and follow-up contribute more to observed R/E differences in cervical cancer incidence and mortality rather than large differences in underlying risks, at least for older women with similar social economic status.

Elders and Racial/Ethnic Differences in Pap Testing

Compared to other cancer screening tests, the Pap screening rates are much higher both in terms of women who have ever had a test and women who have had recent test. Like other cancer tests, however, there are significant age and R/E differences in the utilization of Pap tests. In general, API and Hispanic women have much lower lifetime and recent Pap tests, than either white or AA women. Older R/E minority women are significantly less likely to have ever had Pap test or to have a recent test (Mandelblatt and Yabroff, 1999; Hegarty, Burchett, Gold, et al., 2000; Zambrana, Breen, Fox, et al., 1999; Kagawa-Singer et al., 2000; Blackman, Bennett and Miller, 1999).

Older AA women seem to be less likely to ever use Pap tests although they are just as likely as White women to recent use (CDC 1995; Blackman et al., 1999). Blackman, Bennett and Miller (1999) examined trends in Pap use by age and R/E group and showed that women aged 70 and over, followed by women aged 60-69 were less likely to ever use or to have recent use than the younger women. More recently, Hegarty, Burchett, Gold, et al. (2000) used a follow-up survey design and a stratified probability sample to evaluate rates of Pap test utilization among women from the Piedmont area of North Carolina. They surveyed 4,162 women at baseline in 1986-1987 and 2,846 surveyed in 1992-1993. At time of follow-up survey in 1992-1993 there were 1,486 women aged 70 years and over, 1,246 of these were AA and 966 were white. They found that compared with older whites, older Black persons were 8.5 % less likely to receive Pap test.

Mandelblatt and Yarboff (1999) used a structured telephone survey of a quota sample of 1,420 New York City women from four Hispanic groups (Columbian, Dominican, Puerto Rican, Ecuadorian) and three groups of African descent (U.S., Caribbean, and Haitian) to evaluate R/E patterns of 'ever' and 'recent' self-reported use of Pap smears. The sample included both elders and non-elder women. They found that among these Latinas, women age 65 and older were significantly less likely to have ever had a Pap test by 21% and 33 % less likely to have recently Pap test than younger women.

Follow-Up on Abnormal Pap Tests Racial/Ethnic Differences

R/E minority women are, less likely to be followed up after abnormal Pap smear. Because Pap smear is a screening test and not diagnostic, further tests are needed after an abnormal Pap screen. There is general consensus that women whose Pap test indicate high-grade abnormal cell changes should have follow-up with more definitive diagnostic workup such as colposcopy and cone biopsy of any abnormal areas (Ferenczy, 1997; NCI Cancer facts, 2001). The cost-effective management of minor cervical abnormalities by preventing unnecessary colposcopies and cone biopsies, however, presents a challenge. Disparities may arise in this process. Two options are available for management of patients with mild cervical abnormality such as ASCUS or LSIL. One option is to recommend colposcopy only for those women who present with persistent low-grade abnormalities such as two positive Pap smears within a two-year follow-up period. The other option is to have immediate colposcopy for women with a single abnormal cytology suggestive of LSIL. Additional assessment criteria focus on whether or not a patient is at low or high risk for developing cervical cancer or HSIL. According to Ferenczy (1997), high-risk patients should be followed-up with immediate colposcopy. If appropriate, they should be treated immediately to prevent the development of invasive cervical cancer. If repeat Pap test is positive for LSIL, low risk patients should be followed up with Pap tests at 6-month intervals for up to two years to determine whether the lesion will become persistent or will regress.

To get a sense of the area of cervical cancer prevention, in which each R/E group is lagging, we compared abnormal screening rates to rates of screening (Figure 6.3), incidence and mortality using national level data from various sources collected within a similar period. We compared each racial/ethnic minority group to white women using rate ratios, with the white women as the comparison. Figure 6.3 indicates that AA and white women have comparable screening and abnormal cytology rates. These groups differ on high-risk cervical cytology, incidence and mortality rates. Although AA women have lower rates of high-risk cervical cytology, their incidence of cervical cancer is higher and AA women experience higher mortality rates. According to Bernard. Lee, Piper, et al., (2001), AA women are less likely to be followed up after an abnormal screen. Hispanic women, by contrast, have lower pap screening rates (both ever and in the last two years) lower abnormal Paps and lower high risk Paps but higher incidence of cervical cancer and higher mortality rates than do white women. These data suggests that Hispanic women could benefit from both more careful screening and follow-up after abnormal screening. Similarly, the diverse pan-ethnic API women seem to have the lower levels of Pap screening as well as abnormal and high risk cytology detection rates than white women (lowest over all), but have slightly higher incidence and almost comparable mortality rates as white women. Like Hispanic women, they could benefit from increasing the prevalence of women who have ever screened and those who have had a recent screen. Finally, AN/AI group, have rates of ever screening that are comparable to white women but have slightly lower rates of recent screening much higher rates of abnormal pap tests (highest overall), much lower rates of high risk Pap test and incidence but disproportionately higher mortality rates. Like Hispanic and API women, they could benefit from increasing the prevalence of women who have had a recent screen and more rigorous follow-up of abnormal Pap tests.

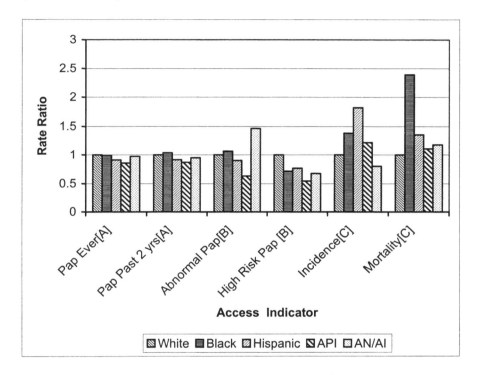

Figure 6.3 Racial/ethnic patterns of Pap tests, abnormal Pap tests, and cervical cancer incidence and mortality: 1991-1998

Data Sources: [A]= Blackman (1999), BRFFS 1991-1997; [B]= Bernard, Lee, Piper, et al., (2001), N=628,085, data is for 1991-1998, rates are per 1000 Pap tests; [C]= Ries et al. (2002) NCI/SEER Statistical review 1973-1999, data is for a period 1992-1998. API=Asian and Pacific Islander, AN/AI= Alaskan Native/American Indian; Rate Ratio of 1=no difference.

The disparity in follow-up after abnormal Pap test suggested by this data is supported by analytic studies. Mandelblatt, Traxler, Lakin, et al., (1993) found that nearly 1/3 of older AA women with abnormal Pap smear did not complete follow-up. This cross-sectional study examined clinical findings from a cervical cancer-screening program at an urban public clinic for poor, elderly, AA women. The sample comprised 491 women aged 65 years and over. In another study, Fox et al.,

(1997) found significant differences in follow-up on cervical cancer screening by R/E and urban/rural residence. About 1,738 women in the California Breast and Cervical cancer Control Program who received an abnormal cervical screening result comprised the sample. Severity of diagnosis was another significant predictor of follow-up.

These data suggest that R/E minorities are less likely to be followed up. Part of this may be due to the complexity of the triage system. Preliminary findings from NCI-funded ASCUS/LSIL Triage Study (ALTS) suggest that testing cervical samples for HPV is an option to help direct follow-up for women with an ASCUS Pap test result. Although once completed the NCI-funded ASCUS/LSIL Triage Study (ALTS) will help practitioners decide what course of action to take when mild abnormalities are found on Pap tests, it may not automatically translate in fewer disparities unless specific barriers facing women from R/E minorities are also eliminated.

Explaining Racial/Ethnic Differences in Pap Screening

Many factors have been associated with R/E disparities in cervical cancer screening and follow-up. These factors may be classified as related to the practitioner, provider institution, ca+re system, individual economic status and individual attitudes. In general, the published studies provide compelling support for the roles of provider, system of care, and individual economic status/insurance in receipt of Pap smear, but less consistent findings for the effects of individual attitudes and beliefs. Women with more adequate insurance coverage, income and education and a usual source of care were more likely to adhere to Pap smear testing and to receive complete follow-up services. Some of the evidence for each of these potential determinants of R/E disparities is described below.

Systems of care and access Having no usual source of care, no regular primary care provider and having and no private health insurance have been strongly and consistently associated with disparities in Pap use. Zambrana, Breen, Fox, et al., (1999) compared the use of Pap smear 3 years prior to interview among five subgroups of Hispanic women. They examined whether socio-demographics, access, health behavior, perception, and knowledge; and acculturation factors predict screening practices for any subgroup. They used data 1990 and 1992 National Health Interview Surveys. The study sample included 2,391 women. Mexican women were the least likely to be screened with any procedure. Logistic regression results for each screening practice showed that having a usual source of care was a positive predictor for obtaining Pap test in the last 3 years. O'Malley, Earp, and Harris (1997) examined R/E patterns of cancer screening for 7 groups: US-born Blacks, English-speaking Caribbean-born Blacks, Haitian Blacks, and Puerto Rican, Dominican, Colombian, and Ecuadorian Hispanics. They found that women with usual source of care and regular provider were more likely to have ever had a Pap smear or to have recently had a Pap smear. Compared with women without a usual site of care, those with a usual site, but no regular clinician, were 1.56 times as likely to ever have received a Pap smear, and 1.84 as likely to report receiving a recent Pap smear.

Hiatt, Pasick, Stewart, et al., (2001) using a multi-ethnic sample (Latina, Chinese, AA) of 1,599 women aged 40-75 found significant R/E variations in the use of Pap smears. They used baseline data from a Breast and Cervical Cancer Intervention Study conducted in San Francisco from 1993 to 1996. They found about 89% had ever had a Pap test. Pap screening in the past 3 years was low among non-English-speaking Latinas (72%) and markedly lower among non-English-speaking Chinese women (24%). They found that the strongest predictors of screening behavior were having private health insurance and frequent use of medical services. Having a regular clinic was also important predictor of having a Pap smear in the past 3 years.

Juon, Choi, and Kim (2000) evaluated factors associated with breast and cervical cancer screening behaviors among Korean-Americans. They used a face-to-face cross-sectional survey of 438 Korean-American women residing in Maryland. About 50% of women age 18 and older had had a Pap smear in the past 2 years. In multiple logistic regression analyses, the strongest predictor of screening behaviors was having a regular medical check-up (Juon et al., 2000). Similarly, Hubbell et al., (1996) conducted a telephone survey of 1,225 English and Spanish speakers age 18 and older using the computer-assisted telephone interview system, random digit dialing, and an instrument adapted from national surveys and a previous ethnographic study. They found that health insurance was associated with using Pap smears within the past 3 years.

Practitioner factors McKee, Schechter, Burton, et al., (2001), collected data by chart abstraction on an historical cohort to examine the level of adherence to recommended follow-up after Pap test screening for a sample of women attending 7 urban community health centers who had an initial ASCUS or atypical Pap test. They found that health care practitioners recommended colposcopy after an initial atypical Pap test results in 12% of cases and repeat cytology in 67%. Failure to document a plan for management was found in 19% of cases, and low adherence to recommended follow-up was documented for 45%. The factors associated with complete versus moderate or low adherence included site of care, description of the abnormality (ASCUS vs. atypia), availability of on-site colposcopy, and discussing the plan with the patient at a visit.

Individual patient factors Several individual factors have been examined in connection with pap screening, including: health insurance, knowledge cultural beliefs/attitudes such as fear and fatalism and the perceptions about the role of sexual behavior in developing cervical cancer as well as acculturation. Kim, Yu, Chen, et al. (1999) offer one example of studies that examined cervical cancer screening knowledge and practices. They studied 159 Korean-American women aged 40 to 69 years. They used the 1987 Cancer Control Supplement questionnaire, translated into Korean. Twenty-six percent of the respondents never heard of the Pap smear test. Only 34% of respondents reported having had a Pap smear test for screening. The most frequently cited reason for not having had a Pap smear test was absence of disease.

Ramirez, Suarez, Laufman, et al., (2000) used a bilingual survey instrument to collect information on attitudes toward cancer, and screening participation. They found that attitudes were not predictive of Pap smear behavior. Attitudes varied across Hispanic subgroups with Mexican Americans and Puerto Ricans having more negative or fatalistic views of cancer than Cuban or Central Americans. In contrast, Suarez, Roche, Nichols, et al., (1997) found that for older Mexican American women with more fatalistic views were less likely to have a recent Pap smear. They interviewed 923 Mexican American women about their knowledge, attitudes, and Pap smear and mammogram screening practices. In another study, Chavez, Hubbell, Mishra, et al., (1997) found that Latina women who had more fatalistic views were less likely to report having a Pap smear in the previous 3 years. They used ethnographic interviews and a cross-sectional telephone survey in Orange County, California. Hubbell and colleagues (1996) found that Hispanic women who believed that cervical cancer had a connection with sexual behavior were less likely to report Pap smear within the past 3 years. They found that Latina immigrants were more likely than US-born Latinas or white women to believe that a variety of behaviors were risk factors for cervical cancer. Logistic regression analysis revealed that Latinas who held such beliefs that certain types of sexual activities were related to cervical cancer were significantly less likely to report receiving a Pap smear within the past 3 years than were women without these views.

Acculturation has been defined as the psychological adjustment to the host country of an immigrant and measures include: length of stay in the host country, language preference for written or oral communication, cultural norms, and English language use. Wu, Wan, and Bernstein(2001) examined patterns of mammogram and Pap screenings among Mexican American women ages 67 and over. They used 1,403 Mexican American women from the Hispanic Established Population for the Epidemiological Study of the Elderly, a cohort study of community-dwelling Mexican Americans ages 65 years or over from the southwestern United States. They found that Mexican American women, age 75 or older were less likely to ever have had cervical screening than women ages 67-74, even controlling for socio-demographic, cultural, and selected health factor. Further, older Mexican Americans, women who were less acculturated and had lower education were less likely to have ever had a Pap smear. Hubbell and colleagues (1996) found acculturation to be negatively associated with receiving a Pap smear in the past 3 years. Juon et al., (2000) evaluated factors associated with cancer screening behaviors among Korean-Americans. In multiple logistic regression analyses, the strongest predictor of screening behaviors was having a regular medical checkup. Acculturation measures were also important predictors of cancer screening: those who had spent substantial amount of time in the US were more likely to have had a Pap smear.

Interventions to Increase Cervical Cancer Screening

There is currently great interest in establishing the efficacy of interventions to increase Pap screening. Three prior reviews conducted between 1998 and 2001 focused on assessing the impacts of interventions to increasing screening participation and adherence for general populations and not on the impacts of interventions specifically targeted to elders of color (Yabroff, Kerner, & Mandelblatt, 2000; Marcus, Kaplan, Crane, et al., 1998). None of these analyses, however, focused on cervical cancer projects or studies that explore the use of explicitly culturally adapted intervention strategies to improve adherence by older women of color to screening guidelines. In the sections, we first provide an overview of findings from prior reviews and then present our meta-analysis of culturally tailored interventions focused on traditionally underserved R/E elders.

Interventions to Increase Pap Screening in General Populations

Interventions to increase the level of cervical cancer screening are similar to those for mammography and can be broadly classified based on: 1) the barriers being addressed (i.e. individual client or community, provider, provider institutional and system of care/financing); 2) communication strategy being used (i.e. direct mail, mass media campaign, social networks or community health worker); 3) recruitment method (inreach, outreach or combined); and 4) desired outcome e.g. screening uptake or adherence. According to each of the systematic reviews, both simple and more complex interventions seem effective in increasing uptake and adherence to screening.

Outreach strategies Patient mailings are among the most successful low cost outreach interventions, especially if they are personalized or if they are used conjunction with other strategies. However, mass mailings without personalized messages tend to be ineffective. The impact of media campaign on increasing Pap screening is mixed (Marcus, et al., 1998). Some studies have found little or no effect. Mass media programs appear more effective when multiple types are used or when tailored to a specific screening program that reduces other access barriers or in combination with other strategies. Use of community health workers (CHWs) as cultural intermediaries has been reported to have some positive impact on Pap use in previous reviews. It has also been observed that the impact of the CHWs is enhanced if they are coordinated with existing community intermediaries. Other community outreach programs include use of outreach clinics and mobile examination rooms. Although mobile clinics are effective, one potential problem with use of mobile clinics among population without usual provider is continuity of care (Marcus, et al., 1998; Shekelle, et al., 2001; Yabroff, et al., 2000).

Inreach strategies Recruiting participants from within the health facility's in-patient and outpatient departments appears to represent an under-utilized opportunity for increasing participation in Pap screening particularly for older women. Studies have shown consistent positive effects of recruiting patients from the inpatient department especially the elderly (Marcus, et al., 1998). Personalized prompts to patients regarding screening done before an encounter with a provider have been found effective especially if they are combined with physician prompts.

In contrast, the impact of physician prompts in the outpatient department is mixed. Some studies have shown positive effects on Pap screening while others have shown no effect, according to these reviews.

Meta-analysis of Culturally Tailored Pap Screening Interventions

Meta-analysis methods Paralleling the search and meta-analysis strategy we used in exploring mammography interventions, studies of culturally tailored projects were sought. We sought reports exploring any of the following interventions: 1) language appropriate education materials or role model media education; 2) use of CHWs of the same R/E and SES as prospective participants; and 3) use of social networks such as church or other community organizations. Articles were searched from various sources, including Medline, prior reviews and the CDC database. Key words for this search included 'interventions and cervical cancer screening, patient support and cervical cancer screening, cervical cancer screening and community health worker, cervical cancer screening and community health advisor, cervical cancer screening and volunteers, cervical cancer screening and lay educators, cervical cancer screening and lay advisor, cervical cancer screening and community interventions.' The databases were also searched using leading author names to identify prior studies on by identified authors. Additional article sources were recommendations by expert consultants, review of bibliographies in prior reviews, and the CMS report on Reducing Disparities in Health Outcomes: Effective and Promising Outpatient Interventions with Underserved Populations.

Twenty-five reports met inclusion criteria, but some of these were multiple papers on a single intervention, while others did not meet minimal methodological standards. To be included, studies needed to report on an experimental or quasi-experimental project. Acceptable control strategies were: 1) Pre-test and post-test (paired control) design with independent concurrent control at each point in time; or 2) independent concurrent controls. In addition, quasi-experimental studies had to have both baseline and follow-up data to be included. Eight programs, yielding 11 comparisons between intervention and comparison groups met these criteria and were included in the meta-analysis.

Measures of adherence were Pap smear rate changes among women who had some prior use, and Pap uptake measures were Pap test changes among women who had some prior use. We used the absolute rate difference as the Effect Size measure. We used comprehensive meta-analysis software developed by Biostat, Inc., to compute fixed effects point and variance measures. For both the control and the intervention group, the change in number of screened women was calculated by subtracting the follow-up number from the baseline number. Thus, the effect measure included in the meta-analysis reflects a so-called difference-in-differences approach. Because we wanted to identify moderator effects, we report the Mantel-Hanszel fixed effects estimates without adjustment for program heterogeneity. Because of the small number of final interventions included, only three control variables were tested: 1) Outreach vs. Inreach recruitment strategy; 2) Individualized vs. Group communication and 3) Screening Uptake vs. Adherence.

Characteristics of the studies The seven studies and 11 intervention arms contributed a total sample of 5271 participants. The target populations included AI/AN, Hispanic/Latina, NHOPI, AA women. The ages of the study participant ranged from 18-97, and all included studies served some elders. Six intervention arms included only patients with low SES while 5 were diverse with respect to patient social class. The studies used two types of designs. Seven intervention arms used controlled community trials and four used randomized controlled trials. Seven studies contributing nine intervention arms used the outreach method to recruit participants; only one study with two intervention arms used the inreach strategy. While three programs used individualized interventions (i.e. CHWs as education/counseling for individual patients), eight programs used group approaches, such as public events or support groups alone or in conjunction with individual interventions. Four programs focused on screening uptake, while 7 focused in screening adherence as their outcomes. Appendix 6.1 provides a summary of these projects and their findings.

Meta-Analysis Findings

Table 6.6 provides a summary of the meta-analysis. The meta-analysis showed that as a group, these programs achieved small but significant impacts on screening rates, achieving a rate difference (RD) of about 11% (RD= 0.107; 95% CI =0. 089, 0.125); Z=11.68, p<. 0001). Nonetheless, the program findings were remarkably heterogeneous (Q=177.41, p<. 0001). That is, these programs did not produce consistent findings but rather there were differences in their designs and populations that influenced outcomes. To determine the proportion of heterogeneity attributable to program features and not chance, we calculated I^2 as described by Higgins et al (2003). The I^2 showed that 88% of the heterogeneity was due to program factors rather than chance (I^2=88).

Table 6.3 Meta-analysis of Pap screening interventions for older women of color

Citation	Recruitment	Strategy	Effect	-0.25	0.00	0.25
Bird, 1998	OutReach	Group	.214			
Bird, 1998	OutReach	Group	.180			
Dignan, 1996	OutReach	Individual	.123			
Gotay, 2000	OutReach	Group	.020			
Gotay, 2000	OutReach	Group	.071			
Margolis, 1998	InReach	Individual	.128			
Margolis, 1998	InReach	Individual	-.038			
Navarro, 1998	OutReach	Group	.093			
Paskett, 1999	OutReach	Group	.209			
Ramirez, 1999	OutReach	Group	.065			
Sung, 1997	OutReach	Individual	-.015			
Fixed Combined (11)			.107			

Negative   Positive

Effect: Absolute rate difference

We found two significant moderator effects: individualized vs. group strategies and uptake vs. adherence. Studies that utilized group strategies produced larger effects, about 13% higher than control (RD=12.7, CI=0.11-14.5, P=0.000); compared to those that utilized individualized strategies -- 7% percentage points higher than the control groups (RD=0.074; 95%). Programs that emphasized screening uptake produced a greater effect, with an average rate difference about 11% points higher for treatment than control groups (RD=0.114; 95% CI=0.086, 0.142; Z=8.01, p<0.000) than did those focusing on screening adherence and follow-up where treatment subjects had rate differences about 10% higher than the controls (RD=0.099; 95% CI=0.077, 0.122); a significant difference, (Z=8.71, p<0.000). In-reach was not significantly different from the control, particularly in adherence arm (RD=-0.038, CI=-.115, 0.039, p=0.335) (Margolis, Lurie, McGovern, et al., 1998). However, this intervention was significantly more effective than control when used to increase Pap uptake (RD=0.128, CI=0.049, 0.208, p=0.005).

To determine stability of effect size estimates we calculated Fail-safe-N (FSN). FSN is defined as the number of unpublished null studies that would render the effect size statistically insignificant. The FSN calculations showed overall 25 additional studies that found no effect of these interventions would be needed to render our estimates statistically insignificant. In stratified analyses the estimate for Group Interventions were the most stable (FSN=45) followed by those for Outreach Interventions (FSN=33). It is unlikely that so many culturally tailored unpublished studies exist. We also examined a funnel plot to determine if there was any publication bias. From the funnel plot, we found no evidence of publication bias. Studies that did not show statistically significant intervention outcomes were just as likely to be published as those that were statistically significant.

We conclude that these findings provide some confidence that culturally tailored strategies for improving cervical cancer screening can be effective. Although the overall impacts on Pap test use were modest, this can be attributed to the fact that some baseline screening levels were fairly high in the participating populations. We found strong evidence for studies that used Group Intervention and Outreach Strategies and fairly strong evidence for both Uptake and Adherence outcomes. More primary studies involving inreach and individualized interventions are needed to improve the estimate's stability for these two approaches. Further, we were unable to test the impact of population attributes such as age, and race/ethnicity because there were relatively few studies and reporting did not support sub-group analyses.

Cervical Cancer Treatment and Racial/Ethnic Disparities

A consensus has emerged on stage-specific treatment protocols for cervical cancer as outlined by the National Cancer Institute (NCIPDQ, 2002c). Treatment for cervical cancer involves surgery and or radiation, depending on extent of the disease. Compared to treatment of invasive cervical cancer, treatment for pre-invasive lesions (SIL, CIN 2 and 3) more effective and may provide a cure (Smith, 2000). As seen earlier, the role of screening is to detect these lesions to prevent progression to invasive disease. Detection of these lesions should be followed-up with appropriate treatment. One advantage of early detection is that treatment for pre-invasive cervical cancer is technically simpler – accomplished using much simpler and lower cost outpatient procedures such as cryotherapy (the destruction of cells by extreme cold), by electro-coagulation (the destruction of tissue through intense heat by electric current), laser ablation, or local surgery (ACS, 2002). Another advantage over breast cancer is that one specialist, i.e. the gynecologist, can deal with these early lesions. The socio-economic complexity of even this apparently simple treatment is in the need for follow-up. There is need for follow-up and to continue screening to monitor and treat recurrences. There are, however, no simple treatments for invasive cervical cancer even at localized stage. The treatments for invasive cervical cancer are complicated and highly individualized. Treatment for invasive cervical cancer also involves other disciplines. Invasive cervical cancer treatment usually involves surgery and/or RT as primary treatment or as adjuvant therapy. Unlike breast cancer where chemotherapy plays a major role in controlling metastasis, chemotherapy is typically used for palliative treatment. For stage I-IIA, RT may be used as adjuvant therapy after radical hysterectomy if there is evident of lymph node involvement or extensive disease. RT, however, may also be used as primary treatment in patients who are deemed clinically inoperable, such as those with co-morbid illnesses. RT has slightly more adverse effects than surgery. For example, serious urological complications are about 1-2% for surgery and about 1.4-5.3% for RT. Like treatment of pre-invasive lesions, surgical treatment of localized disease (stage I-IIA) may also provide a cure (Lopez et al, 1997).

The treatment of choice for regional disease (stage IIB-III) and distant metastasis (IV) is RT and chemotherapy (NCI-PDQ, 2002c). Further, treatment failure for regional disease and distant metastases seem to be common. For example according to the ACS (2002) and Ries, Eisner, and Kosary, (2002), the survival rate for pre-invasive lesions and carcinoma – in-situ is 100%; for localized disease 92%; for regional disease, 42% and for distant metastasis, 15%.

The need to individualize the treatment based on the extent of the disease, and other clinical contra-indications are meant to ensure optimal treatment with minimal adverse effects. These features of disease management, unless carefully managed themselves, however, also leave room for disparities in treatment even for localized disease.

Racial/Ethnic Disparities in Cervical Cancer Care

Evaluation of the impact of treatment should distinguish between treatment efficacy and treatment effectiveness. Efficacy refers to impact of treatment on outcomes under controlled experimental conditions while effectiveness refers to the effect of treatment on outcomes under normal clinical conditions. Differences in cervical cancer outcomes are not due to differential efficacy. A review by Shavers and Brown (2002) found that there was no evidence of differences in treatment efficacy for R/E minorities compared to White women who received similar treatment for similar disease characteristics.

In contrast to efficacy studies, observational studies have consistently found differences in treatment effectiveness between white and R/E women. Reasons for the observed differences in treatment effectiveness are multiple. Much of this evidence has been on AAs. AA women are less likely to be treated for cervical cancer. When treated, contrary to recommendations, AA are more likely to receive fertility sparing treatment for early stage cancer (Shavers and Brown, 2002). Factors that influence differences in treatment according to this review were differences in the prevalence of co-morbidities, poor health, patient's refusal of treatment and lack of physician recommendation for treatment.

We found additional factors associated with R/E disparities in treatment outcomes to be lack of adhering to radiation therapy (Formenti, Meyerowitz, Ell, et al., 1995) and prolonged treatment duration (Han, Orton, Shamsa, et al., 1999; Formenti, et al., 1995) found inadequate adherence to radiotherapy among Latina immigrants to be significantly associated with poor survival for cervical cancer. They examined records of 69 consecutive Latina patients with cervical cancer who received RT at Los Angeles County Hospital. They also found that a large subset of patients (20%) elected to discontinue treatment without a medical reason. Han, et al., (1999) examined the role of duration of treatment in survival differences in 216 patients treated radically with external beam radiation (EBRT) and low-dose-rate brachytherapy for cervical cancer between 1980 and 1991 at Wayne State University. Racial comparisons showed White women having more extended treatment and better survival than AA.

No studies were identified that explored methods for reducing R/E disparities in follow-up on suspicious cervical cancer screening. No studies that explored reducing disparities in treatment and aftercare were identified.

Cervical Cancer and Racial/Ethnic Disparities

Our review of R/E differences in cervical cancer outcomes, detection, and treatment yielded several major findings. Hispanics and AAs are at greater risk for getting cervical cancer. They also have lower potential for surviving cervical cancer. Evidence for the role of late stage at diagnosis and R/E differences in survival was mixed, because Whites maintained a survival advantage at both early and advanced stages. Consensus recommendations for use of screening methods are available. Screening rates for cervical cancer are lower than desirable for all Medicare beneficiaries, but notably lower for R/E minorities. Traditionally underserved R/E group members are also less likely to be followed up after abnormal screening. Our findings suggest that differences in stage-at-diagnosis could be attributed to lack of follow-up on high-risk abnormal screens. Unlike other cancers, however, higher mortality for AA and Hispanic women with early stage-at-diagnosis also points to failure to complete treatment planning and implementation for these women. As for other cancers, final diagnosis and staging of cervical cancer requires a multi-step process involving multiple tests, procedures, and professional consultations. There is evidence that older R/E minorities are less likely to complete the cervical cancer diagnostic process. There is evidence that AA women are less likely to receive complete diagnostic work-ups and valid clinical staging. These disparate practice patterns seem to be an important factor in survival and mortality outcome differences.

We found a number of reports on culturally tailored interventions to increase screening. These programs typically involved use of community health workers to conduct educational programs using culturally and linguistically adapted materials. Some programs used group strategies to help overcoming barriers to uptake and adherence to Pap screening. Our meta-analysis of these studies shows that overall cervical cancer screening interventions aimed at women of R/E minorities and employing lay health workers and other cultural tailoring components produce modest significant impacts on screening rates, although extremely heterogeneous in their impact. We however found strong and stable associations for outreach strategies that use group strategies, and for both Uptake and Adherence outcomes. These findings are consistent with several observations from emerging programs as described in Chapter 8: site leader emphasized the importance of using community members as staff and communal planning and implementation as crucial cultural tailoring tools.

Equally important as screening, complete diagnosis work-ups is receipt of appropriate treatment. Studies that examined the impact of 'equal treatment for equal disease' suggest that differences in treatment may be a factor in R/E differences in survival especially for stage II and III and to some extent stage I disease. We also found evidence for prolonged treatment period, lack of adherence to radiation therapy and advanced stage at time of diagnosis influenced R/E disparities in cervical cancer treatment. We also found that elder R/E minorities were more likely to be treated with only radiation therapy than with surgery.

Our reviews suggest that interventions aimed at both reducing R/E disparities in cervical cancer detection and treatment have the potential to influence overall differences in outcomes. The available research shows the role of both differences in stage-at-diagnosis and differences in treatment influence cancer and health outcomes. Improving screening participation and adherence for R/E elders are clearly worthwhile goals in light of these findings. Although the evidence could be stronger, it appears that culturally tailored screening interventions that focus on adherence and interventions based on group strategies have somewhat greater potential to influence R/E differences in pap screening. Further, some of the differences in survival appear to be due to differences in stage-at-diagnosis, treatment and aftercare that arise from barriers such as health insurance, difficult access to care, and lack of physician recommendation for treatment that could be addressed through detection and treatment facilitation interventions.

These findings underscore the potential to improve cancer survivorship by ensuring that patient and practitioners complete the process. A treatment management intervention that draws upon a community health worker serving as a patient navigator holds the potential to increase the share of elders of color who receive the current standard of care. Although demonstrations and evaluations of cancer treatment management services were not identified in the literature, this review highlights treatment management as a potential area for important and cost-effective reductions in cancer care disparities.

References

ACS (2002). *Cancer Facts and Figures 2002*. American Cancer Society. Available: http://www.cancer.org.

ACS (2004). *Cancer Facts and Figures 2004*. American Cancer Society. Available: http://www.cancer.org.

Bernard, V.B., Lee, N.C., Piper, M. et al. (2001). Race-specific results of Papanicolaou testing and the rate of cervical neoplasia in the National Breast and Cervical Cancer Early Detection Program, 1991-1998 (United States). *Cancer Causes Control*, 12(1): 61-68.

Bird, J.A., McPhee, S.J., Ha, N.T. et al. (1998). Opening pathways to cancer screening for Vietnamese-American women: lay health workers hold a key. *Preventative Medicine*, 27(6):821-829.

Blackman, D.K., Bennett, E.M. and Miller, D.S. (1999). Trends in self-reported use of mammograms (1989-1997) and Papanicolaou tests (1991-1997) – Behavioral Risk Factor Surveillance System. *MMWR-Morbidity and Mortality Weekly Report, CDC Surveillance Summary, 1999*. 48(6): 1-22.

Chavez, L.R., Hubbell, F.A., Mishra, S.I. et al. (1997). The influence of fatalism on self-reported use of Papanicolaou smears. *American Journal of Preventive Medicine*, 13(6): 418-424. (Center for Health Care Quality, 2002).

Cole, P. and Morrison, A.S. (1978). Basic Issues in Cancer Screening. In A. B. Miller (Ed.), *Screening in Cancer*. Geneva: UICC.

Dignan, M., Michielutte, R., Blinson, K. et al. (1996). Effectiveness of health education to increase screening for cervical cancer among eastern-band Cherokee Indian women in North Carolina. *Journal of the National Cancer Institute*, 88(22):1670-1676.

Ferenczy, A. (1997) Optimal Management of Cervical Cancer Precursors: Low Grade Squamous Intraepithelial Lesions. Chapter 10 in Franco, E. and Monsonego, J., New (Eds.) Developments in Cervical Cancer Screening and Prevention. Blackwell Science Ltd: Australia.

Formenti, S.C., Meyerowitz, B.E., Ell, K. et al. (1995). Inadequate adherence to radiotherapy in Latina immigrants with carcinoma of the cervix. Potential impact on disease free survival. *Cancer*, 75(5): 1135-1140.

Fox, P., Amsberger, P. and Zhang, X. (1997). An examination of differential follow-up rates in cervical cancer screening. *Journal of Community Health*, 22(3): 199-209.

Gotay, C.C., Banner, R.O., Matsunaga, D.S. et al. (2000). Impact of a culturally appropriate intervention on breast and cervical screening among native Hawaiian women. *Preventative Medicine*, 31(5):529-537.

Han, I., Orton, C., Shamsa, F. et al. (1999). Combined low-dose-rate brachytherapy and external beam radiation for cervical cancer: experience over ten years. *Radiation Oncology Investigation*, 7(5): 289-296.

Hegarty, V., Burchett, B.M., Gold, D.T. et al. (2000). Racial differences in use of cancer prevention services among older Americans. *Journal of the American Geriatric Society*, 48(7): 735-740.

Hiatt, R.A., Pasick, R.J., Stewart, S. et al. (2001). Community-based cancer screening for underserved women: design and baseline findings from the Breast and Cervical Cancer Intervention Study. *Preventive Medicine*, 33(3): 190-203.

Higgins, J.P., Thompson, S.G., Deeks, J.J. et al. (2003). Measuring inconsistency in meta-analyses. *British Medical Journal*, 327(7414): 557-560.

Hubbell, F.A., Chavez, L.R., Mishra, S.I. et al. (1996). Differing beliefs about breast cancer among Latinas and Anglo women. *Western Journal of Medicine*, 164(5): 405-409.

Juon, H.S., Choi, Y. and Kim, M.T. (2000). Cancer screening behaviors among Korean-American women. *Cancer Detection and Prevention*, 24(6): 589-601.

Kagawa-Singer, M. and Pourat, N. (2000). Asian American and Pacific Islander breast and cervical carcinoma screening rates and healthy people 2000 objectives. *Cancer*, 89(3): 696-705.

Kim, K., Yu, E.S., Chen, E.H. et al. (1999). Cervical cancer screening knowledge and practices among Korean-American women. *Cancer Nursing*, 22(4): 297-302.

Lin, S.S., Clarke, C.A., Prehn, A.W. et al. (2002). Survival differences among Asian subpopulations in the United States after prostate, colorectal, breast, and cervical carcinomas. *Cancer*, 94(4): 1175-1182.

Lopez, A., Kudelka, P. and Edwards L. (1997). Medical Oncology Comprehensive Review Carcinoma of the Uterine Cervix. http://www.cancernetwork.com/textbook/morev24.htm.

Mandelblatt, J., Traxler, M., Lakin, P. et al. (1993). Targeting breast and cervical cancer screening to elderly poor black women: who will participate? The Harlem Study Team. *Preventive Medicine*, 22(1): 20-33.

Mandelblatt, J.S. and Yabroff, K.R. (1999). Effectiveness of interventions designed to increase mammography use: a meta-analysis of provider-targeted strategies. *Cancer Epidemiology, Biomarkers, and Prevention*, 8(9): 759-767.

Marcus, A.C., Kaplan, C.P., Crane, L.A. et al. (1998). Reducing loss-to-follow-up among women with abnormal Pap smears. Results from a randomized trial testing an intensive follow-up protocol and economic incentives. *Medical Care*, 36(3): 397-410.

Margolis, K.L., Lurie, N., McGovern, P.G. et al. (1998). Increasing breast and cervical cancer screening in low-income women. *Journal of General Internal Medicine*, 13(8): 515-521.

McKee, M.D., Schechter, C., Burton, W. et al. (2001). Predictors of follow-up of atypical and ASCUS papanicolaou tests in a high-risk population. *Journal of Family Practice*, 50(7): 609.

Miller, B.A., Kolonel, L.N., Bernstein, L. et al. (eds.) (1996). *Racial/Ethnic Patterns of Cancer in the United States 1988-1992*. NIH Pub. (96-104). National Cancer Institute: Bethesda, MD.

Miller, B., Kolonel, L.N., Bernstein, L.Y., Jr. et al. (1996). *Racial/Ethnic Patterns of Cancer in the United States 1988-1992: Cervix Uteri Cancer – U.S. Racial/Ethnic Cancer Patterns*: National Cancer Institute: Bethesda, MD.

Navarro, A.M., Senn, K.L., McNicholas, L.J. et al. (1998). Por La Vida model intervention enhances use of cancer screening tests among Latinas. *American Journal of Preventative Medicine*, 15(1):32-41.

NCI (2001). Cancer Facts. *http://cis.nci.nih.gov/fact/3_20.htm*.

NCI-PDQ (2002a). *Cancer screening overview: Scientific basis for cancer screening*, [Website]. National Cancer Institute: Bethesda, MD.

NCI-PDQ (2002b). *Cervical Cancer Prevention*. NCI. Available: http://www.cancer.gov.

NCI-PDQ (2002c). *Cervical Cancer PDQ^R Treatment*. NCI. Available: http://www.cancer.gov.

O'Malley, M.S., Earp, J.A., Harris, R.P. (1997). Race and mammography use in two North Carolina counties. *American Journal of Public Health*, 87(5): 782-786.

Paskett, E.D., Tatum, C.M., D'Agostino, R et al. (1999). Community-based interventions to improve breast and cervical cancer screening: results of the Forsyth County Cancer Screening (FoCaS) Project. *Cancer Epidemiology Biomarkers and Prevention*, 8(5):453-459.

Ragland, K.E., Selvin, S., Merrill, D.W. (1991). Black-White differences in stage-specific cancer survival: Analysis of seven selected sites. *American Journal of Epidemiology*, 133(7): 672-682.

Ramirez, A.G., Villarreal, R., McAlister, A. et al. (1999). Advancing the role of participatory communication in the diffusion of cancer screening among Hispanics. *Journal of Health Communication,* 4(1): 31-36.

Ramirez, A.G., Suarez, L., Laufman, L. et al. (2000). Hispanic women's breast and cervical cancer knowledge, attitudes, and screening behaviors. *American Journal of Health Promotion,* 14(5): 292-300.

Ries, L., Eisner, M.P., Kosary, C.L. et al. (eds). (2004). SEER Cancer Statistics Review, 1975-2001. National Cancer Institute: Bethesda, MD. *http://seer.cancer.gov/ Publications/CSR.*

Ries, L., Eisner, M.P., Kosary, C.L. et al. (eds). (2001). *SEER Cancer Statistics Review, 1973-1999 Statistical Supplemental Material #1, Rates and Trends for Top 15 Cancer Sites by Sex and Race/Ethnicity for 1992-1998.* National Cancer Institute: Bethesda, MD.

Shavers, V.L. and Brown, M.L. (2002). Racial and ethnic disparities in the receipt of cancer treatment. *Journal of the National Cancer Institute,* 94(5): 334-357.

Shekelle, P., Stone, E., Mangolione, M. et al. (2001). Healthy Ageing Initiatives Evidence Reports: Interventions that Increase the Utilization of Medicare-Funded Preventive Services for Persons Age 65 and Older. *http://www.hcfa.gov/healthyaging/2a.htm.*

Smith, R., Mettlin, C.J., Davis, K.J. et al. (2000). Articles – American Cancer Society Guidelines for the Early Detection of Cancer. *Cancer,* 50(1): 34-49.

Suarez, L., Roche, R.A., Nichols, D. et al. (1997). Knowledge, behavior, and fears concerning breast and cervical cancer among older low-income Mexican-American women. *American Journal of Preventive Medicine,* 13(2): 137-142.

Sugarman, J.R., Dennis, L.K. and White, E. (1994). Cancer survival among American Indians in western Washington State (United States). *Cancer Causes Control,* 5(5): 440-448.

Sung, J.F., Blumenthal, D.S., Coates, R.J. et al. (1997). Effect of a cancer screening intervention conducted by lay health workers among inner-city women. *American Journal of Preventative Medicine,* 13(1):51-57.

Vickie L. Shavers, Martin L. Brown (2002). Racial and Ethnic Disparities in the Receipt of Cancer Treatment. *Journal of the National Cancer Institute,* 94: 334-357.

Wang, S.S., Sherman, M.E., Hildesheim, A. et al. (2004). Cervical adenocarcinoma and squamous cell carcinoma incidence trends among White women and Black women in the United States for 1976-2000. *Cancer,* 100(5): 1035-1044.

Wu, A., Wan, P., Bernstein, L. (2001). A multiethnic population-based study of smoking, alcohol, and body size and risk for adenocarcinomas of the stomach and esophagus (United States). *Cancer Causes and Control,* 12(8): 721-732.

Yabroff, K.R., Kerner, J.F. and Mandelblatt, J.S. (2000). Effectiveness of interventions to improve followup after abnormal cervical cancer screening. *Preventive Medicine,* 31(4): 429-439.

Zambrana, R.E., Breen, N., Fox, S.A. et al. (1999). Use of cancer screening practices by Hispanic women: analyses by subgroup. *Preventive Medicine,* 29(6): 466-477.

Appendix 6.1 Culturally tailored Pap screening interventions

Author	Disparity	Design	Setting	Age
Bird (1998)	Adherence	CPT	Community based	40+
Bird (1998)	Uptake	CPT	Community Based	40+
Dignan (1996)	Uptake [C2]	RCT [A2]	Cherokee tribal area	18+
Gotay (2000)	Uptake	CPT	Population based [A3]	40+
Gotay (2000)	Adherence	CPT	Population based [A3]	40+
Margolis (1998)	Uptake	CCT	In reach [A4]	40+
Margolis (1998)	Adherence	CCT	In reach [A4]	40+
Navarro, 1998	Adherence	RCT [D5]	Community based	18-72 [A5]
Paskett (1999)	Adherence	CPT	Outreach [A6]	40+
Ramirez (1999)	Adherence	Quasi-exp.	Population based	[A7]
Sung (1997)	Adherence	RCT	Community based	18-97

Pap Screening Intervention Studies Notes

CHW: Community Health Worker; CCT: Controlled clinical trial; RCT: Randomized clinical trial; CCBT: Controlled community based trial; RD: Rate absolute rate difference; BLN: Baseline sample; CGBL Rate: Control group baseline sample; MD: Medical doctor; NP: Nurse practitioner.

[A1] Small group education session by CHW plus education material distribution, promotional events. CPT=Controlled Population Trial.

[A2] Solomon four-group design. [B2] Baseline rates were not available. [C2] The groups with/without pre-test were combined for this analysis.

[A3] Random digit telephone sampling. Control communities were identified by census tracts. [B3] CHW led the Kokua groups. Native Hawaiians conducted interviews. There was no information about community participation in the planning process. The intervention was a Kokua group, which were composed of community women gathered by friends or colleagues. The groups were led by female CHW.

Target Group	Intervention	BL N	CGBL Rate	RD
Vietnamese American	CHW, education materials, events[A1]	645	25	22
Vietnamese American	CHW, education materials, events [A1]	645	42	18
Cherokee	CHW Individualized education	815[B2]		9.2
NHOPI	Volunteer CHW group [B3]	642	96	2
Native Hawaiian	Volunteer 1 CHW led group [B3]	415	63	7
Native American[B4]	CHW invite and NP [C4]	590	na [D4]	12.9
Native American[B4]	CHW invite and NP[C4]	377	na[D4]	-3.8
Latina	Poor La Vida Model [B5]	361	51.6[E5]	9.1
AA and White	Multiple outreach tools, CHW [B6]	248	67	21
Latina	Peer networks [B7]	212	46.8	6.2
AA	CHW in-home education [A8]	321	51.9	-3.4

[A4] Women, including AI/ANs, were recruited from clinics by CHW and supervised by coordinator. [C4] CHWs assessed participants' cervical cancer screening status and offered appointments with a female nurse practitioner at cancer screening clinic to women who were due. Each clinic visit was linked to pelvic exam and mammography on the same day so screening could be completed in one visit. [D4] Sample sizes for each group were calculated from the baseline percentage for each group and the total sample from Table 2 of the article.

[A5] Age range in text is 18-72 but the table for baseline shows age stratified as <40 and 40-49 yrs. [B5] The Poor La Vida model involved 36 CHWs (Consejeras) who conducted educational sessions. [C5]. Median income: 12k, median education: 7 yrs. [D5] CHWs recruited participants through social networks. Randomization was by CHW. [E5] Results are for participants who completed pretest and posttest. Original Ns were238 for the control group and 274 for the experimental group.

[A6] Education brochures to address identified barriers: e.g. where to get a pap. [B6] Multifaceted education and promotional intervention, including community events with educational classes and information booths, prizes, cholesterol and diabetes screening.

[A7] Repeat use in women that were highly adherent at baseline defined as having a pap smear in past year at baseline or at follow-up and intended to have one in future. [B7] This was a tailored mass media campaign including 'mobilization of communication networks to promote the positive health behavior'. Campaign included 82 television segments, 67 newspaper stories, and 48 radio programs. Intervention also included 175 volunteer CHWs who distributed 11 educational pamphlets monthly to family friends and neighbors.

[A8] Lay health workers visited from a community-based women's health organization.

Chapter 7

Racial/Ethnic Disparities in Colorectal, Lung and Prostate Cancer

Introduction and Approach

This chapter continues the examination of evidence regarding racial/ethnic (R/E) disparities in cancer outcomes and receipt of appropriate screening, diagnostic, and treatment services. Also examined is available evidence on interventions to address these gaps. In this chapter, we focus on three of the most prevalent cancers among elders: colorectal, lung, and prostate cancers. Although R/E differences in stomach, oral (neck and throat), and pancreatic cancers as well as leukemia have been documented, the available literature provides few clues on how screening, detection, diagnosis, or treatment factors explain these outcomes. As was the case for breast and cervical cancers, we sought to identify R/E differences among Medicare beneficiaries or elders, but published studies often did not focus on this population segment. For this reason, we also examined reports on older adult populations (age 50 and above) and general adult populations. Another parallel with the reviews of breast and cervical cancer research is our focus on stage of the disease at the time of diagnosis, since stage has been linked to survival, discomforts of care, costs of treatment, and other outcomes for all three of the cancer sites emphasized here.

The reviews for colorectal, lung, and prostate cancer each begins with a discussion of current data on R/E differences in prevalence and outcomes and then turns to data on the role of stage at diagnosis in group differences in survival. The remainder of each review follows the sequential models of cancer detection and treatment consensus for these cancer sites. In each case, we tried to identify where there was agreement about what care an individual Medicare beneficiary should receive to detect cancer as early as possible and to treat it effectively. Each review also sought specific evidence that observed differences in care patterns accounted for additional variance in outcomes beyond that associated with stage at diagnosis or co-morbid health conditions. Since our findings did demonstrate disparities in diagnostic completeness, treatment, and follow-up services, we sought evidence for interventions aimed at reducing R/E disparities at these later stages in the cancer care process. Although recently initiated research by NCI and AHRQ is supporting scholars in exploring reasons for such treatment differences, this review was largely unsuccessful in identifying any published reports focused on reducing R/E differences among Medicare or other populations in receipt of colorectal, lung, and prostate cancer services subsequent to screening or detection.

The potential to influence outcomes through Medicare and other health financing programs is notably enhanced when there is a consensus on what services promote survival and well-being. For all three sites of cancer explored in this chapter, there remains considerable debate about the most appropriate detection and diagnostic approaches and/or the relative efficacy and effectiveness of alternative treatment strategies. As a result of these less well-developed technologies of care, there has also been less opportunity for – and attention to – the causes and consequences of R/E disparities in the utilization or quality of cancer detection and treatment services. The complex issues around the roles of individual, practitioner, and care system influences on participation in cancer detection and treatment services have not been examined in detail comparable to studies of breast and cervical cancer. Similarly, for each of these cancers, cancer epidemiology and care differences between African Americans (AA) and whites are particularly dramatic, and whites have received the lion's share of research attention even though there is evidence that major sub-populations within other R/E groups are experiencing inadequate care and poor outcomes.

Identification and Selection of Reports for Systematic Reviews

We conducted electronic searches of Medline and the NCI Cancer Lit from 1985 to 2002, supplemented by backward citation searches using Social Science Citation Index/Web of Science for selected papers. Searches were performed for colorectal, lung and prostate cancers. These terms and their variants (e.g. 'colon', 'rectal', 'prostatic' etc.) were used in each search. All searches used the following key words to locate reports on cancer among persons of color, 'minority elderly, race, elders of color, elders, minority, older adults, adults, African-American, Black, Hispanic, Latino, Spanish surname, American Indian, Native American, Alaskan Native, Hawaiian Native, Pacific Islanders, Chinese, Vietnamese, Japanese and Asian American.' Additional key words included 'prevalence, incidence, mortality, survival, screening, diagnosis, treatment, surgery, chemotherapy, radiotherapy, radiation, quality of life, relapse, monitoring, culture, intervention, RCT, community health worker, case management, quality improvement.' Other sources of information were Interventions that Increase the Utilization of Medicare-Funded Preventive Services for Persons Age 65 and Older, prepared for CMS by RAND and the reviews supporting the AHRQ Task Force on Clinical Preventive Services guidelines.

Colorectal Cancer

Cancer Prevalence and Mortality Differences by Race/Ethnicity

Colorectal cancers (CRCs) have the second highest incidence and associated mortality overall (lung cancer is highest) and are the third most prevalent for both men and women. Adenomatous polyps or other lesions generally precede colorectal cancer and their treatment prevents progression to invasive disease. In part because of improvements in detection and treatment of these pre-cancerous lesions, colorectal cancer incidence and mortality declined during the early 1990s and have stabilized since then. An average annual mortality rate of 21.9/100,000 was estimated from SEER data for 1996-2000 (Weir, Thun, Hankey, et al., 2003). Data from the early 1990s indicates that CRCs are more common for men than women in all racial/ethnic groups. These same data indicate that Alaska Natives, Japanese Americans and AAs have both higher incidence and mortality than whites, while Latinos, Pacific Islanders, and some American Indian groups experience these diseases at lower rates, although estimates for some groups are based on relatively small numbers (Miller, Kolonel, Bernstein, et al., 1996). Both prevalence and mortality were higher for African Americans than any other group in both genders, lower for American Indian/Alaska Native, Asian and Pacific Island, and Hispanic groups, and rates varied notably by state during 1996-2000 but sub-population analyses were not provided (Weir, Thun, Hankey, et al., 2003). Although about 75% of CRCs are in persons with no family history of the disease and generally diagnosed in persons age 60 and older, the remaining 25% of patients have a family history of colorectal cancer. A small proportion of CRCs (5-6%) are associated with specific syndromes with known genetic components and much younger age at diagnoses. For most cases in persons with a family history of CRC, onset appears to occur as in non-familial CRC and thus suggests a combination of genetic factors and shared exposures. There appear to be no studies that demonstrate R/E differences in risk for genetically linked CRC.

Review of 1998 age-adjusted CRC incidence and mortality with a focus on differences between AAs and whites shows for both men and women larger racial disparity for mortality than for incidence. While the findings of Table 7-1 are not as dramatic as those for breast cancer, where AA women have lower incidence of the disease but higher associated mortality, they still indicate that some aspects of the prevention, detection, and treatment of CRCs are being implemented with differential success across R/E groups.

Consistent with the findings of greater racial disparities in mortality than incidence are the results of several studies that link R/E differences in CRC mortality to differences in stage at the time of diagnosis. Several studies demonstrate the importance of R/E in stage at diagnosis. For example, Mandelblatt and colleagues matched New York State (NYS) Tumor Registry with US Census area-level social class indicators to examine the relationship of gender, race, and SES on stage of disease at diagnosis (Mandelblatt, Andrews, Kao, et al., 1996). Controlling for other predictors, the odds of late-stage cancer increased with lower age and for women and AAs. Living in low SES areas was the strongest predictor of late-stage diagnosis for all groups. Further, these differences in stage matter for survival. Lee-Feldstein and colleagues compared disease stage at initial diagnosis of colorectal cancer and survival rates for 1,329 Northern California Medicare beneficiaries (Lee-Feldstein, Feldstein, and Buchmueller, 2002). Diagnosis in early stage was greater for whites than Blacks, while whites had lower all-cause and CRC mortality by 10 years. Once stage at diagnosis and insurance factors were considered in a multivariate survival analysis, race was no longer significant. A study of the tumors of 703 newly identified cases of invasive colon adenocarcinoma in the AA/White Cancer Survival Study found that more advanced stage at the time of diagnosis accounted for most of the 60% excess mortality among AAs (Chen, Fenoglio-Preiser, Xu, et al., 1997; Mayberry, Coates, Hill, et al, 1995). Similarly, an analysis of records of 1,245 CRC patients at an urban medical center found that local patients (who were more likely to be older and people of color) were more likely to have advanced disease at the time of presentation than patients from distant communities (Neugut, Fleischauer, Sundararajan, et al., 1991).

Table 7.1 Comparison of 1998 colorectal cancer incidence and mortality rates by race and gender*

	White Male	Black Male	W/B	White Female	Black Female	W/B
Incidence	64.8	67.4	.96	47.7	53.6	.75
Mortality	25.1	33.4	.89	17.7	25.3	.69

* Incidence and mortality rates are per 100,000 persons in each group and based on 1998 SEER and National Center for Health Statistics data.

Source: Cancer Progress Report 2001, National Cancer Institute, NIH Publication 02-5045, http://progressreport.cancer.gov.

Colorectal Cancer Detection Methods

Several methods for detecting CRC have been developed. Most authors agree that there is potential efficacy of screening using a non-invasive procedure, fecal occult blood testing (FOBT) along with appropriate subsequent more intensive examinations. But others believe that two procedures, that are both more invasive and more expensive, flexible sigmoidoscopy and colonoscopy may be more efficacious. Unlike flexible sigmoidoscopy that permits only partial views of the colon, colonoscopy permits a complete view and can be followed by immediate excision of polyps. There is consensus that removal of polyps is an effective approach to prevention of CRC, although patients need to be carefully monitored for recurrence. Because of cost, availability, and acceptability of these procedures, the CRC screening regimen recommended by the American Cancer Society (ACS) and the American Gastroenterological (AGA) Association for persons with average risk profiles includes:

- Annual digital rectal exam at 40;
- Annual Fecal Occult Blood Testing (FOBT) beginning at age 50;
- Sigmoidoscopy every 5 years beginning at 50 or;
- Colonoscopy every 10 years beginning at 50.

As noted below, several other professional and research organizations are recommending similar multi-pronged approaches to screening. Experimental evidence shows the benefit of FOBT, and evidence from observational studies supports the other recommendations. Simulation models also suggest that flexible sigmoidoscopy and colonoscopy cost-effectively reduce CRC mortality. However, because of the relative costs, risks, and effectiveness of the various screens, and because of low rates of population participation in any screening, which CRC screening test(s) should be used and the frequency of testing are still being debated.

One simulation study used a Markov decision model to examine alternative screening strategies: FOBT alone and in combination with flexible sigmoidoscopy, flexible sigmoidoscopy alone, and colonoscopy alone (Vijan, Hwang, Hofer, et al., 2001). Data were drawn from colonoscopic screening studies for prevalence of polyps and the SEER data for the incidence and mortality rates of CRC. The modeling varied the timing and frequency of screenings to assess optimal screening intervals, and sensitivity analyses were conducted to assess the factors that have the greatest effect on the cost-effectiveness of screening. The authors conclude that all strategies are cost-effective in comparison to no screening, at less than $20,000 per life-year saved, but colonoscopy is the preferred test because of its greater effectiveness and because it obviates the need for follow-up testing.

Colonoscopy alone is by no means the consensus approach to screening, however. The US Preventive Services Task Force, 3rd Edition, indicates that all of the CRC screening strategies appear efficacious and cost-effective. But as Pesce (2001) notes the US Preventive Services Task Force found, 'there is fair evidence that annual FOBT and/or flexible sigmoidoscopy every 3-5 years be considered in a periodic health exam.' Screening with colonoscopy receives a 'C' recommendation (defined as: 'there is insufficient evidence to recommend for or against the inclusion in a periodic health exam, but recommendations may be made on other grounds'). Pesce concludes that there is reliable data from randomized controlled trials to recommend the effectiveness of FOBT. This conclusion rests in part on a study that showed a statistically significant reduction in death from CRC with biennial testing over an 18-year follow-up period (Mandel, Church, Ederer, et al., 1999). Their 1993 study of 46,000 men and women aged 50-80 documented a significant 33% reduction in deaths from CRC with annual FOBT and a non-significant 6% reduction with biennial screening (the latter not statistically significant).

The effectiveness of flexible sigmoidoscopy as a screening tool has been questioned since follow-ups with full colonoscopies show that cancer in the rest of the colon can be missed. One cross-sectional study of asymptomatic adults over 50 who underwent colonoscopy in a university setting in Indianapolis, Indiana from 1995-1998 (Imperiale, Wagner, Lin, et al., 2000) found that depending on the criteria for referring (type of polyps in the distal colon) either 61% or 79% of those with cancer in the proximate colon would have been referred with a flexible sigmoidoscopy. Similarly, a study of 1,321 asymptomatic persons, at VA medical facilities, who underwent screening colonoscopy (Lieberman, Weiss, Bond, et al., 2000) found that 10.5% had advanced neoplasms, and 52% of those with advanced proximal neoplasms had no distal adenomas, again suggesting that flexible sigmoidoscopy has limited sensitivity.

In summary, although FOBT has been studied the most, recommending large-scale application of FOBT is still problematic. FOBT is not effective in detecting polyps which can be precursors to CRC (colonoscopy is a better choice), adherence rate is about 50%, and the predictive value of a positive test is no more than 10% (Lowenfels, 2002). Colonoscopy is the gold standard for visualizing the entire colon and is used when abnormal findings are noted on FOBT and flexible sigmoidoscopy (Inger, 1999). However, even if the literature does not support one screening test over another, Pesce notes that the real issue is the low screening rates for CRC and that 'physicians, the media, and educators, must be more diligent in recommending screening for early detection of colorectal cancer' (Pesce, 2001). One expert concludes that screening rates are so low that the test the patient wants is the best one (Barry, 2002).

Screening and Follow-up for Medicare

Although there are debates as to the most appropriate follow-up after an abnormal FOBT, it is generally agreed that a complete examination of the colon and rectum using one or more of the accepted procedures is appropriate. In order for screening methods other than colonoscopy to be effective in detecting cancer, these methods must be used. An additional challenge for Medicare in supporting appropriate screening was identified in an analysis of follow-up testing among 24,246 aged Medicare beneficiaries receiving FOBT testing in 1995 (Lurie and Welch, 1999). Only 34% received the follow-up testing recommended by the American College of Physicians. Older beneficiaries were somewhat less likely to get appropriate follow-up testing. The study did not examine R/E differences in rates of appropriate follow-up. The study concluded that covering FOBT screening is likely to be less cost-effective for Medicare than paying for colonoscopies. Although there appear to be no studies specifically addressing R/E differences in appropriate follow-up after a suspicious FOBT, Cooper et al (1996) found that among 81,579 Medicare beneficiaries, that Blacks had lower rates of all colorectal diagnostic and treatment procedures, perhaps indicating less aggressive FOBT follow up.

Factors that hold back screening for clinic patients A number of variables have been found to affect screening rates, including place of treatment, knowledge among providers, and resistance to the screening procedures. First, individuals with public insurance, Medicaid and Medicare, are seen in larger numbers at ambulatory clinics in teaching hospitals. Patients receiving care at teaching facilities see residents in training for the bulk of their medical care. Residents in training rotate during their residency program, so patients seldom have continuity of care with a single provider. Further, patients seen in teaching clinics wait longer to see health care providers and specialists. Arranging a colonoscopy or flexible sigmoidoscopy becomes a more arduous process because the patients must be scheduled for the specialty clinic before receiving the procedure. Getting an appointment in many specialty clinics can be a 3-6 month wait, and then the appointment for the procedure can be another long wait. For example, Zack and colleagues conducted a retrospective analysis of 108 medical charts of patients who received primary care at University of Nebraska Medical Center and found that residents overstated their actual screening rates for FOBT (88%) and flexible sigmoidoscopy (78%). Actual rates for FOBT and flexible sigmoidoscopy were 13% and 16% respectively. Another study also found that resident physicians adhered poorly to CRC screening recommendation for both Black and White patients (Borum, 1999).

Race/Ethnicity Differences in Colorectal Cancer Screening

There is extensive evidence for differences by R/E and other dimensions in CRC screening. An examination of data from the National Health Interview Survey (NHIS), Cancer Control Supplements (1987-1992) found that higher income and education were positively associated with screening for colorectal cancer across R/E groups, but older Blacks reported less screening than whites, controlling for age and gender (Hoffman-Goetz, Breen, and Meissner, 1998). Breen, Wagener, Brown, et al., (2001) examined R/E and gender differences using 1998 NHIS data and found that while both AAs and Hispanics had lower rates of CRC screening, the differences were not statistically significant after controlling for usual source of care, age, and insurance coverage. Overall screening rates were 35% for whites over age 65 and had increased rapidly since 1992, but remained lower and had not grown as rapidly for other groups. Our analysis of un-weighted 2000 NHIS data found that while 44% of white persons age 65 and older recall ever having had a CRC cancer screen, rates for AAs and Hispanics were notably lower at 31% and 30% respectively. AI/AN and Asian self-reported CRC screening was intermediate between whites and AAs. Ioannou, Chapko, and Dominitz (2003), examined all persons aged 50 and older in the NHIS and concluded that Hispanics and Asian/Pacific Islanders had the lowest overall rates of CRC screening, but were more likely to receive colonoscopy than whites or AAs. These data suggest that while screening rates for whites continued to increase, rates for elders of color remained relatively constant and the disparity in screening rates had increased (Cancer Progress Report, 2001; Swan, Breen, Coates, et al., 2003). While these data must be viewed with some caution since they are from self-reports, Freeman, Klabundne, Schussler, et al., (2002), note that measures of colorectal cancer screening derived from the Medicare claims data probably underestimate use because of reimbursement incentives for providers to use diagnostic rather than screening codes. Nonetheless, Richards and Reker (2002) analyzed 1999-2000 billing records for 5% sample of Medicare beneficiaries and found that AA men had a 25% lower rate of colonoscopy and 50% lower rate of flexible sigmoidoscopy than white men. Similar, though less pronounced differences were found for female Medicare beneficiaries.

A small group of studies has examined why elders of color have lower rates of CRC screening. Holmes-Rovner, Williams, Hoppough, et al., (2002) conducted focus groups with older people in Michigan. They found that while most white and Black participants were knowledgeable about screening procedures and considered them potentially efficacious, Black respondents were particularly likely to report that physicians had either not offered them the tests or failed to provide follow-up information. In a Georgia qualitative study, AAs reported little knowledge of CRC screening and having been offered little information by practitioners (Beeker, Kraft, Southwell, et al., 2000). Local surveys in AAs and Whites in Michigan (Janz, Wren, Schottenfeld, et al., 2003), Korean elders in Baltimore (Juon, Han, Shin, et al., 2003), AA and white elders in low-income housing (Paskett, Rushing, D'Agostino, et al., 1997), AAs in North Carolina (James, Campbell and Hudson, 2002), Korean and Filipino elders in Los Angeles (Maxwell, Bastani, and Warda, 2000), Mexican American men in Texas (Coronado and Thompson, 2000) and AAs in Seattle (Taylor, Lessler, Mertens, et al., 2003) all support the conclusion that differences in knowledge, physician recommendations, and attitudes towards the procedures explain R/E differences in participation. For example, in the Taylor study, 39%, 57% and 60% reported never having received a recommendation for FOBT, colonoscopy, or sigmoidoscopy respectively from their physician These recommendations were the strongest predictor of use. Ioannou, Chapko, and Dominitz (2003), came to a similar conclusion from a national telephone survey of over 61,000 persons aged 50 and over. They found that having regular appointments with a physician was the modifiable factor most associated with CRC screening participation. From a rather different perspective, Powe (1995) argued that an attitude of fatalism explained AA/white differences in older women's use of CRC screens after controls for age, income and education, based on data from a sample of 192 congregate meal site participants. None of these studies adequately controlled for measures of access, coverage, availability, or independently measured practitioner behaviors, thus the relative importance of patient, practitioner and care system factors in CRC screening remains poorly understood.

Interventions to Reduce Race/Ethnicity Disparities in CRC-Screening

A recent meta-analysis of approaches to increasing immunizations and cancer screening conducted for CMS found that organizational changes (e.g. prevention clinics, using a care visit for prevention, or using non-physician staff to promote prevention) were most effective in increasing screening, including FOBT (adjusted OR 17.6) (Shekelle, Stone, Manglione, et al., 2001). Provider education (OR 3.01) and patient reminders (OR 2.75) were also effective. Approaches that combined multiple strategies were found more effective than any single method alone. None of the published studies provided separate data on impacts for elders of color.

Our review identified several additional studies that report results of efforts to enhance FOBT use by elders of color, but no studies focused on increasing colonoscopy or flexible sigmoidoscopy use for these populations were identified. Several of the FOBT studies explored system level interventions and/or reminders in settings that served persons of color. For example, researchers worked with a Chicago HMO to train and support primary care physicians in 47 practices serving low-income – largely AA and Latino – areas to increase cancer screening rates (Manfredi, Czaja, Freels, et al., 1998). Reviews of patient charts before (N=2,316) and after (N=2,238) the intervention showed increases in the proportion of patients with a FOBT for HMO (14.1%) and FFS panels (20.2%). Another study randomized 49 physicians (and their 7,397 adult patients) in a university-based clinic setting for a one-year test of computer-generated reminders for preventive services (Ornstein, Garr, Jenkins, et al., 1991). Increases in FOBT use were highest when both physicians and patients received personalized reminder letters (from 19.5% to 38.1%), and increases were greater for Blacks and for patients with insurance. Other studies adopted more culturally tailored intervention strategies. Cargill and colleagues report on an effort to use nurse clinicians having in-person contact with patients to increase FOBT screening among a largely AA patient population (n=359) served by a medical clinic at a university hospital (Cargill et al., 1991). The percent of patients given FOBT kits increased from 4.1% to 46.6% in the experimental group compared to 9.9% to 13.0% in the control group, who were reminded through a letter to promote screenings. The experimental group patients were also much more likely to return their kit (69.8% vs. 20.0%).

Powe has been involved in a series of culturally tailored efforts to increase CRC screening (Powe and Weinrich, 1999; Powe, 1995). Most recently, a repeated measures pre/post experiment tested the effectiveness of a culturally relevant intervention to increase the rates of FOBT use in a population of elderly, rural AA females attending senior centers (Powe, 2002). One intervention group received both a short video intervention to address fatalism with respect to CRC as well as information and contacts over several months, a second group only watched the video, and the controls received traditional senior center services. After controlling for family history of CRC, provider visits, age and insurance, study group predicted FOBT at 1-year follow-up. Both intervention groups had higher screening than controls and rates were higher in the intensive intervention than in the video only group. Weinrich and colleagues report on an intervention to increase FOBT with a similar rural elderly senior center population (n=135) in a pre/post design (Weinrich, Weinrich, Boyd, et al., 1994). There was a substantial increase in screening after education sessions conducted by a community health worker (OR=6.2).

Colorectal Cancer Treatment and Race/Ethnicity Differences

According to the National Cancer Institute's PDQ, the consensus view on treatment of CRC calls for surgical resection of the primary and regional lymph nodes for localized disease, though other techniques are being evaluated. It is now believed that adjuvant chemotherapy with a combination of fluorouracil (5-FU) and leucovorin increases disease free survival for stage II or higher patients. Other combination chemotherapies, radiotherapy and other approaches continue to be explored because of high recurrence rates that vary by site and stage. For example, Sandler, Halabi, Baron, et al., (2003) examined the effects of daily doses of aspirin on recurrence of colorectal cancer in a randomized trial with 517 patients. Recurrence rates were 17% and 27% at one year for the aspirin and customary care groups respectively. Although lower rates of recurrence have been observed in other studies, such findings have lead to recommendations for long-term surveillance of CRC patients to detect recurrence or metastasis.

Race/Ethnicity disparities in treatment As noted by Shavers and Brown (2002) available studies find no evidence for differential efficacy of CRC treatments between African Americans and whites in clinical trials or in equal access care systems such as the Veterans Administration. More recently, Dignam et al (2003) found that for the 104 AA and 1070 white rectal cancer patients participating in the National Surgical Adjuvant Breast and Bowel Project (NSABP) there were no statistically significant differences in recurrence or disease-free survival by race. But the relatively small number of AA in the sample was associated with large confidence intervals. When examining literature regarding differences between whites and AAs or Latinos in access/use of specific cancer treatments, Shavers and Brown located 7 studies. They found evidence that AAs and/or Latinos were less likely to receive definitive primary therapy, conservative therapy, or adjuvant therapy in six large studies. Several of these studies also indicate that differences in treatment in part explain differences in survival. We did not find more recent studies relevant to these questions. Research reflecting current practice, studies focused on other R/E groups, and explorations of the determinants of unequal treatment are notably lacking. No interventions that address R/E differences in receipt of appropriate CRL care were identified.

Lung Cancer

Lung cancer offers a distinct contrast to CRC with respect to screening, treatment and treatment efficacy from the perspectives of both scientific consensus and our current understanding of how to address R/E disparities. Unlike other cancers, most forms of lung cancer are primarily linked to tobacco use, there is little consensus on cost-effective or efficacious strategies for early detection, and treatment appears to have less impact on survival. Nonetheless, like other cancers, there are R/E differences in stage at the time of detection, completion of appropriate treatments, and survival even after controlling for any group differences in prevalence. As shown below, available research is consistent with two different hypotheses about AA/white differences in lung cancer survival: a) AAs are diagnosed with lung cancer after the disease and other co-morbid conditions have already reduced their likelihood of survival even with state-of-the art treatment and b) AA are less likely to receive appropriate treatment services once diagnosed with lung cancer. In sharp contrast to breast and cervical cancer, there appear to be no studies that demonstrate mechanisms for eliminating R/E differences in detection. Like other cancers, however, there appears to be an absence of studies on reducing treatment disparities.

Cancer Prevalence and Mortality Differences by Race/Ethnicity

Lung cancer is the leading cause of cancer deaths in both genders, with an estimated 157,200 deaths in 2003 (ACS, 2003). According to SEER data, the age-adjusted incidence of non-small cell lung cancer (NSCLC) was 53.9/100,000. NSCLC is an aggregate of cancers with distinct histologies including squamous carcinoma, adenocarcinoma, and large cell carcinoma. Because all three forms of lung cancer have the potential for cure with surgical resection if detected in the localized stage, they are grouped together. By contrast, SEER data indicated an age-adjusted incidence of 8.6/100,000 for small cell carcinoma of the lung. This form of lung cancer is more likely to be widely spread by the time of diagnosis and is associated with median survival times of less than 6 months without treatment. Because of the high probability of metastases, chemotherapy is the usual treatment.

Available research primarily addresses prevalence and mortality for lung cancer in AA and White groups. The SEER Cancer Statistics Review 1975-2000 (Ries, Eisner, Kosary, et al., 2003) shows that incidence and mortality associated with invasive lung cancer on an age-adjusted basis is highest for AAs and whites, followed in decreasing rates by American Indians/Alaska Natives, Asian and Pacific Islanders, and Hispanics. Among older people, five-year relative survival rates for persons diagnosed 1992-1999 were significantly lower for AAs than for whites, but unlike the findings for CRC, overall lung cancer incidence and mortality rates are comparably disparate. In an older review of lung cancer patterns based on SEER data, the prevalence rate is 73.39 per 100,000 for AAs and 54.31 per 100,000 for whites (Stewart, 2001). Local studies show similar patterns. For example, Gadgeel and colleagues (2001) analyzed temporal trends in the impact of race on lung cancer using SEER data. The authors used data on 48,318 individuals from the Metropolitan Detroit Cancer Surveillance System (MDCSS), diagnosed 1973-1998. Lung cancer rates were found to be comparable for women but Black males had a 37% higher rate of lung cancer than white males. In terms of survival rates during 1986-1998, Blacks had significantly lower two and five-year survival rates than whites. Overall stage of lung cancer at diagnosis was the largest predictor of survival.

The national cancer statistics for Hispanics, based on SEER data, show that Hispanics had a lower incidence of lung cancer, 27.1 per 100,000 as opposed to 58.4 per 100,000 for whites without age adjustment (ACS, 2002b). Mortality rates were reported at 19.8 per 100,000 versus 50.3 per 100,000 for whites. Specific data for Latino elders were not reported, and the younger average age of the Latino population may have influenced these findings. ACS attributes the difference to less cigarette smoking among Hispanics. Specifically, rates of lung cancer were 70% lower than those for non-Hispanics, but the reliability of R/E coding (not based on self-report) and sample design (selects for some but not all Latino subgroups) have both been challenged for these data.

There are studies that examine other population groups. For example, one study looked at all cancers of American Indians in several western states, using Indian Health Service data and other sources and found that American Indians in New Mexico had lower rates of lung cancer than whites while American Indians in Montana had lung cancer rates comparable to whites (Bleed, Risser, Sperry, et al., 1992). Similarly, in an analysis of SEER data, Clegg, Li, Hankey, et al., (2002) concluded that despite lower incidence of lung cancer among Native Hawaiians and American Indians/Alaska Natives, these groups had higher risks of dying within five years of diagnosis.

Lung Cancer Screening and Diagnosis: Evidence for Race/Ethnicity Differences

There is no consensus on the efficacy of screening for lung cancer. The most broadly used approach to screening combines chest x-rays and sputum cytology. But NCI's PDQ review group concludes that there is insufficient evidence on the efficacy of these methods to support a broadly based screening program. Similarly, the ACS, does not recommend general screening for lung cancer (Smith, Cokkinides,. von Eschenbach, et al., 2002). Aberle et al (2001), in a consensus statement of the Society of Thoracic Radiology concurred that routine screening is not appropriate at this time.

Screening has not been recommended because randomized controlled trials conducted in the 1970's failed to show reduced mortality rates. There are ongoing debates about the relative efficacy of chest X-rays vs. more sophisticated but also more costly new methods. Strauss (2002) reexamined one of the largest of these older studies, applying Cox proportional hazards regression to data for 9,192 individuals who participated in the Mayo Lung Cancer Project. The Mayo researchers had concluded that screening with chest x-ray and sputum cytology was ineffective and this is the view that has lead to current recommendations. But the Strauss re-analysis accounted for lead-time bias, length bias, and over diagnosis bias and showed that screening did significantly reduce mortality rates. Lead time bias was excluded by comparing survival among cases from the time of randomization, instead of from the time of detection; length bias was excluded by conducting an intent-to-treat analysis that considered screening-detected and symptom detected cases, and over-diagnosis bias was excluded by multivariate analyses that showed that resection was the only significant predictor of survival in this study.

There have been several advances in screening technology over the past few years, including Positron Emission Tomography (PET) and Low-Dose helical Computed Tomography (LDCT) both of which use multiple x-ray images and computer technology to create a three-dimensional image of a patient's lungs and may thus increase the likelihood of detecting cancer. PET scans may detect smaller tumors than LDCT scan (Coleman, 2002). They can also determine whether or not the tumor is malignant because malignant tumors take up glucose faster than non-malignant tumors and this shows up on the PET scan. Medicare pays for work-ups including diagnoses and staging of NSCLC (Coleman, 2002; McCann, 1998). However there are only 75 PET scanners in the United States at this time and evidence for the cost-effectiveness of this approach has been seen as controversial. Randomized controlled trials of LDCT are only now underway. Henschke, McCauley, Yankelevitz, et al., (1999) described the design and baseline results from the Early Lung Cancer Action Project (ELCAP), an effort aimed at assessing the use of LDCT in screening for lung cancer. In their study, 1000 symptom-free volunteers, over age 60, who had a history of smoking and no previous cancer, were given chest radiographs and LDCT. Malignant nodules were detected in 2.7% of individuals through use of LDCT versus .7% by chest radiography.

Race/Ethnicity differences in lung cancer detection Data from SEER (Ries, Eisner, Kosary, et al., 2003) indicate that during 1992-1999, AA of both genders (14%) are only slightly less likely than whites (16%) to be diagnosed at the most curable localized stage. Earlier data had shown that African Americans are more likely than whites to be diagnosed with lung cancer at later stages (Graham, Geitz, Byhardt, et al., 1992). Shavers and Brown (2002) also found evidence in three studies based on SEER data that Blacks were more likely than whites to have metastases by the time they are diagnosed.

Additional studies support the conclusion that social factors are associated with stage at diagnosis for lung cancer. Bradley and colleagues (2000) analyzed disparities in lung and other cancer diagnoses and survival based on three Michigan databases 1996-1998. Total sample size was 51,296. The majority of the participants with lung cancer were >65 years of age. The mean age group at cancer diagnosis was 65-69 across R/E. The authors found that seniors with Medicare were less likely to receive late stage diagnosis while elders with Medicaid had higher risk for late stage diagnosis. Risk of death from lung cancer was highest in the Medicaid population under age 65 and in AA women regardless of age or insurance status. The authors concluded that the disparities in diagnosis and mortality rates found in the study were primarily due to poverty, although AA were disproportionately poor in this sample. Another Michigan study, however, drew a different conclusion. Gadgeel, Severson, Kau, et al., (2001) analyzed metropolitan Detroit SEER data for 1973-1998 and concluded that AAs were more likely to be diagnosed at distant stage than whites and that this difference was a strong predictor of racial differences in survival. A similar conclusion was reached in a comparison of Asian immigrants and white lung cancer patients in Boston. Finlay, Rodrigues, Griffith, et al., (2002) conducted a 5-year retrospective case-control study and reported that Asians were significantly more likely to present with advanced stage lung cancer and that this difference was associated with lower 5-year survival.

The recent NCI analyses of SEER data appear to suggest that age-adjusted differences between AA and whites in stage at diagnosis for lung cancer may be moderating, but these broad statistics may not provide as full a picture as indicated by the more detailed analyses of local and regional registry data. None of the studies that found R/E or other social factor disparities in stage at diagnosis for lung cancer explored the potential causes. Authors simply hypothesized that the discrepancy was due to access to care, low income or education. The access to care hypothesis deserves special attention, since a larger proportion of lung cancers are detected by practitioner-initiated screening tests with high-risk patients than for other reasons (Strauss, 2002). There do not appear to be studies that explore mechanisms for increasing participation by African Americans in screening or other early detection for lung cancer, and there is a particular shortage of research on screening participation, stage at diagnosis, or improving detection of lung cancer for other racial/ethnic groups.

Lung Cancer Treatment and Race/Ethnicity Differences

Shavers and Brown (2002) note than that while about one-third of NSCLC patients can receive surgical resection and have fair prognoses, the remaining NSCL patients and those with SCLC are less often recommended for surgery because the disease is broadly disseminated at the time of diagnosis. In these cases, adding chemotherapy to the treatment regimen does increase the median survival rate. Consensus on efficacious lung cancer treatments has not progressed notably in the last decade and participation in several ongoing clinical trials is recommended for many patients.

Shavers and Brown (2002) reviewed five studies of R/E differences in treatment for lung cancer and three studies of lung cancer treatment effectiveness. They conclude that no significant differences in treatment responses were found between Black and white patients in the Veterans Administration Chemotherapy Trial or other equal treatment settings. They also reported on two other studies that found Blacks and whites had similar five-year survival rates after receiving surgical resection and radiation therapy. This is evidence that efficacy of treatment does not vary by R/E group. But, Shavers and Brown report that five population studies show that Blacks were less likely to receive surgical resection, radiation therapy, chemotherapy, or any other treatment. All of these studies utilized population databases with large sample sizes. Among these studies was the Bach, Cramer, Warren, et al., (1999) analysis of linked SEER-Medicare data for 1985-1993 on 10,984 patients with early stage NSCLC. They found that surgery rates were 12.7% lower for Blacks and, that these differences partially explained lower survival for Blacks.

Stewart (2001) also reviewed literature that lead to the hypothesis that excess mortality of lung carcinoma in Blacks was due to inadequate access to care. Blacks undergo surgery for Stage I NSCLC at lower rates than whites. He cites the Bach, Cramer, Warren, et al., (1999) finding that if Blacks underwent resection at rates similar to whites the excess mortality in Blacks with NSCLC would be lowered by 57%. Consistent with Stewart's analysis, Earle, Venditti, Neumann, et al., (2000) in a retrospective study using Medicare data examined socio-demographic and disease characteristics of individuals who received chemotherapy for lung cancer. All individuals were age 65 or older. They found that younger, healthier patients were more likely to receive chemotherapy. Whites and other non-Blacks, those of higher socioeconomic status and those treated at teaching hospitals were more likely to receive chemotherapy.

Yet the Earle et al study, and a study by Blackstock, Herndon, Paskett, et al., (2002) might also be consistent with the hypothesis that because of inadequate primary care, AAs, were more likely to present both with more developed disease and lower overall health status. Blackstock et al investigated survival rates for 504 patients with advanced NSCLC. Subjects included 458 White and 46 Black patients who were receiving chemotherapy for advanced NSCLC between 1989 and 1998 and were part of the Lung Cancer and Leukemia Group B studies. Fifty nine percent of the subjects were older than age 60. Their aim was to see if disparities in survival would persist if patients were receiving the same treatments. They found a significantly different unadjusted one-year survival rate of 22% for Blacks and 30% for whites. However, differences in survival rates narrowed with control for performance status and weight loss, signifying that the Black patients were sicker when diagnosed. Black patients were more likely to be unemployed, unmarried, disabled, present with poor performance status and weight loss, and more likely to be on Medicaid. They suggest that poor social circumstances lead to poor prognosis even in clinical trial contexts.

There appear to be no published studies that seek to explain these differences in treatment patterns between AAs and whites or how to resolve them. There appear to be no published studies on treatment and outcome disparities for lung cancer focused on other R/E groups.

Prostate Cancer

Prostate cancer presents still a different story about R/E and health disparities. The risk factors and pre-cancerous processes for this male cancer are poorly understood and yet it does seem to be more prevalent among AAs than in any other group. Further, although there are established, non-invasive and low-cost screening mechanisms for prostate cancer, the cost effectiveness of screening and its ethical appropriateness are highly debated. This debate reflects findings that prostate cancer is slow in its development in many but not all cases and potential cures often have negative side effects that are not outweighed by improvements in survival. Nonetheless, white men are more likely to be screened and more likely to receive aggressive treatment than AA men. Both R/E group differences in stage at diagnosis and receipt of treatment are associated with the much higher mortality for AA men. While a few studies demonstrate that screening participation can be improved with culturally tailored approaches, there is no body of literature on improving access to more effective treatment patterns. Experiences for other traditionally excluded R/E groups fall somewhere between these extremes, but there is much less evidence available.

Prostate Cancer Prevalence and Mortality Differences by Race/Ethnicity

African American men carry the highest burden in terms of morbidity, survival rates and mortality of prostate cancer. AAs experience a 62% higher incidence and a 137% higher mortality rate than whites. Between 1992 and 1997, the 5-year survival rate for AAs was 92%, five percent lower than for whites (Jemal, Thomas, Murray, et al., 2002). For any stage category, the 5-year survival rates are poorer for African American than for whites (Wingo, Ries, Parker, 1998). A central question for prostate cancer researchers is whether these differences in disease outcomes reflect underlying biological differences, different patterns of risk behavior, or differential access to appropriate screening or treatment. There is some evidence for a genetic explanation for these differences. Families with high risk of prostate cancer share a genetic marker and this feature is more prevalent among AA families with at least three members with prostate cancer than whites with the same family history (Powell and Meyskens, 2001). Similarly, prostatic intraepithelial neoplasia (PIN), considered the most probable precursor of invasive prostate cancer, is higher in AAs. These differences might explain the development of more aggressive cancer among this group (Montironi, Mazzucchelli, Marshall, et al., 1999).

R/E disparities in stage at the time of prostate cancer diagnosis have been reported consistently in analyses of SEER data. Between 1984 and 1991, 85% of prostate cancer cases in whites, registered in SEER and with known stage, had a local or regional stage while only 74% of AA were in the least severe stage (Harlan, Brawley, Pommerenke, et al., 1995). Similarly, based on SEER data, between 1992 and 1996, 5.9% of whites and 9.5% of AAs had a distant stage disease (Merrill, Capocaccia, Feuer, et al., 2000). Significantly, in the Veterans Administration equal access setting, no racial differences in prostate cancer stage at diagnosis was observed for 477 men diagnosed with prostate cancer (Freedland, Sutter, Naitoh, et al., 2000). These data parallel those for other cancers in suggesting that elders from traditionally excluded groups are less likely to obtain early detection and diagnosis.

Consistent with the other diseases, there is a broad consensus that stage and grade at diagnosis for prostate cancer is a crucial determinant of survival (Alexander and Brawley, 1998; Wingo, Ries, Parker, et al, 1998; Merrill and Brawley, 1997; Clegg, Li, Hankey, et al., 2002; Bianco, Wood, Grignon, et al., 2002). For example, Chu, Tarone, and Freeman, (2003) analyzed SEER data for 1976-1999, and note that a primary determinant of survival was stage at diagnosis, and that the findings of later stage at diagnosis for AAs were the primary factor in continuing racial differences in prostate cancer survival.

Cancer Screening and Diagnosis: Evidence for Race/Ethnicity Differences

Prostate cancer detection methods   The most commonly used methods for early detection of prostate cancer are digital rectal examination (DRE) and prostate-specific antigen (PSA) testing. Their combined use increases the positive predictive value of an abnormal result over either test alone (Crawford, 1997). The effectiveness of DRE in detecting clinically significant intracapsular tumors is questioned, and so is its ability to reduce mortality rates. Nonetheless, the presence of an abnormal DRE can be indicative that cancer has spread outside the prostate and this can be confirmed with a biopsy. In a study of 2,425 men, aged 55-70, without history of prostate cancer, overall sensitivity and specificity of DRE were 57.9% and 96.3% respectively (Mettlin, Lee, Drago, et al., 1991) but positive predictive value of DRE was higher for older men and those who also had elevated PSA.

The PSA is the most reliable non-invasive test available for the early detection of prostate cancer (Miller, Diefenbach, Kruus, et al., 2001). The introduction and diffusion of the use of the PSA test have played a major role in the detection of this cancer. Incidence of prostate cancer has followed a parallel trend with first-time use of PSA testing, with a rise and then a decline during 1990s (Legler, Feuer, Potosky, et al., 1998). It has more sensitivity but lower specificity than DRE. Positive predictive value depends on the levels of PSA: the higher the level the larger the positive predictive value, but the higher the level, the higher the chance of advance disease. Further, it may be appropriate to set different PSA cut-off points for AAs than other groups, though adequate assessments of this question have not been performed. PSA levels do appear higher in Blacks than in whites both among men without clinical evidence of prostate cancer and among men at the time of prostate cancer diagnosis (Abdalla, Ray, Ray, et al., 1998; Moul, Sesterhenn, Douglas, et al., 1995). Other suggestions for increasing the predictive value of PSA tests have been advanced (Crawford, 1997; DeAntoni, 1997) and it is possible that some of these measures may be more sensitive for AAs than those in common use (Catalona, Partin, Slawin, et al., 2000).

Even after receipt of suspicious PSA findings, it is a complex, multi-step process to achieve a definitive diagnosis of prostate cancer. Most often, diagnosis is made by needle biopsy and histologic confirmation. Transrectal ultrasound is often used to guide needle biopsies. However, among patients with a suspicious PSA and/or DRE, one time biopsy can miss up to 23% of clinically significant prostate cancer cases. A serial biopsy study of 2,526 volunteer men aged 40 or older with abnormal PSA and/or DRE demonstrates the following cumulative cancer detection rate: one biopsy 77%, two biopsies 91%, three biopsies 97%, and four biopsies 99% (Roehl, Antenor, and Catalona, 2002).

Screening for prostate cancer: Debated efficacy   The goal of screening is to diagnose prostate cancer at an early, localized stage, with the goal of potential cure, thus reducing or eliminating morbidity and mortality. The classical principles of screening are: the disease has a natural history which is well understood, should represent a serious public health problem and be able to be detected in an early stage; a simple, valid, harmless and acceptable test must be available; diagnosis and treatment in an early stage must be more beneficial than in an late stage and, the program must be cost-effective (Wilson and Junger, 1968; Moffat, 2000). Without information from randomized trials, population-based mass screening will continue to be controversial. Currently, there are two prospective randomized trials underway to test the efficacy of PSA screening for reducing prostate cancer mortality and improving quality of life (Maattanen, Auvinen, Stenman, et al., 1999; Canadas, Cusan, Gomez, et al., 2000).

Major professional organizations have published guidelines on screening for prostate cancer. They are: American College of Physicians-American Society of Internal Medicine (ACP-ASIM)(American College of Physicians, 1997), American College of Preventive Medicine (ACPM, 1998), American Cancer Society (Smith, Mettlin, Davis, et al., 2000; Smith, Cokkinides, von Eschenbach, et al., 2002), American Urological Association (AUA, 1999), and U.S. Preventive Services Task Force (USPSTF, 1996). Among them, the ACP-ASIM, the ACPM, and the USPSTF do not recommend routine population screening for prostate cancer. The main reasons stated against routine screening include low specificity of DRE and PSA, leading to relatively high biopsy rate. They argue that these biopsies are not free of complications and that the known and significant risk of adverse effects associated with prostate cancer treatment as well as the lack of conclusive evidence of effectiveness of treatments on survival rates all outweigh any possible positive impacts on survival. This argument against prostate cancer screening arises from the most common course of the disease and the risks of treatment. Autopsy studies have shown that prostate cancer is very common among men who are 50 years old and above, and its prevalence increases with age. There is an overall 30% histologic prevalence of latent cancer among elders (Coley, Barry, Fleming, et al.,

1997). However, the lifetime risk of clinical prostate cancer is only 17% (Jemal, Thomas, Murray, et al., 2002). Screening leads to over-diagnosis that can be as high as 275% of cancers that might be clinically insignificant or never diagnosed without screening (Ciatto, 2000). When these types of biases are not taken into account, comparison of survival rates between screened and unscreened groups can erroneously suggest a benefit of cancer screening in survival rates (Coley, Barry, Fleming, et al., 1997). Over-diagnosis is associated with over-treatment. Treatment is associated with very frequent adverse effects: such as incontinence and impotence or even death. Thus patients with indolent cancer can end up receiving unnecessary treatments that are not only ineffective and costly but also both deleterious to their quality of life (Alexander, 2000).

Despite this absence of definitive evidence for screening, both the ACS and the AUA nevertheless recommend the routine use of DRE and PSA testing among men 50 and older who have a life expectancy of at least 10 years. They also recommend earlier screenings for higher risk men such as AAs or those with a first-degree relative diagnosed with prostate cancer at a younger age. For these groups, the ACS guidelines suggest that screening should begin at age 45 (Smith, Cokkinides, von Eschenbach, et al., 2002). Their recommendations are based on the fact that prostate cancer mortality among white men has declined to levels below those existing before the PSA measurement that started in 1986. Moreover, populations that undergo annual PSA testing have higher rates of organ-confined diseases (Catalona, Richie, Ahmann, et al., 1994; Etzioni, Legler, Feuer, et al., 1999). Early-stage disease is associated with better survival than late-stage disease. (Coley, Barry, Fleming, et al., 1997; Jemal, Thomas, Murray, et al., 2002), and metastasic disease at the time of diagnosis is almost eliminated (Labrie, Candas, Cusan, et al., 1996). Some authors, even while in favor of routine screening, doubt the benefit of an annual screening without targeting only those with a higher risk of prostate cancer. Those men with low PSA levels are expected to have a very slow progression to higher levels, making them an unnecessary target for annual screening (Carter, 2001; Fang, Metter, Landis, et al., 2001; Brawer, 2000).

Increasing use of screening and attention to informed consent One of the most important factors that influence the use of PSA testing is the recommendation from a health care provider. There is general consensus that given the uncertainties related to prostate cancer screening, patients should participate actively in that decision and provide informed consent. It might be argued that having informed consent around prostate cancer screening, rather than receipt of the test is the best measure of appropriate services, and thus studies of informed consent issues take on special importance. Informed consent requires that patients be knowledgeable about risks and benefits from testing and potential treatment. Primary care providers play a key role in both educating and getting patient consent. Many information aids have been developed and tested for men to foster informed decisions about prostate cancer screening such as videotapes, scripted verbal information, pamphlets, written information and, group presentation, (Chan, 2001; Schapira and VanRuiswyk, 2000).

When men receive information about PSA screening, they usually show less interest in having the test according to a study that explored the effects of educational videotape on short-term knowledge and attitude toward prostate cancer screening. About half of 372 men seeking a free PSA test were assigned to watch the educational videotape, while the other half watched a non-educational video. Although those in the intervention group reported a significantly better knowledge about prostate cancer, they also showed significantly less interest in having another PSA test within the next two years. Similar findings emerged in a series of studies by Wolf and colleagues (Volk, Cass, and Spann, 1999; Wolf and Schorling, 1998; Wolf, Philbrick, and Schorling, 1997; Wolf, Nasser, Wolf, et al., 1996), but no separate analyses by race/ethnicity are reported.

Although there is a distinct absence of studies that explore PSA testing informed consent and impacts on screening participation in elders of color, Barber and colleagues (Barber, Shaw, Folts, et al., 1998; Abdalla, Ray, Ray, et al., 1998) indicate that lack of information was a clear factor in the lower participation by AAs in screening. A community based screening program in Michigan recruited 944 men 40 years of age and older for DRE and PSA testing. About 39% of the men screened were AAs. Although AAs reported less knowledge of prostate cancer before the program, the racial gap disappeared after the intervention. According to Barber, Shaw, Folts, et al., (1998) African Americans' lower level of knowledge, and in particular their low awareness of the early symptoms of prostate cancer, could explain delayed screening, but neither this nor other existing studies include specific multivariate analyses that explore the effects of primary care participation, insurance status, and prostate cancer knowledge on testing.

Racial/Ethnic differences in prostate cancer screening   Although informed decision-making around prostate cancer screening, rather than screening participation, may be the best indicator of appropriate care, the potential to increase early detection for those with more aggressive tumors has sparked continued interest in R/E differences in screening. Nonetheless, no published data on PSA utilization based on clinical or billing records for men of all ages at national level appear to be available to date (Smith, Cokkinides, von Eschenbach, et al., 2002). Analyses of NHIS and BRFSS data can partially address this gap, but as many as 31% of PSA recipients do not recall having had the test (Federman, 1999). For Medicare beneficiaries, billing records do allow for more reliable investigation of demographic factors in screening participation, although Freeman, Klabundne, Schussler, et al., (2002) caution that providers may face incentives not to bill these procedures as screens. In this population, AAs have been tested at a lower and slower rate than whites. Based on analysis of claims, in 1992, 34% of White and 25% of AA men received a PSA test in that year. In 1998, an analysis of Medicare claims found that 38% of white and 31% of AA men received at least one PSA test (Legler, Feuer, Potosky, et al., 1998). Among those who received the test, about 80% of them had received a PSA test in the past year. Our analysis of self-reported data from the NCHS National Health Interview Survey also found broad R/E differences in recent PSA use among elders. While 55% of white elders reported receipt of a PSA in the last two years, the comparable proportions were 42%, 43%,

42%, and 46% for AAs, AI/AN, Asian, and Hispanics respectively. Rates for 'others' were even lower at 33%. Further, utilization rates and race differences in rates are very heterogeneous across regions (Etzioni, 2002).

It is noteworthy, that there are no differences by R/E group in PSA testing among VAMC users aged 65 and older, so these findings may say more about the functioning of health systems than individual preferences (Freedland, Sutter, Naitoh, et al., 2000). Consistent with this conclusion are findings that the type of primary health care facility and insurance status seem to influence screening rates. A small survey study of 142 men over 40 years of age showed differences in DRE and PSA testing rates depending on the setting in which patients were seen (Perez and Tsou, 1995). Patients seen in an internal medicine clinic were compared to those seen in a private practice. Seventy two percent of men from each of the settings received a DRE. However, only 10% of patients seen in the clinic received a PSA testing alone or combined with DRE in comparison with 68% of patients in the private setting. While most of the patients in the clinic were Medicare/Medicaid beneficiaries (91%), the majority of the patients in the private setting had private insurance supplements to Medicare (82%). Beyond these studies, no reports have explicated the underlying reasons for differences in screening.

Interventions to increase PSA use by African Americans   Several studies demonstrate that educational programming about prostate cancer conducted in work sites, churches, and housing projects can recruit large numbers of men for prostate cancer education and screening. But large-scale general prostate cancer screening programs have failed in recruiting AAs. The Washington University Study recruited 22,000 men but only 4% Blacks. The ACS National Prostate Cancer Detection Project recruited 2,999 men, but only 7.2 % were African Americans. The Prostate Cancer Awareness Week is arguably the largest cancer-screening program focused on men. Since 1989, this program has reached more than 3 million men, yet less than 6% were of African descent (Crawford, 1997; DeAntoni, 1997). By contrast, smaller initiatives have targeted mainly AAs. Although these efforts have shown that AA, Latino and AI/AN men can be engaged in PSA testing, reports have typically not provided information on screening rates prior to the intervention or offered community data on the number of persons who might have participated in programs, thus it is impossible to fully assess the success of these interventions.

The Detroit Education and Early Diagnosis program was initiated in 1993. Churches have played a key role in this program. An outreach coordinator sought support from ministers, who announced the educational session weeks in advance during services. The target population was Black men, aged 40-70. The educational component, provided at the conclusion of Sunday services, used an AA team, a physician and a prostate cancer survivor, to reach participants. Participants completed a brief questionnaire and informed consent. The session included information regarding prostate cancer natural history, staging, diagnostic methods, and treatment options. After the session, participants had the chance to get PSA tests. The lab result was mailed two weeks later; if the test results were suspicious, a nurse would call the patient to coordinate follow-up visits. More than 1,000 men participated in the program in its first 17 months. Of the 647 men who received a PSA screening, 8% had a suspicious result. The cancer detection rate was 2.5% among men tested (Powell, Gelfand, Parzuchowski, et al., 1995; Powell, Heilbrun, Littrup, et al., 1997).

A quasi-experiment design was used in South Carolina to analyze the effect of an educational intervention on PSA testing among 1,717 men aged 40-70 years old without history or current diagnostic evaluation for prostate cancer. The sample had 71% AA men. Men were recruited from a variety of sites. Participants were randomly assigned to receive one of four interventions: traditional, peer-educator only, client navigator only, or a combined intervention. The peer-educator intervention presented a testimony on the importance of screening, and was conducted by a man whose race was the same as that most represented in the site. The client-navigator condition consisted of a follow-up phone call by a social worker to help the man overcome potential barriers to screening and move through the health care system. After completion of the educational session, each man received a voucher for a free prostate cancer screening including a DRE and PSA test, to be used with his primary care physician. The physicians were reimbursed for their services. Participants' prior screening behavior was reported, and differences between races were significant. Among AAs, 37% did not have a prior DRE and 77% did not have a prior PSA test. Among whites, the proportions were 23% and 33% respectively. Screening participation rates depended on the race and the type of interventions. Despite the educational intervention and access to free prostate cancer screening, 39% of AAs and 25% of whites who participated in the educational interventions chose not to get screened, a significant difference. Regarding type of interventions, Blacks were 90% more likely to receive screening under the client navigator intervention than after receiving the traditional intervention. Among whites, none of the interventions produced higher screening rates than the traditional approach (Weinrich, Holdford, Boyd, et al., 1998).

Even very simple interventions are useful in increasing screening participation. For example, 413 Black men between 40-70 years old without a history of prostate cancer attending a university health service were randomized in two groups after completion of a phone survey. One group received a reminder letter inviting them to a urology clinic for education and screening. The other group received a letter, plus printed informational material about prostate cancer as well as a phone call from a lay health worker. While only 21% of the men who received only a letter accepted the invitation, 51% of men called by the lay health worker responded (Myers, 1999).

Prostate Cancer Treatment and Race/Ethnicity

Currently there are three primary approaches for the treatment of clinically localized prostate cancer: radical prostatectomy, radiotherapy and expectant management (watchful waiting). Recommended approaches differ by cancer stage. The relative efficacy of these approaches is not known, but ongoing clinical trials may provide needed answers. In the meantime, both, radical prostatectomy and radiotherapy are associated with serious complications. Radical prostatectomy is associated with mortality (1.1%), incontinence (any 26.6%, and complete 6.8%), impotence (85%) bowel injury (any 2.7%, and injury requiring long-term treatment or colostomy 1.3%), and urethral stricture requiring long-term treatment (12.4%). External beam radiation is also associated with similar complications but occurring at different rates (Office of Technology Assessment, 1995).

Lu-Yao and Yao (1997) analyzed long-term survival in 57,876 patients with clinically localized prostate cancer aged 50-79 using SEER data. Ten-year survival depended on the cancer grade. Patients with Stage I disease had better survival and those with Stage III had the worst. There were no statistically significant differences in survival by treatment among men with Stage I cancer. In this study, men with Stages II or III who underwent surgery had significantly better survival than those who received radiotherapy or watchful waiting. The authors emphasized the possibility of selection bias, since patients who are healthier are more likely to receive an aggressive treatment. Further, this study tracked all localized prostate cancer patients in the registry, not only those who received treatment, and yielded substantially lower survival benefit than prior studies. Lu-Yao and Yao's findings suggest that other comparisons of prostatectomy with conservative treatments may have over-stated the value of surgery.

Race/ethnicity differences in treatment   The Shavers and Brown (2002) review found 17 equal treatment studies that examined whether or not there are R/E differences in the efficacy of prostate cancer interventions, and found that 11 of them concluded that R/E was not an independent predictor of treatment failure. Further, in 5 of the remaining studies, R/E differences in survival or cause-specific mortality were eliminated after controls for age, stage and/or tumor grade. The one exception, Shekarriz, Tiguert, Upadhyay, et al., (2000) focused on a small group of men who received surgery but not adjuvant therapy, and found that AA men had shorter survival rates. Consistent with the bulk of the evidence through 2001 reviewed by Shavers and Brown, among the 11 more recent equal treatment studies of prostate cancer survival (not included in their review), nine found no evidence that R/E is an independent predictor of survival or treatment failure after control for disease features and other demographic features (Man, Pickles, and Chi, 2003; Ray, Dunn, Cooney, et al., 2003; Koff, Connelly, Bauer, et al., 2002; Roach, Lu, Pilepich, et al., 2003; Cross, Shultz, Malkowicz, et al., 2002; Kupelian, Buchsbaum, Elshaikh, et al., 2002; Kupelian, Elshaikh, Reddy, et al., 2002b; Kupelian, Reddy, Carlson, et al., 2003c; Lee, Barnswell, Torre, et al., 2002). The two equal treatment studies that did find either higher disease recurrence or higher mortality in AA (Grossfeld, Latini, Downs, et al., 2002; Powell, Dey, Dudley, et al., 2002) focused on men with localized prostate cancer who received radical prostectomy but no adjuvant therapies. While the predominant finding from these studies is that prostate cancer treatments are equally efficacious across R/E lines, prostate cancer is unlike any of the other cancers we examined in that there are several studies that conclude that African Americans have worse outcomes in equal treatment context.

The evidence for racial/ethnic differences in treatment patterns is also more complex for prostate cancer than for other cancers. Shavers and Brown (2002) found 5 observational studies. In these studies, AAs and Hispanic men were consistently more likely to have received no treatment/watchful waiting or conservative treatment (hormones or radiation without surgery), but findings on rates of prostatectomy and other surgical treatments varied by disease features and study catchment area and period. For instance, a study of all invasive prostate cancer cases in Connecticut between 1988 and 1992 observed that when the cancer was at a local/regional stage, radical prostatectomy was performed less frequently in AAs but no significant racial differences in surgery were observed among patients 75 years and above (Polednak, 1998). In an analysis of 98,377 SEER patients diagnosed with prostate cancer between 1992 and 1996, however more African Americans (46%) received watchful waiting as treatment compared to Whites (40%). Shavers and Brown also concluded that white men were more likely than non-whites to receive more expensive or innovative treatments, and none of these differences in treatment could be explained by racial differences in clinical factors. Three additional observational studies that appeared more recently provided additional evidence for unequal treatment of African American and Hispanic men with prostate cancer. Harlan, Potosky, Gilliland, et al., (2001) studied 30,373 men with clinically localized disease. Among men 60 and older, after adjustment for age, stage, grade, and baseline PSA, AA men underwent aggressive treatment less often than did white men or Hispanic men. Similarly, Hoffman, Harlan, Klabunde, et al., (2003) examined treatment patterns using SEER data from Connecticut, Los Angeles and Atlanta for 1,144 men with clinically localized disease and found an interaction between race and tumor aggressiveness. Among men with more aggressive cancer, AAs were less likely to undergo radical prostatectomy than non-Hispanic whites, but among the 71% of subjects with less aggressive cancers, AAs and non-Hispanic whites were equally likely to receive either radical prostatectomy or radiation therapy. Hall, Satariano, Thompson, et al., (2002) argue that apparent R/E differences in treatment patterns are complexly related to co-morbid health conditions. Among 1,075 Kaiser Permanente patients diagnosed during the late 1970's and 1980's, there were interactions between R/E and co-morbid conditions, such that AA men with co-morbid heart disease, diabetes, or prior heart attacks were less likely to receive aggressive treatment for clinically localized prostate cancer. The inconsistencies among these study findings suggest that because of relatively less developed consensus on the efficacy of prostate cancer treatments, care patterns are associated with clinical and non-clinical factors that play out in different ways across settings and communities.

Race/Ethnicity differences in treatment and survival Several authors indicate the need to disentangle the relative roles of R/E and socioeconomic class as pervasive risk factors as compared with other determinants of treatment access in explaining survival of prostate cancer patients (Dale, Vijayakumar, Lawlor, et al., 1996; Robbins, Whittemore, and Thom, 2000). A multivariate analysis of SEER data on 146,979 prostate cancer patients diagnosed from 1973 to 1990 showed that AAs have a 35% higher risk of cancer specific mortality among patients with non-distant prostate cancer after controlling for age and type of treatment (Robbins, Whittemore, and Thom, 2000). This suggests that some correlate of R/E other than age, stage at diagnosis or treatment is associated with higher mortality. Nevertheless, a recent meta-analysis has estimated the overall and cancer-specific survival differences for prostate cancers between Blacks and whites when receiving comparable treatment for similar stage cancer. To calculate the overall survival and the cancer specific survival, a total of 30 cohort studies for average survival and 27 cohort studies for cancer specific survival were included. Blacks were at a significant excess risk of death due to a greater burden of co-morbidities, but there were no differences in the risk of prostate cancer specific death after controlling for population mortality (Bach, Schrag, Brawley, et al., 2002).

More recently, Godley, Schenck, Amamoo, et al., (2003) examined merged SEER and Medicare billing data for 5747 Black and 38,242 white patients diagnosed at age 65-84 years with clinically localized prostate cancer between 1986 and 1996. They found that Black patients were less likely to have undergone surgery as their primary prostate cancer treatment (24% versus 33%) and were more likely to have had non-aggressive treatment (38% versus 27%). But among those who received surgery, Black patients had more co-morbid conditions and more advanced tumors. After adjustment for age, co-morbidity score, SEER site, census tract education and income level, marital status, and pathologic stage and tumor grade, the racial disparity in survival remained significant for those treated with surgery but not for those who received radiation or non-aggressive treatment. The effects of race on overall mortality were larger than those on cancer specific mortality, but the interaction of treatment approach and race on survival was consistent over time, suggesting that changes in screening, diagnostic and treatment norms were not explanatory. Godley et al's findings are consistent with several conclusions, including worse overall health and more aggressive disease for AAs who received surgery and less adequate care for co-morbid conditions for AA men with prostate care. The primary conclusion, however, seems to be that unequal treatment either of the prostate cancer or of co-morbid health conditions explains some but not all of the Black/white disparity in prostate cancer and that we know very little about the relative efficacy of treatment or treatment equity for other groups of men.

Summary and Discussion

The review of epidemiological and health services research evidence on R/E and colorectal, lung, and prostate cancers suggests important differences between these three cancer sites and in comparison to breast and cervical cancer. For these three cancer sites, there is less detail and precision in current knowledge and less consensus on the extent and causes for disparities in incidence, mortality, detection, and treatment.

Our literature review found that AAs faced a greater chance of developing and lower chances of surviving all three cancers than whites. One or more other racial/ethnic groups experienced higher rates of disease or worse survival for each of these cancers, but there was evidence that Latino, Asian American, NHOPI, American Indian/Alaska Native pan-ethnic groups may experience a lower overall burden from these cancers than do whites. Research that disaggregates these pan-ethnic groups, focuses on older people, and examines regional variations is lacking. For CRC, the R/E differences in incidence are much smaller than in mortality, more closely approximating the breast cancer situation. For lung and prostate cancers, survival after diagnosis is consistently lower for AAs, Hispanics and other groups than for whites but the differences are less dramatic than in the case of CRC. Across each of the cancers, cancer stage and other clinical features at the time of diagnosis are important determinants of outcomes, and R/E differences in survival are at least partially explained by differences in stage at diagnosis. There is little evidence for R/E differences in the underlying disease process that accounts for later stage at diagnosis for CRC and lung cancers and differences in stage at diagnosis seem to represent less access to appropriate screening. For prostate cancer, the greater frequency and more advanced stage at diagnosis observed for AA men may still indicate some R/E differences in the etiology and natural history of this condition. It seems that whites have better access to informed consent initiatives around prostate cancer screening, are screened at higher rates, and receive more aggressive treatment.

Our findings on cancer detection and R/E disparities in these three cancers also contrasted with findings for breast and cervical cancer. For all three of these cancers, there is considerable ongoing debate surrounding the efficacy and cost-effectiveness of screening. For CRC, the debate focuses on choice among several tests and their timing, while for prostate cancer the focus is on the advisability of screening particularly in older men. Attention has now turned to increasing informed consent around testing. In the case of lung cancer, attention is now focused on the potential cost-effectiveness of new imaging techniques for general or targeted screening. For CRC and prostate cancer, there is clear evidence for lower than desirable screening rates among all elders and disproportionately lower rates for African Americans and other traditionally underserved groups. Further, the debate around CRC screening remains important because of the potential to remove pre-cancerous lesions identified through colonoscopy. As in the case of breast cancer, obtaining a definitive diagnosis requires a multiple step process for each of these cancers that may involve visits to multiple practitioners over time. Also paralleling the breast cancer findings, African Americans are at higher risk for not receiving a definitive and complete diagnostic work-up for both CRC and prostate cancer. There is insufficient data on R/E groups other than whites and African Americans about screening participation for all three of these cancers.

For both CRC and prostate cancer there is evidence from a small number of studies that various cultural tailoring and care coordination strategies can be effective in improving screening participation for elders of color. The paucity of these studies underscores the need for new thinking and research on engaging traditionally underserved elders in a broad range of cancer screening and diagnostic services. The community health worker interventions that we found to be effective in increasing breast and cervical cancer screening participation have not been broadly adapted to reaching out to men, nor has there been the development through qualitative studies of a sufficient understanding of individual and cultural influences on best approaches for communicating practitioner recommendations for screening.

Our findings highlight treatment consensus for these cancers with the exception of SCLC and prostate care. While some combination of primary and adjuvant treatments of prostate cancer appears helpful for many men, there are troublesome side effects that reduce quality of life and small improvements in survival with treatment. Similarly, for small-cell lung cancer, many patients are referred to ongoing clinical trials as the search continues for efficacious treatment strategies. Having noted these debates and areas for continued technological improvements, much more striking is the observation that across all three cancers, recommended treatment regimens require multiple interventions over an extended time frame and careful monitoring for disease recurrence. This aspect of cancer care provides enormous opportunities for practitioner and health system failures in managing patient adherence to complicated regimens and noteworthy challenges in ensuring continuity of treatment particularly for elders with lower socioeconomic status or other barriers to care. We found almost no evidence outside of breast cancer navigation studies for systematic attention to ensuring that traditionally underserved patients succeed in making their ways through these systems.

We found that there are consistent patterns of less than complete treatment for African Americans across all three cancers. In the case of lung cancer, some studies may suggest that co-morbid conditions and other clinical features explain differences in treatment by R/E, but even here, it appears that differences in access to complete treatment is an important factor in racial differences in survival after controlling for co-morbid conditions. For CRC and prostate cancer, available studies appear to indicate that clinical factors do not account for R/E differences in treatment, although a number of non-clinical factors such as co-insurance and residential location account for some of the R/E differences in treatment.

These findings extend our observations based on the review of evidence for breast and cervical cancer in documenting clear patterns of R/E disparity in cancer-related survival that are not explained by prevalence or available technology. In particular, for CRC, lung, and prostate cancer, African Americans have lower survival relative to whites independent of differences in disease prevalence. Further, African Americans and whites typically have similar outcomes for all three cancers when they are participants in clinical trials or in other equal-disease/equal-care settings. These findings suggest that R/E differences in access to appropriately coordinated and culturally tailored primary care (for screening) and tertiary care (for definitive diagnosis, treatment, aftercare) are causal factors in disparate health outcomes. There are important questions about the nature and causes of unequal care in this context that need to be addressed, such as the patient, practitioner, and care system factors that can be harnessed to ensure greater adherence to screening recommendations or the determinants of less than recommended cancer treatments among Medicare patients.

Evidence supports the conclusion that interventions aimed at both reducing R/E disparities in cancer detection and R/E disparities in cancer treatment have the potential to influence overall differences in outcomes. Improving screening participation and adherence for R/E elders are clearly worthwhile goals in light of these findings. Unlike prior efforts that have focused primarily on breast and cervical cancer, new demonstrations might focus on programming that specifically targets screening adherence across the range of cancer sites. Because of the importance of co-morbid health conditions in cancer treatment and outcomes, such a model could also be extended to adherence to other recommended and Medicare-reimbursed screening and preventive services. A major challenge, in light of existing research gaps, is how best to develop screening adherence programming that engages men and that is responsive to cultural and health service access variations across the full range of racial/ethnic groups. For cancers without accepted screening mechanisms, however, it appears that addressing the stage at diagnosis differences requires ensuring medical care use and attention on the part of both patients and practitioners to health risk management.

Finally we found evidence that underscores the need for interventions to ensure timely completion of all recommended components of cancer diagnosis and primary and adjuvant treatments. These findings indicate that there is a significant potential to improve cancer survivorship by ensuring that patients and practitioners work together to complete the process. A treatment management intervention that draws upon a community health worker serving as a patient navigator holds the potential to increase the share of elders of color who receive the current standard of care. Although demonstrations and evaluations of cancer treatment management services were not identified in the literature, this review highlights treatment management as a potential area for important and cost-effective reductions in cancer care disparities.

References

Abdalla, I., Ray, P., Ray, V. et al. (1998). Comparison of serum prostate-specific antigen levels and PSA density in African-American, White and Hispanic men without prostate cancer. *Urology*, 51(2): 300-305.

Aberle, D., Gamsu, G., Henschke, C. et al. (2001). A consensus statement of the Society of Thoracic Radiology: Screening for lung cancer with helical computed tomography. *Journal of thoracic imaging*, 16(1): 65-68.

ACS – American Cancer Society. (2002b). *Cancer Facts and Figures for Hispanics: 2000-2001*. Atlanta, GA: ACS.

ACS – American Cancer Society. (2003). *Cancer Facts and Figures: 2003*. Atlanta, A: ACS. http://www.cancer.org/downloads/STT/CAFF2003PWSecured.pdf.

Alexander, G. and Brawley, O. (1998). Prostate cancer treatment outcome in blacks and whites: a summary of the literature. *Seminars in Urologic Oncology*, 16(4): 232-234.

Alexander, F. (2000). Prostate cancer screening. *Microscopic Research Technology*, 51(5): 419-422.

American College of Physicians. (1997). Screening for prostate cancer. *The Annals of Internal Medicine*, 126(6): 480-484.

American College of Preventive Medicine. (1998). Screening for prostate cancer in American men. *American Journal of Preventive Medicine*, 15(1): 81-84.

American Urological Association. (1999). *Prostate-Specific Antigen (PSA) Best Practice Policy*. Baltimore (MD): American Urological Association, Inc.

Bach, P., Cramer, L., Warren, J. et al. (1999). Racial differences in the treatment of early-stage lung cancer. The *New England Journal of Medicine*, 341(16): 1198-1205.

Bach, P., Schrag, D., Brawley, O. et al. (2002). Survival of blacks and whites after a cancer diagnosis. The *Journal of the American Medical Association*, 287(16): 2106-2113.

Barber, K., Shaw, R., Folts, M. et al. (1998). Differences between African American and Caucasian men participating in a community-based prostate cancer screening program. *Journal of Community Health*, 23(6): 441-451.

Barry, M. (2002). Fecal occult blood testing for colorectal cancer: a perspective. *The Annals of Oncology*, 13(1): 61-64.

Beeker, C., Kraft, J., Southwell, B. et al. (2000). Colorectal cancer screening in older men and women: Qualitative research findings and implications for intervention. *Journal of Community Health*, 25(3): 263-278.

Bianco, F., Wood, D., Grignon, D. et al. (2002). 'Prostate cancer stage shift has eliminated the gap in disease-free survival in black and white American men after radical prostectomy.' *Journal of Urology*, 168(2): 479-482.

Blackstock, A., Herndon, J., Paskett, E. et al. (2002). Outcomes among African-American/Non-African-American patients with advanced non-small-cell lung carcinoma: Report from the cancer and leukemia Group B. *Journal of the National Cancer Institute*, 94: 284-290.

Bleed, D., Risser, D., Sperry, S. et al. (1992). Cancer incidence and survival among American Indians registered for Indian health service care in Montana, 1982-1981 *Journal of the National Cancer Institute*, 84: 1500-1505.

Borum, M.L. (1999). Colorectal cancer surveillance in African-American and white patients at an urban university medical center. *Journal of the National Medical Association*, 91(9): 505-508.

Bradley, C., Given, C. and Roberts, C. (2000). Disparities in cancer diagnosis and survival. *Cancer*, 91(1): 178-188.

Brawer, M. (2000). Screening for prostate cancer. *Seminars in Surgical Oncology*, 18(1): 29-36.

Brawley, O. (2002). Disaggregating the effects of race and poverty on breast cancer outcomes. *Journal of the National Cancer Institute*, 94(7): 471-473.

Breen, N., Wagener, D., Brown, M. et al. (2001) Progress in cancer screening over a decade: Results of cancer screening from the 1987, 1992, and 1998 National Health Interview Surveys. *Journal of the National Cancer Institute*, 93(23): 1704-1713.

Campbell, J. and Hudson, M. (2002) Perceived barriers and benefits to colon cancer screening among African Americans in North Carolina: how does perception relate to screening behavior? *Cancer, Epidemiology, Biomarkers, and Prevention*, 11(6): 529-534.

Canadas, B., Cusan, L., Gomez, J. et al. (2000). Evaluation of prostatic specific antigen and digital rectal examination as screening tests for prostate cancer. *Prostate*, 45(1): 19-35.

Cargill, V., Conti, M., Neuhauser, D. et al. (1991). Improving the effectiveness of screening for colorectal cancer by involving nurse clinicians. *Medical Care*, 29(1): 1-5.

Carter, H. (2001). Rationale for earlier and less frequent prostate cancer screening. *Urology*, 58(5): 639-641.

Catalona, W., Richie, J., Ahmann, F. et al. (1994). Comparison of digital rectal examination and serum prostate specific antigen in early Detection of Prostate Cancer: Results of Multicenter Clinical Trial of 6,630 Men. *The Journal of Urology*, 151(5): 1283.

Catalona, W., Partin, A., Slawin, K. et al. (2000). Percentage of free PSA in black versus white men for detection and staging of prostate cancer: A prospective multi-center clinical trial. *Urology*, 55(3): 372-376.

Chan, E. (2001). Promoting informed decision making about prostate cancer screening. *Comprehensive Therapy*, 27(3): 195-201.

Chen, V., Fenoglio-Preiser, C., Xu, X. et al. (1997). Aggressiveness of colon carcinoma in blacks and whites. National Cancer Institute Black. White Cancer Survival Study Grou *Cancer Epidemiology, Biomarkers, and Prevention*. 6(12): 1087-1093.

Chu, K. Tarone, R. and Freeman, H. (2003). Trends in prostate cancer mortality among black men and white men in the United States. *Cancer*, 97(6): 1507-1516.

Ciatto, J. (2000). Screening for prostate cancer by PSA determination: A time for caution. *International Journal of Biological Markers*, 15(4): 285-287.

Clegg, L., Li, F., Hankey, B. et al. (2002). Cancer survival among US whites and minorities: A SEER (Surveillance, Epidemiology, and End Results) Program population-based study. *Archives of Internal Medicine*, 162(17): 1985-1993.

Coleman, R. (2002). Value of FDG-PET scanning in management of lung cancer. *Lancet*, 359(9315): 1361-1362.

Coley, C., Barry, M., Fleming, C. et al. (1997). Early detection of prostate cancer. *Annals of Internal Medicine*, 126(6), 394-406.

Cooper, G., Yuan, Z., Landefeld, C. et al. (1996). Surgery for colorectal cancer: Race-related differences in rates and survival among Medicare beneficiaries. American journal of public health, 86(4): 582-586.

Coronado, G. and Thompson, B. (2000). Rural Mexican American men's attitudes and beliefs about cancer screening. *Journal of Cancer Education*, 15(1): 41-45.

Crawford, E. (1997). Prostate cancer awareness week: September, 22-28, 1997. *Cancer*, 47(5): 288-296.

Crespi, M. and Lisi, D. (2002). Is colorectal cancer screening by fecal occult blood feasible? *The Annals of Oncology*, 13(1): 47-50.

Cross, C., Shultz, D., Malkowicz, S. et al. (2002). Impact of race on prostate-specific antigen outcome after radical prostatectomy for clinically localized adenocarcinoma of the prostate. *Journal of Clinical Oncology*, 20(12): 2863-2868.

Dale, W., Vijayakumar, S., Lawlor, E. et al. (1996). Prostate cancer, race, and socioeconomic status: inadequate adjustment for social factors in assessing racial differences, *The Prostate*, 29(5): 271-281.

DeAntoni, E. (1997). Eight years of 'Prostate Cancer Awareness Week': Lessons in screening and early detection. *Cancer*, 80(9): 1845-1851.

Dignam, J., Colangelo, L., Smith, R. et al. (2003). Prognosis after rectal cancer in blacks and whites participating in adjuvant therapy randomized trials. *Journal of Clinical Oncology*, 21(3): 13-420.

Earle, C., Venditti, L., Neumann, P. et al. (2000). Who gets chemotherapy for metastatic lung cancer? *Chest*, 117(5): 1239-1246.

Etzioni, R., Legler, J., Feuer, E. et al. (1999). Cancer surveillance series: interpreting trends in prostate cancer – part III: Quantifying the link between population prostate-specific antigen testing and recent declines in prostate cancer mortality. *Journal of the National Cancer Institute*, 91(12): 1033-1039.

Etzioni, R., Berry, K., Legler, J. et al. (2002). Prostate-specific antigen testing in black and white men: An analysis of medicare claim form 1991-1998. *Urology*, 59(2): 251-255.

Fang, J., Metter, E., Landis, P. et al. (2001). Low levels of prostate-specific antigen predict long-term risk of prostate cancer: results from the Baltimore Longitudinal Study of Aging. *Urology*, 58(3), 411-416.

Federman, D., Goyal, S., Kamina, A. et al. (1999). Informaed consent for PSA screening: Does it happen? *Effective clinical practice*, 2(4): 152-157.

Finlay, G., Rodrigues, J., Griffith, C. et al. (2002). Advanced presentation of lung cancer in Asian immigrants – a case-control study. *Chest*, 122(6): 1938-1943.

Flood, A., Wennberg, J., Nease, Jr., R. et al. (1996). The importance of patient preference in the decision to screen for prostate cancer. *Journal of General Internal Medicine*, 11(6): 342-349.

Freeman, J., Klabundne, C., Schussler, N. et al. (2002). Measuring breast, colorectal, and prostate cancer screening with Medicare claims data. *Medical Care*, 40(8): Suppl. IV 36-42.

Freedland, S., Sutter, M., Naitoh, J. et al. (2000). Clinical characteristics in black and white men with prostate cancer in an equal access medical center. *Urology*, 55(3): 387-390.

Gadgeel, S., Severson, R., Kau, Y. et al. (2001). Impact of race in lung cancer: analysis of temporal trends from a surveillance, epidemiology, and end results database. *Chest*, 120(1): 55-63.

Godley, P., Schenck, A., Amamoo, M. et al. (2003). Racial differences in mortality among Medicare recipients after treatment for localized prostate cancer. *Journal of the National Cancer Institute*, 95(22): 1702-1710.

Graham, M., Geitz, L., Byhardt, R. et al. (1992). Comparison of prognostic factors and survival among black patients and white patient treated with irradiation for non-small cell lung cancer. *Journal of the National Cancer Institute*, 84: 1731-1735.

Grossfeld, G., Latini, D., Downs, T. et al. (2002). Is ethnicity an independent predictor of prostate cancer recurrence after radical prostatectomy? *Journal of Urology*, 168(6): 2510-2515.

Hall, H., Satariano, W., Thompson, T. et al. (2002). Initial treatment for prostate carcinoma in relation to comorbidity and symptoms. *Cancer*, 95(11): 2308-2315

Harlan, L., Brawley, O., Pommerenke, F. et al. (1995). Geographic, age, and racial variation in the treatment of local/regional carcinoma of the prostate. *Journal of Clinical Oncology*, 13(1): 93-100.

Harlan, L., Potosky, A., Gilliland, F. et al. (2001). Factors associated with initial therapy for clinically localized prostate cancer: Prostate cancer outcomes study. *Journal of the National Cancer Institute*, 93(24): 1864-1871.

Henschke, C., McCauley, D., Yankelevitz, D. et al. (1999). Early lung cancer action project: overall design and findings from baseline screening. *Lancet*, 354(9173): 99-105.

Hoffman, R., Harlan, L., Klabunde, C. et al. (2003). Racial differences in initial treatment for clinically localized prostate cancer: Results from the prostate cancer outcomes study. *Journal of General Internal Medicine*, 18(10): 845-853.

Hoffman-Goetz, L., Breen, N. and Meissner, H. (1998). The impact of social class on the use of cancer screening within three racial/ethnic groups in the United States. *Ethnicity and Disease*, 8(1): 43-51.

Holmes-Rovner, M., Williams, G., Hoppough, S. et al. (2002) Colorectal cancer screening barriers in persons with low income. *Cancer Practice*, 10(5): 240-247.

Imperiale, T., Wagner, D., Lin, C. et al. (2000). Risk of advanced proximal neoplasms in asymptomatic adults according to the distal colorectal findings. *New England Journal of Medicine*, 343(3): 169-174.

Inger, D. (1999). Colorectal cancer screening. *Primary Care*, 26(1): 179-187.

Ioannou, G., Chapko, M. and Dominitz, J. (2003). Predictors of colorectal cancer screening participation in the United States. *American Journal of Gastroenterology*, 98(9): 2082-2091.

James, A., Campbell, M. and Hudson, M. (2002). Perceived barriers and benefits to colon cancer screening among African Americans in North Carolina: how does perception relate to screening behavior? *Cancer epidemiology biomarkers and prevention*, 11(6): 529-534.

Janz, N., Wren, P., Schottenfeld, D. et al. (2003). Colorectal cancer screening attitudes and behavior: A population-based study. *Preventive Medicine*, 37(6): 627-634.

Jemal, A., Thomas, A., Murray, T. et al. (2002). Cancer Statistics, 2002. *Cancer*, 52(1): 23-48.

Juon, H., Han, W., Shin, H. et al. (2003). Predictors of older Korean American's participation in colorectal cancer screening. *Journal of Cancer Education*, 18(1): 37-42.

Koff, S., Connelly, R., Bauer, J. et al. (2002). Primary hormonal therapy for prostate cancer: Experience with 135 consecutive PSA-ERA patients from a tertiary care military medical center. *Prostate Cancer and Prostatic Diseases*, 5(2): 152-158.

Kupelian, P., Buchsbaum, J., Elshaikh, M. et al. (2002). Factors affecting recurrence rates after prostatectomy or radiotherapy in localized prostate carcinoma patients with biopsy Gleason score 8 or above. *Cancer*. 95(11): 2302-2307.

Kupelian, P., Elshaikh, M., Reddy, C. et al. (2002b). Comparison of the efficacy of local therapies for localized prostate cancer in the prostate-specific antigen era: A large single-institution experience with radical prostatectomy and external-beam radiotherapy. *Journal of Clinical Oncology*, 20(16): 3376-3385.

Kupelian, P., Reddy, C., Carlson, T. et al. (2002c). Preliminary observations on biochemical relapse-free survival rates after short-course intensity-modulated radiotherapy (70 Gy at 2.5 Gy/fraction) for localized prostate cancer. *International Journal of Radiation Oncology, Biology, and Physics*. 53(4): 904-912.

Labrie, F., Candas, B., Cusan, L. et al. (1996). Diagnosis of advanced or non-curable prostate cancer can be practically eliminated by prostate-specific antigen. *Urology*, 47(2): 212-217.

Lee, L., Barnswell, C., Torre, T. et al. (2002). Prognostic significance of race on biochemical control in patients with localized prostate cancer treated with permanent brachytherapy: multivariate and matched-pair analyses. *International Journal of Radiation Oncology, Biology, and Physics*, 53(2): 282-289.

Lee-Feldstein, A., Feldstein, P. and Buchmueller, T. (2002). Health care factors related to stage at diagnosis and survival among Medicare patients with colorectal center. *Medical Care*, 40(5): 362-374.

Legler, J., Feuer, E., Potosky, A. et al. (1998). The role of prostate-specific antigen (PSA) testing patterns in the recent prostate cancer incidence decline in the United States. *Cancer Causes and Control*, 9(5): 519-527.

Lieberman, D., Weiss, D., Bond, J. et al. (2000). Use of colonoscopy to screen asymptomatic adults for colorectal cancer. Veterans Affairs Cooperative Study Group 380. *New England Journal of Medicine*, 343(3): 162-168.

Lowenfels, A. (2002). Fecal occult blood testing as a screening procedure for colorectal cancer. *The Annals of Oncology*, 13(1): 40-43.

Lurie, J. and Welch, H. (1999). Diagnostic testing following fecal occult blood screening in the elderly. *Journal of the National Cancer Institute*, 91(19): 1641-1646.

Lu-Yao, G. and Yao, S. (1997). Population-based study of long-term survival in patients with clinically localized prostate cancer. *The Lancet*, 349(9056): 906-910.

Maattanen, L., Auvinen, A., Stenman, U. et al. (1999). European randomized study of prostate cancer screening: First-year results of the Finnish trial. *The British Journal of Cancer*, 79(7): 1210-1214.

Man, A., Pickles, T. and Chi, K. (2003). Asian race and impact on outcomes after radical radiotherapy for localized prostate cancer. *Journal of Urology*, 170(3): 901-904.

Mandel, J., Church, T., Ederer, F. et al. (1999). Colorectal cancer mortality: effectiveness of biennial screening for fecal occult blood. *Journal of the National Cancer Institute*, 91(5): 434-437.

Mandelblatt, J., Andrews, H., Kao, R. et al. (1996). The late-stage diagnosis of colorectal cancer: demographic and socioeconomic factors. *American Journal of Public Health*, 86(12): 1794-1797. *Journal of Gerontology*.

Manfredi, C., Czaja, R., Freels, S. et al. (1998). Prescribe for health. Improving cancer screening in physician practices serving low-income and minority populations. *Archives of Family Medicine*, 7(4): 329-337.

Mayberry, R., Coates, R., Hill, H. et al. (1995). Determinants of black/white differences in colon cancer survival. *Journal of the National Cancer Institute*, 87(22): 1686-1693.

Maxwell, A., Bastani, R. and Warda, U. (2000). Demographic predictors of cancer screening among Filipino and Korean immigrants in the United States. *Women Health*, 27(3): 89-107.

McCann, J. (1998). PET scans approved for detecting metastic non-small-cell lung cancer. *Journal of the National Cancer Institute*, 90: 94-96.

Merrill, R. and Brawley, O. (1997). Prostate cancer incidence and mortality rates among white and black men. *Epidemiology*, 8(2): 126-131.

Merrill, R., Capocaccia, R., Feuer, E. et al. (2000). Cancer prevalence estimates based on tumor registry data in the Surveillance, Epidemiology, and End Results (SEER) Program. *International Journal of Epidemiology*, 29(2): 197-207.

Mettlin, C., Lee, F., Drago, J. et al. (1991). The American Cancer Society National Prostate Cancer Detection Project: Findings on the detection of early prostate cancer in 2425 men. *Cancer*, 67(12): 2949-2958.

Miller, B., Kolonel, L., Bernstein, L. Jr., J. et al. and Eds. (1996). *Racial/Ethnic Patterns of Cancer in the United States 1988-1992*. (Vol. NIH Pub. No. 96-4104). Bethesda, MD: National Cancer Institute.

Miller, D. and Edwards, B. (1998). Cancer incidence and mortality 1973-1995: A report card for the U.S. *Cancer*, 82(6): 1197-1207.

Miller, S., Diefenbach, M., Kruus, L. et al. (2001). Psychological and screening profiles of first-degree relatives of prostate cancer patients. *Journal of Behavioral Medicine*, 24(3): 247-258.

Moffat, L. (2000). Screening for early prostate cancer: What is the problem? *Journal of the Royal College of Surgeons of Edinburgh*, 45(2): 127-131.

Montironi, R., Mazzucchelli, R., Marshall, J. et al. (1999). Prostate cancer prevention: review of target populations, pathological biomarkers, and chemopreventive agents. *Journal of Clinical Pathology*, 52(11): 793-803.

Moul, J., Sesterhenn, I., Douglas, T. et al. (1995). Prostate-specific antigen values at the time of prostate cancer diagnosis in African-American men. *Journal of the American Medical Association*, 274(16): 1277-1281.

Myers, R., Chodak, G., Wolf, T. et al. (1999). Adherence by African American men to prostate cancer education and early detection. *Cancer*, 86(1): 88-104.

Neugut, A., Fleischauer, A., Sundararajan, V. et al. (2002). Use of adjuvant chemotherapy and radiation therapy for rectal cancer among the elderly: A population-based study. *Journal of Clinical Oncology*, 20(11): 2643-2650.

Ornstein, S., Garr, D., Jenkins, R. et al. (1991). Computer-generated physician and patient reminders. Tools to improve population adherence to selected preventive services. *Journal of Family Practice*, 32(1): 82-90.

Paskett, E., Rushing, J., D'Agostino, R. et al. (1997). Cancer screening behaviors of low-income women: the impact of race. *Women's Health*, 3(3-4): 203-226.

Perez, N. and Tsou, H. (1995). Prostate cancer screening practices: Differences between clinic and private patients. *The Mount Sinai Journal of Medicine*, 62(4): 316-322.

Pesce, A. (2001). Selections from current literature. Colorectal cancer screening. *Family Practice*, 18(4): 457-460.

Peterson, D. and J. D'Ambrosio. (1992). Diagnosis and management of acute and chronic oral complications of nonsurgical cancer therapies. *Dental Clinics of North America*, 36(4): 945-966.

Polednak, A. (1998). Prostate cancer treatment in black and white men: The need to consider both stage at diagnosis and socioeconomics status. *Journal of the National Medical Association*, 90(2): 101-104.

Powe, B. (1995). Cancer fatalism among elderly Caucasians and African Americans. *Oncology Nurses Forum*, 22(9): 1355-1359.

Powe, B. (2002). Promoting fecal occult blood testing in rural African American women. *Cancer practice*, 10(3): 139-146.

Powe, B. and Weinrich, S. (1999). An intervention to decrease cancer fatalism among rural elders. *Oncology Nursing Forum*, 26(3): 583-588.

Powell, I., Gelfand, D., Parzuchowski, J. et al. (1995). A successful recruitment process of African American men for early detection of prostate cancer. *Cancer*, 75(7): 1880-1885.

Powell, I., Heilbrun, L., Littrup, P. et al. (1997). Outcome of African American men screened for prostate cancer: Detroit Education and Early Detection Study. *The Journal of Urology*, 158(1): 146-149.

Powell, I.J. and Meyskens, F. (2001). African American men and hereditary/familial prostate cancer: Intermediate-risk populations for chemoprevention trials. *Urology*, 57(4): 178-181.

Powell, I., Dey, J., Dudley, A. et al. (2002). Disease-free survival difference between African Americans and whites after radical prostatectomy for local prostate cancer: A multivariable analysis. *Urology*, 59(6): 907-912.

Ray, M., Dunn, R., Cooney, K. et al. (2003). Family history of prostate cancer and relapse after definitive external beam radiation therapy. *International Journal of Radiation, Oncology, Biology, and Physics*, 57(2): 371-376.

Richards, R. and Reker, D. (2002). Racial differences in use of colonoscopy, sigmoid-oscopy, and barium enema in Medicare beneficiaries. *Digestive Diseases and Sciences*, 47(12): 2715-2719.

Ries, L., Eisner, M., Kosary, C. et al. (eds). (2003). *SEER Cancer Statistics Review, 1975-2000*, National Cancer Institute. Bethesda, MD, http://seer.cancer.gov/csr/1975_2000, 2003.

Roach, M., Lu, J., Pilepich, M. et al. (2003). Race and survival of men treated for prostate cancer on radiation therapy oncology group phase III randomized trials. *Journal of Urology*, 169(1): 245-250.

Robbins, A., Whittemore, A. and Thom, D. (2000). Differences in socioeconomic status and survival among white and black men with prostate cancer. *American Journal of Epidemiology*, 151(4): 409-416.

Roehl, K., Antenor, J. and Catalona, W. (2002). Serial biopsy results in prostate cancer screening study. *Journal of Urology*, 167(6): 2435-2439.

Sandler R., Halabi, S., Baron, J. et al. (2003). A randomized trial of aspirin to prevent colorectal adenomas in patients with previous colorectal cancer. *The New England Journal of Medicine*, 348(10): 883-890.

Schapira, M and VanRuiswyk, J. (2000). The effect of an illustrated pamphlet decision-aid on the use of prostate cancer screening tests. *The Journal of Family Practice*, 49(5): 418-424.

Shavers, V. and Brown, M. (2002). Racial and ethnic disparities in the receipt of cancer treatment. *Journal of the National Cancer Institute*, 94(5): 334-357.

Shekarriz, B., Tiguert, R., Upadhyay, J. et al. (2000). Impact of location and multifocality of positive surgical margins on disease-free survival following radical prostectomy: A comparison between African-American and white men. *Urology*, 55(6): 899-903.

Shekelle, P., Stone, E., Mangolione, M. et al. (2001). Healthy aging initiatives evidence reports: Interventions that increase the utilization of Medicare-Funded preventive services for persons age 65 and older. HCFA. Available: http://www.hcfa.gov/healthy aging/2a.html.

Smith, R., Mettlin, C., Davis, K. et al. (2000). Articles – American Cancer Society guidelines for the early detection of cancer. *Cancer*, 50(1): 34-49.

Smith, R., von Eschenbach, A., Wender, R. et al. (2001). American Cancer Society guidelines for the early detection of cancer: Update of early detection guidelines for prostate, colorectal, and endometrial cancers. Also: Update 2001 – testing for early lung cancer detection. *Cancer Journal for Clinicians*, 51(1), 38-75: Quiz 77-80.

Smith, R., Cokkinides, V., von Eschenbach, A. et al. (2002). American Cancer Society guidelines for the early detection of cancer. *Cancer Journal for Clinicians*, 52(1): 8-22.

Stewart, J. (2001). Lung carcinoma in African Americans. *Cancer*, 91(12): 2476-2482.

Stone, E., Morton, S., Hulscher, M. et al. (2002). Interventions that increase use of adult immunization and cancer screening services: A meta-analysis. *Annals of Internal Medicine*, 136(9): 641-651.

Strauss, G. (2002). The Mayo lung cohort: A regression analysis focusing on lung cancer incidence and mortality. *Journal of Clinical Oncology*, 20(8): 1973-1983.

Swan, J., Breen, N., Coates, R. et al. (2003). Progress in cancer screening practices in the United States: Results from the 2000 National Health Interview Survey. *Cancer*, 97(6): 1528-1540.

Taylor, V., Lessler, D., Mertens, K. et al. (2003). Colorectal cancer screening among African Americans: The importance of physician recommendation. *Journal of the National Medical Association*, 95(9): 806-812.

U.S. Preventive Services Task Force. (1996). Screening for prostate cancer. *Guide to clinical preventive services: Report of the U.S. Preventive Services Task Force*. (119-134). Baltimore, MD: Williams and Wilkins, Edition: 2nd ed.

Vijan, S., Hwang, E.W., Hofer, T. et al. (2001). Which colon cancer screening test? A comparison of costs, effectiveness, and compliance. *American Journal of Medicine*, 111(8): 593-601.

Volk, R. Cass, A. and Spann, S. (1999). A randomized controlled trial of shared decision making for prostate cancer screening. *Archives of Family Medicine*, 8(4): 333-340.

Weinrich, S., Weinrich, M., Boyd, M. et al. (1994). Teaching older adults by adapting for aging changes. *Cancer Nurses*, 17(6): 494-500.

Weinrich, S., Holdford, D., Boyd, M. et al. (1998). Prostate cancer education in African American churches. *Public Health Nursing*, 15(3): 188-195.

Weir, H., Thun, M., Hankey, B. et al. (2003). Annual report to the nation on the status of cancer 1975-2000, featuring the issues of surveillance data for cancer prevention and control. *Journal of the National Cancer Institute*, 95(17): 1276-1299.

Wilson, J. and Junger, G. (1968). *Principles and practice of screening*. Geneva: WHO.

Wingo, P.A., Ries, L.A.G., Parker, S.L. et al. (1998). Long term cancer patient survival in the United States. *Cancer Epidemiology, Biomarkers, and Prevention*, 7: 271-282.

Wolf, A., Nasser, J., Wolf, A. et al. (1996). The impact of informed consent on patient interest in prostate-specific antigen screening. *Archives of Internal Medicine*, 156(12): 1333-1336.

Wolf, A., Philbrick, J. and Schorling, J. (1997). Predictors of interest in prostate-specific antigen screening and the impact of informed consent: What should-we tell our patients? *The American Journal of Medicine*, 103(4): 308-314.

Wolf, A. and Schorling, J. (1998). Preferences of elderly men for prostate-specific antigen screening and the impact of informed consent. *The Journals of Gerontology*, 53(3), M 195-200.

Chapter 8

Emerging Interventions to Reduce Racial/Ethnic Disparities in Cancer

Introduction

The reviews of published reports on racial/ethnic disparities in cancer, their causes, and potential solutions in the preceding chapters have demonstrated the depth and breadth of literature in this area. Important gaps in available reports were also shown. More information is needed on cancer prevalence, treatment, and outcome for the full range of underserved populations and cancer types. More information is also needed on the practitioner, service setting and delivery system factors that may cause disparities along each of these dimensions. Most notably, the reviews suggested lacunae in knowledge of successful methods for engaging racial/ethnic (R/E) minority populations in programs with the potential to reduce cancer prevention, care, and outcome disparities. These gaps may reflect a period when many efforts to reduce R/E cancer and health disparities are ongoing and not yet included in the scientific literature. At the same time, the traditional model of translation of evidence-based interventions into broad-scale practice remains powerful and thus there has been insufficient attention to organizational and contextual determinants of health services delivery change (Glasgow et al, 2003).

We sought to learn more about emerging strategies for addressing R/E cancer disparities and the lessons for program design that derive from implementation experiences. Case studies were completed on programs that modeled cancer care disparity elimination strategies that had either received inadequate descriptive attention in the published literature or had not yet produced broadly available reports. Since the universe of potential sites was not established, we first sought to identify programs that (1) have a high probability of reducing cancer risk factors, increasing appropriate use of Medicare services, and improving health-related outcomes for R/E groups or (2) could offer insights into the design and operations of such programs. We sought program sites for case studies that could showcase variations in interventions and contexts. The case studies had three related goals:

- Describe the emerging programs' perspectives about the causes of – and solutions for- R/E disparities in cancer prevention, treatment, and outcomes;
- Describe emerging programs' goals, operations, and outcomes within the constraints of available data; and

- Understand the programs' implementation learning about key intervention components, such as cultural tailoring, engagement strategies, and use of community health workers.

After describing the methods used in developing the case studies, we present site characteristics, analyses of the causes of cancer care and outcome disparities and approaches to addressing them. Attention then turns to what case study programs learned during implementation about cultural tailoring, engaging participants, and community health workers.

Methods

In order to identify emerging models for inclusion in case studies, we first identified an inclusive set of programs, organizations, and contacts with potential relevance to our study. We excluded programs from the case study sample universe if they had been the subjects of comprehensive published reports. We wished to develop a national sample of initiatives from which to draw case study sites that varied with respect to four basic features: community context; organizational context; population target; and primary prevention or cancer target. We conducted screening calls to categorize projects along these dimensions. Screening calls also assessed whether or not programs could provide information about their experiences with program effectiveness and achievements, program costs, and program sustainability. Based on these data, we selected 25 case study sites that appeared to offer models that could be incorporated in public policy and adopted in diverse settings while also reflecting the broad range of program contexts and targets.

Identification of sites   The process of identifying sites included: multiple nationwide out-reach initiatives, selective screening to eliminate sites that were no longer active or subjects of prior reports, and finally, targeted screening to ensure that our sample was both representative and inclusive. Multiple out-reach incorporated following up referrals generated by word-of-mouth, phone contacts, and other sources identified by the team. To ensure comprehensive networking at this stage, a list of organizations and contacts was generated and conference proceedings were screened for relevant contacts. This list included:

- Federal Agencies and Federally-Sponsored Programs, such as the Center for Disease Control's (CDC) Racial and Ethnic Approaches to Community Health (REACH 2010) and Breast and Cervical Cancer Prevention (BCCP) replication projects, Disparity and Quality Initiatives, and NCI ongoing cancer disparities studies.
- Health Payer/Delivery System Organizations, such as Blue Cross/Blue Shield, and the National Association of Community Health Centers, among others.

- R/E identity and professional organizations, such as the National Indian Council on Aging, National Hispanic Council on Aging, National Association for the Advancement of Colored People, and National Council of La Raza.
- Conference Proceedings Since 1997, including the American Public Health Association, Gerontological Society of America, Association of Health Services Research, cancer conferences, and health disparities conferences.
- Foundation Initiated Programs, like the Robert Wood Johnson Foundation's Last Acts Campaign, and the Access Program.
- Cancer Centers, such as the Moffitt Center in Tampa FL, Sloan-Kettering in New York, NY, and the Dana-Farber Cancer Institute in Boston, MA.

To solicit recommendations of potential sites, telephone calls, letters and e-mails were addressed to individuals and networks associated with each of these sources. Additional referral sources and projects were identified in the literature reviews. Participation in the Inter-Cultural Cancer Council meetings Feb 6-10, 2002 was another source of contacts. Additional federal government sources were identified in telephone conferences with disparities program leaders and experts within all relevant federal agencies. Over time, this open networking process resulted in recurring referrals, indicating out-reach saturation and the reduced potential of missed programs models.

Sample development and screening calls We sought a sample that reflected the heterogeneity of programs to address R/E disparities in cancer prevention and care (Blankerz, 1998). We wished to identify program models from which to select programs for case studies that were diverse with respect to targeted populations, cancer prevention and care targets, regional locations, organizational types, and intervention approaches. Even as we continued to conduct outreach efforts to identify potential examples of cancer prevention and cancer care disparities initiatives, we also conducted screening interviews by telephone and mail with prospective sites. Screening calls helped us classify sites with respect to these broad context and goal differences. As gaps were identified, we sought additional sources of input on potential sites to make sure our sample represented the heterogeneity of existing programs. We also made preliminary assessments of how potential sites might provide new learning: screening calls gathered addressed the innovation being explored, feasibility and replication potential as indicated by implementation experiences, and evidence of effectiveness from preliminary research and stakeholder reports. Eventually, 115 initiatives nationwide were screened. Although this sample probably over-represents initiatives aimed at R/E groups, cancer prevention and care targets, and contexts that have received less attention nationally, it does provide a strong sense of the variability in programs and does point to contexts, populations, and health issues where innovations might be directed.

A national sample of cancer prevention and care disparities initiatives Table 8.1 provides a description of the programs screened by type of cancer and R/E group. It demonstrates the broad range of efforts to improve cancer prevention and care for traditionally underserved groups. Approximately one-third of the programs targeted African Americans (AA) and about one-quarter targeted multiple R/E groups, typically in urban low-income communities. Slightly over one-fifth targeted Latinos, 10% American Indians/Alaska Natives, and 10% Asian American and/or NHOPI groups. The focus on AA populations may well reflect the pervasiveness and intensity of the healthcare disparities they face. When separated by type of cancer program, 64% (n=74) addressed breast and cervical cancer. These programs were evenly distributed between African American and Latina groups (27% for each group). Fewer programs addressed prostate, lung, and colorectal cancers, other types of cancer (pancreas, lung, oral etc.) or multiple cancer and primary prevention targets. These findings suggest that cancer prevention, colorectal cancer screening, and continuity of cancer care targets may have yet to receive programmatic attention that parallels demonstrated disparities.

Table 8.1 Screened programs by population group and cancer care target

Population Group	Total N=115	Breast and Cervical Cancer N=74	Prostate, Lung, Colorectal, N=24	Primary Prevention, N=10	Other Cancers/ Multiple N=7
African Americans	33%	27%	58%	40%	10%
Latino	21%	27%	11%	20%	10%
Asian American/NHOPI	10%	4%	0%	0%	10%
American Indian/Alaska Natives	10%	9%	11%	13%	30%
Multiple Groups	26%	33%	20%	27%	40%

Table 8.2 presents the distribution of screened programs by region and by the type of organization where the program was housed. One third of the programs were located in the Southeast or Texas and the remainder came about equally from other regions. Most of the programs were sponsored or located at community-based organizations (36%), community health centers and public health organizations, including state departments of health (30%) or in networks that combined hospitals and other providers with linkages to academic health programs (26%). Fewer programs were faith-based or private initiatives.

Table 8.2 Screened programs by regions and sponsoring organization

Organization Type	Total, N=115	Northeast/ Mid-Atlantic N=24	Southeast/ Texas N=38	Midwest/ Mid-South N=26	West N=27
Hospital Systems/ Academic Health Centers	26%	12	40%	18%	28%
Community Health Centers/Public Health Programs	30%	44%	20%	29%	33%
Faith based Organizations	5%	0%	4%	18%	0%
Community Coalitions/Advocacy Programs	36%	38%	36%	29%	39%
Private/Philanthropic Initiatives	3%	6%	0%	6%	0%

Selection of case study sites   The 25 sites selected for case studies reflected variability in R/E target population, cancer type or primary prevention addressed, cancer experience phase addressed (e.g. prevention, screening adherence, service management), organizational host, region and urban/rural status. In sharp contrast to the screening sample, many of the programs targeted elders. Several programs that did not target elders were visited because they offered unique possibilities to learn about cultural tailoring and/or primary prevention. In other respects, the case study sites parallel the variability in the screening sample.

Conducting and analyzing case studies   We met with the two-person case study teams before site visits to review screening forms, site documents (applications, marketing materials, interim reports), and areas of special interest in order to develop site-specific interview guides. In general, the interview guides addressed: program context, theory of intervention, and primary objectives; cultural tailoring and participant engagement; availability of data to assess impacts and costs; and assessment methods and preliminary findings on utilization, costs, and outcomes.

The case study teams generally spent 2 days with each project. While the exact set of respondents varied by site, most case studies included interviews with program developers, champions, and current leadership as well as program staff at all levels. We also tried to meet with fiscal and MIS managers, local sponsors and collaborators, and program evaluators. Case study teams prepared draft site reports using a standardized outline. When needed, we re-contacted sites to ask for additional information. We sent draft case studies to site leadership for review, discussed any feedback, and amended the case study as needed. Cross-case analyses used a grounded theory framework: concepts for describing site differences in overall objectives, intervention models, and major findings were developed and revised as individual case experiences were reconsidered with revised categories in an iterative process. The concept map Figure 8.1 emerged from this analysis.

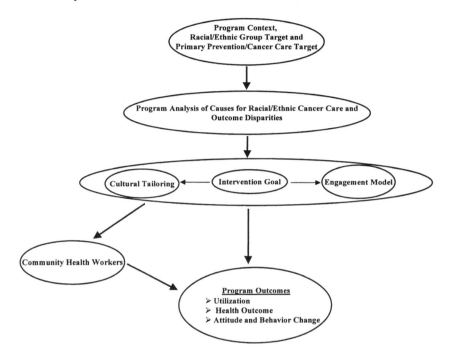

Figure 8.1 Case study concept map

As shown in Appendix 8.1: Summary of Case Study Site Characteristics, the sites targeted a variety of populations, with some interventions focusing on multiple underserved groups. Almost all sites targeted traditionally under-served R/E groups: 14 served AA communities, 11 Hispanic communities, 6 Asian communities, 2 Alaskan Native communities, and 2 Native American communities. Rural communities were targeted by 4 of the interventions, and 10 of the interventions dealt specifically with immigrant communities. As Figure 8.2 shows, case study sites came from across the country. Only 7 of the interventions exclusively targeted elders. The majority of the sites addressed breast and cervical cancer. One program each addressed prostate cancer and lung cancer. Nine interventions addressed multiple cancer types. Although all sites provided strong evidence for the need to improve patterns of prevention, screening, or treatment for the targeted conditions and population groups, internal resources for program development and availability of external funding appeared as the strongest factors in selection of these targets.

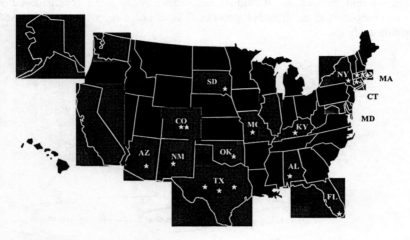

Figure 8.2 Case study site locations

Understandings of Racial/Ethnic Cancer Disparities

The programs that sought to address R/E and other socio-economic disparities in cancer reported learning a great deal about the nature and extent of barriers that prevent underserved communities from accessing and utilizing services. As displayed in Table 8.3, the programs consistently identified several barriers that their target populations faced. These perceptions offer a close parallel to factors highlighted by published research. Program staffs often used language that appeared to attribute barriers to use exclusively to the characteristics of persons in underserved groups. With more discussion, we learned that each of the barriers they identified needed to be understood as a product of both the system of care and group experiences with that system. Many shared the view that these challenges were more closely tied to R/E and social class oppression than cultural artifacts.

Culture and attitude Most programs perceived a disconnection between the target populations' cultural perspectives on cancer and health services and current health care practices. Many sites reported the R/E elders were unlikely because of past experiences of discrimination to challenge (primarily white, high-status, young) practitioners. Also, these elders were less likely to adhere to medical recommendations when providers appeared disrespectful of their worldviews. Grace Hill Centers' ASHES and MAP initiatives offered examples of such attitudinal differences, finding that some AA elders held a belief that cancer is a punishment for 'not believing enough.' In another example, the University of Colorado Native American Women's Wellness Through Awareness program pointed to the deficit of culturally relevant information that would incorporate and disarm some Native American cultural beliefs such as the view that screening invites the cancer spirit into the body. Both projects reported that practitioners were rarely respectful of these beliefs and missed opportunities to address feelings of shame, reflect on a moral obligation to protects one's own health, and reinforce the influence of external and behavioral risk factors in ways that engaged elders.

Table 8.3 Perceived barriers to care for elders of color

Perceived Barriers	Number of programs
Culture and attitudes	19
Poverty and social consequences	15
Lack of transportation/long distances	13
Language and translation services	12
Mistrust of medical system	12
Lack of insurance/inadequate insurance	11
Lack of knowledge about cancer	10
Practitioner attitudes	9
Intimidating system/bureaucracy	7

Poverty and its social consequences   Poverty, unemployment and associated problems constituted another barrier identified by many sites. Program staff reported that cancer education and screening were often viewed as expensive luxuries, not high on the list of priorities for elders and others struggling to meet daily needs. Following through on cancer detection and treatment or dealing with time-consuming medical recommendations may be particularly demanding for individuals facing intergenerational family responsibilities and other practical barriers to using care. For rural Appalachian elders in the Kentucky Homeplace and SKYCAP programs and rural Latino and immigrant elders in the University of Arizona's Juntos Contra el Cáncer, site extreme poverty for individuals and scarce community resources often compounded co-morbid physical and mental health conditions, complicated every aspect of accessing care, and contributed to low adherence to practitioner recommendations.

Lack of transportation Particularly in low-income communities, individuals in the target population often did not have cars or access to affordable transportation to get themselves to services. Huge distances between where people lived and health facilities that offered cancer screening or treatment services were emphasized by sites such as Seattle Indian Health Board's Breast and Cervical Cancer Health Program, and the Indian Health Service Community Health Representative Program in Alaska. Transportation barriers were also noted in urban areas where neither public transport nor neighborhood streets were seen as elder-friendly. Seattle's Senior Wellness program found that even though its programs were within walking distance of some participants' homes, elders were not keen on walking to the center fearing being shot or mugged.

Linguistic and cultural translation of materials Not being able to communicate with providers, read program materials and insurance documents, or understand educational sessions kept many in the R/E populations from getting effective care. The Asian American and Pacific Islander Tobacco Education Network (APITEN) offered striking evidence of this barrier. They found that only six programs in California – strikingly few given the size of Asian American and NHOPI populations in this huge state – tailor their smoking cessation programs to these groups, for example, by offering group programs or materials in relevant languages. Similarly, the American Cancer Society Heartland Division's Patient Navigator program found that printed discharge information was only available in English. Patients with limited English proficiency were often discharged with little knowledge of follow-up expectations.

Mistrust of medical system Deep-seated mistrust of the U.S. health care system ran rampant among the R/E communities served and posed a real obstacle to getting target populations to utilize services. Historical maltreatment of group members and personal experiences of healthcare discrimination were reported to site staffs. The Chicago REACH 2010 program as well as the Deep South Network for Cancer Control program found that for AAs, the Tuskegee syphilis experiments still loomed as a striking example of the medical system's institutional racism and potential for abuse. At the same time, the Latino groups targeted by Chicago REACH 2010 and the Clinica Tepeyac Reach and Teach program often mistrusted the medical system for other reasons. Many in these communities were undocumented immigrants or family members of undocumented immigrants, who worried that their 'illegal status' would be discovered and reported if they sought medical care. Many male recent immigrants in these sites also had little positive prior experience of healthcare and expected to be fleeced by providers. The Native American communities served by the Elder Voices, Inc. Public Benefits Counseling program often expressed a deep mistrust of government, vividly recalling a history of broken agreements, betrayals, and disruptive federal policies.

Lack of adequate insurance Among non-elders served by study sites, lack of any insurance was a notable barrier to care. Limited public financing of care for the uninsured was noted by the Chicago REACH 2010 because of their difficulties securing care for cancer treatment for uninsured persons. Yet even programs serving large proportions of elders, such the Planned Parenthood's Witness Project of Connecticut and some sites in the Baltimore City Cancer Plan noted the need to assist Medicare beneficiaries in finding sources of funding for medications, co-payments, or deductibles. Some of these programs also found that elders without Medicare supplements had been steered to safety net providers, even when these sites were over-subscribed and lacking resources (equipment, expertise) to manage cancer prevention and detection.

Lack of knowledge about cancer Since target communities had not been offered useful data on cancer in the past so many persons held misconceptions about cancer and cancer screening. For example, Connecticut Planned Parenthood's Witness Project reported the great difficulty convincing older AA women that they needed a Pap smear test because of the widely held belief that if one is no longer sexually active, then these tests are not needed. Few reported having ever discussed this belief with practitioners.

Practitioner attitudes Programs identified practitioner attitudes as another barrier to health service access and appropriate utilization. In 9 sites, program staff concluded that target community members had experienced institutional racism because health care providers did not offer cancer-related services at all or offered different (i.e. substandard) services or treatments. For example, the North General Hospital and BECH Patient Navigator programs found that practitioners often were more focused on technical expertise in performing a specific procedure than ensuring that patients completed all needed detection, diagnosis, treatment, and aftercare processes. In other cases, elders of color were found to receive treatments that were more invasive than necessary apparently because practitioners did not believe they would complete less invasive but more complex or extended regimens.

Intimidating and bureaucratic care systems The U.S. health care system is difficult to navigate under the best of circumstances. Elder Voices staff and other state-certified out-reach workers in the Public Benefits Counseling program found that some American Indian elders were eligible for the Medicare Savings Program, a state buy-in initiative that could cover Medicare co-payments and deductibles. The bureaucratic nature of the eligibility determination system posed a formidable barrier to accessing benefits. The local office of the Social Security Administration (SSA), which processed all applications was concerned only with Social Security eligibility and did not pursue Medicare or Medicaid eligibility. Additionally, elders counseled to apply for benefits reported that Medicaid staff would not rule on their applications. It seems that, perhaps due to inadequate training about the eligibility status of Indian elders, the Medicaid workers incorrectly judged the elders ineligible. Adding insult to injury, in some instances the Medicaid workers reportedly treated Native American elders curtly and inhospitably.

Intervention Goals

As sites sought to craft responses to these multiple challenges to equitable access and quality of cancer prevention and care for the elders of color, they developed intervention goals that reflected their understanding of barriers. We found that project goals could be categorized in four groups: health risk management, screening education, screening adherence management, or treatment management. Programs often pursued more than one of these goals.

Health Risk Management

Several sites sought to reduce the risk of cancer by engaging elders and near-elders in programs to reduce specific risk factors (tobacco use, lack of physical activity, high fat diets etc.) or comprehensively promote health. The Senior Services of Seattle King County's Senior Wellness program and Lahey Clinic's Senior Wellness Program both engaged elders in health promotion and chronic disease management activities. Although Lahey targeted a more affluent, primarily white community: both programs enlisted senior managed care members and others in ongoing, individualized health promoting programs and group activities. Although these programs cited impressive impacts on individuals' behaviors as well as cardiovascular disease and diabetes measures, they shared an ongoing questioning of whether or not behavioral changes in late life can overcome the effects of lifetime cumulative risk exposures on cancer.

In contrast to senior wellness programs, the Asian American and Pacific Islander National Cancer Survivors Network (APICSN) developed a network of cancer survivors, their family members, health care providers, and community members concerned about the issues of cancer in the Asian American and NHOPI communities. The network helped survivors manage post-treatment issues and emergent risks by linking them with peers and coordinating referrals to services and providers. In a different vein, Elder Voices Public Benefits Counseling program worked with Native American elders at sites throughout New Mexico in understanding supplements to Medicare insurance, coordinating benefits among public payers, and access to usual care. The thinking was that reducing the impacts of lack of adequate insurance and associated poor continuity of primary care can produce better health outcomes.

Screening Education

The largest group of programs identified nationally sought to reduce R/E disparities in cancer care by educating women from traditionally underserved groups about the value of breast and cervical cancer screening. Sites that adopted this overall goal exclusively were the most likely to be located in community-based settings with weaker ties to primary care providers or other health system components. Among the case studies, there were no cases of screening education programs aimed at other cancers or at men in traditionally excluded R/E groups. This pattern was consistent with the findings of our literature reviews that found a noteworthy shortage of published evaluations of culturally tailored screening programs aimed at colorectal, oral, and prostate cancers. In the Connecticut and Oklahoma sites of the Witness program, community health advisors and Witness Role Models, women survivors of breast and cervical cancer empowered to offer inspirational talks about their own experiences, performed out-reach in AA churches and community facilities such as senior centers. The teams sought to teach AA women about breast and cervical cancer and to promote screening. With goals of making data about cancer screening more accessible and addressing patient attitude barriers, the Chicago REACH 2010 trained volunteers to provide breast and cervical cancer awareness education and information resources in their respective communities.

While screening education programs reported success developing and communicating culturally appropriate cancer prevention messages, they also consistently expressed frustration that they did not have the resources or necessary infrastructure to perform activities aimed at improving screening adherence. For example, many of the programs had no way of tracking program participants to know how many actually participated in screening, while others lacked resources to schedule screening appointments or assist persons in attending. Even when programs did have data on the number of individuals seeking screening as a result of out-reach activities, the results were sometimes disappointing. For example, the Deep South Network for Cancer Control's Community Health Advisor program trained volunteers as Community Health Advisor Research Partners (CHA-RPs) to provide cancer awareness messages and resources to their communities. By the program's second year, CHA-RPs made approximately 3,189 contacts, but only 11% of these contacts resulted in screening referrals, and fewer actually received screening. Compounding the difficulties in turning community contacts into improved adherence to cancer detection guidelines, screening education programs often found that even if they sufficiently motivated people to get screened, their participants often were unable to access care after a suspicious screening findings. For example, during our site visit, the Chicago REACH 2010 program staff complained that the program only had funds for out-reach and education, but not for related services. They felt that this situation put them in the uncomfortable position of educating people about their cancer risk and not offering any help managing risks or treating disease.

Screening Adherence and Detection Management

Some programs focused primarily on ensuring screening adherence and managing the process of cancer detection and diagnosis for screening participants. These programs also tended to focus on breast and cervical cancer, though some focused on colorectal, prostate or lung cancer screening. Yet unlike *Screening Education* initiatives, these programs brought not only information but also concrete care management assistance to under-served persons to improve participating in screening at recommended intervals and completing the complex multi-step processes associated with cancer detection, diagnosis, and treatment planning. The Texas Cancer Council's African American Breast Cancer Outreach program, and programs centered at community health centers, such as the Seattle Indian Health Board's Breast and Cervical Health program, hoped to insure that women follow-through on a desire to participate in cancer screening by assisting in scheduling appointments and addressing coverage, co-payment, or other insurance barriers. In addition, some screening adherence and detection management efforts, such as the BECH Patient Navigation program and the MGH/Chelsea Health Center Avon Breast Cancer project also included establishment of systems to contact persons who missed screening appointments to reschedule. These sites also helped women with suspicious screening findings complete the process of cancer detection and treatment planning. All cases were tracked to resolution. Community Health Workers (CHWs) arranged for follow-up primary care and specialty appointments, made sure that test results were available in the patient's record, and helped patients understand cancer detection procedures. Many of these programs also helped women address other issues that might prevent them from following up suspicious screens by providing emotional support, addressing family issues, or arranging transportation to appointments.

Treatment Management

Typically provided by hospital-based health systems, programs that adopted this goal sought improvements in the continuity and quality of cancer treatment and follow-up services for members of traditionally underserved groups. The American Cancer Society Heartland Division's Patient Navigator program at Truman Medical Center in Kansas City, the hospital-based case management component of the Boston City Health Commission REACH 2010, and Harlem's North General Hospital colorectal cancer Patient Navigation program are examples of treatment management programs. Unlike *Screening Adherence and Detection Management* initiatives, these sites work with patients from the time of cancer detection through the treatment and aftercare process to assist them in overcoming practical barriers to service use (transportation, grandchild care), benefits coordination, and scheduling services in a timely manner. They seek to avoid missed or rescheduled appointments for post-surgical outpatient therapies and work to overcome problems in treatment completion or relapse monitoring. In addition, treatment management programs provided counseling, cultural and linguistic translation, and cancer education throughout the treatment and aftercare process to empower patients in advocating for their own care.

Although several programs addressed multiple goals through inter-related components, the four types of goals described here appear to flow from rather different understandings of the causes and consequences of R/E cancer care and outcome disparities. All programs asserted that elders of color and others from underserved populations had heightened needs associated with current and cumulative exposures to both risky environments and inaccessible, inadequate, and culturally or personally disrespectful health services. Programs focused on primary prevention and screening education, however, were primarily concerned with changing the health-related attitudes, knowledge, and behaviors of target population members. Most explicitly assumed that education and empowerment would be enough to overcome barriers to care. By contrast, the programs that sought to better manage the screening, detection, treatment and aftercare process understood disparities as the joint product of prospective patients' attitudes and behavior and inadequate continuity or quality of accessible care. These programs directed new resources to assisting elders make it through complex healthcare programs that were poorly equipped to meet heightened needs associated with cumulative and current disadvantage.

Cultural Tailoring

Our meta-analysis of 'culturally tailored' programs to increase breast and cervical cancer adherence among women of color showed that program strategies were diverse and produced heterogeneous impacts. There is a clear need to develop consensus on the range of cultural tailoring approaches and their relative merits. Table 8.4 indicates the number of case study sites that included specific strategies as part of their cultural tailoring activities. Cultural tailoring strategies were often closely tied to programs' bi-directional (match of system to patient features) understandings of the causes of cancer disparities even when intervention goals seemed to place most of the burden for eliminating disparities on attitude and behavior change by persons in underserved groups. As with the understandings of causes for disparities, many of these solutions seem as much directed to consequences of R/E and social class oppression as to specific cultural features. Not surprisingly, many of the strategies have clear relevance for improving the continuity and quality of cancer prevention and care for other groups.

Community Members as Staff

The most frequently adopted cultural tailoring strategy was using community members as staff (in paid or volunteer roles). This approach reflected case study programs' shared learning that established medical care organizations and practitioners were rarely deeply engaged with R/E minorities and others in traditionally excluded communities, and thus did not typically approach elders from these communities with the same degree of enthusiastic attention and care that was offered to more affluent white healthcare consumers. The programs were consistently convinced of the need to provide target communities with a responsive, approachable, trustworthy human interface to the healthcare system. The vast majority of programs perceived that staffing the intervention with members of the community represented the most effective option for overcoming barriers created by culture and attitudes, mistrust, lack of information, and myriad practical barriers, such as inadequate insurance and bureaucratic malfunction. Fully 22 of the 25 programs chose to design their programs such that co-ethnic community members with strong ties to targeted communities played key roles.

Using community members as staff reflected a theory of intervention that community members know their communities best. These programs found that individuals from the target populations were best prepared to engage the myths, symbols, and language they shared with elders in their communities and thus could disseminate information, dispel misconceptions, and influence behavior. From this perspective, only when programs engage community representatives do they achieve much-needed credibility and access to community members. Several sites highlighted the potential for program staff that were members of the target community to develop meaningful, ongoing relationships with participants. For example, Grace Hill Community Centers' ASHES and MAP programs both relied upon a 'neighbors-helping-neighbors' approach. Volunteer coaches helped their

Table 8.4 Case study sites and cultural tailoring strategies

Methods of Culturally Tailoring Programs	Number of programs
Community members as staff	22
Communal planning and delivery	18
Provide/arrange transportation	13
Provides benefits counseling	8
Address disconnect with medical establishment	7
Focus on health promotion, not disease prevention	5
Uses IT to track recommendations and follow-through	5
Reduce financial barriers/Provide financial assistance	4
Use ethnic media	3

neighbors quit smoking (ASHES) or have mammograms and pap smears (MAP). In the Native Sisters program, community health workers were encouraged to build on existing relationships and take enough time to become familiar and trusted by elders in the communities they serve. They often extended their process of gaining trust and familiarity with elders over a month or more before specifically recommending cancer services. In a similar vein, the American Cancer Society's Heartland Division Patient Navigator program found that with time nurses could understand patients' needs and activate services to help them get care. One of the nurses described an incident in which one of her patients, a Latino man, refused cancer treatment, viewing receipt of treatment as a sign of weakness. Because the nurse came from the same closely-knit Latino neighborhood, she recognized that, as a woman, she did not have the cultural power to reframe this man's view of what treatment meant. Although she was a native Spanish speaker, she deliberately requested that the male translator come to assist her. She asked the translator to tell the patient that refusing treatment was a sign of weakness: without treatment, the man would not be able to be strong and support his family. Within minutes, the patient requested that treatment begin.

Communal Planning and Delivery

In addition, 18 of the programs used another response to the lack of connection between the health system and elders in underserved R/E communities. They created opportunities for members of targeted communities to come together to help shape program goals and share program activities. Group meetings were also used to bring community members together in familiar settings to discuss health care system issues and explore how project resources be could best be directed to community needs. Group settings were also used in implementing program activities. Projects brought community members together to share cancer information, or to undergo screening. Case study leaders often likened this approach to the power sharing models found successful in political organizing, school-and-community partnerships, or neighborhood economic development. Our meta-analysis of culturally-tailored breast and cervical cancer screening education programs also found that communal delivery was associated with stronger average impacts on screening uptake and adherence.

All of the sites with community health centers as sponsors or collaborators and all of the sites based in advocacy organizations reported some use of community participatory models for establishing program goals, planning program events, production of cancer related information, and other functions. Nonetheless, the extent to which programs used such inclusive program planning and implementation varied. For example, AAPCHO's CARE and the Texas Cancer Council's African American Breast Cancer Outreach offered participating sites specific guidance on what cancer-related information their staffs should be prepared to communicate to target communities. They also encouraged sites to seek input from their communities on the most effective ways to improve cancer detection and care. In other sites, such as Seattle Indian Health Board's Breast and Cervical Cancer Health program, community members' envisioned the project as one component of a larger plan to reduce the scourge of cancer in their community, helped select project leadership, and participated in crafting culturally appropriate cancer-related message.

Communal planning and delivery often meant figuring out how to integrate program activities into existing community organizations and gathering places. At least 14 programs implemented program activities in churches or other central community settings that inspired trust and were easily accessible to community members. The coordinator of the Seattle Indian Health Board's Breast and Cervical Cancer program, for example, conducted out-reach campaigns at powwows and other significant community events that bring together many members of a geographically dispersed community. The Connecticut and Oklahoma City Witness programs exemplify combining group meetings in familiar settings with the use of community members as ways to make culturally meaningful connections. These programs ask community volunteers who are cancer survivors to speak in their own words to groups of women about their experiences with detection, diagnosis, treatment, and aftercare for breast and cervical cancer. The AA women who become Witness Role Models address groups of their peers in a non-intimidating and engaging way. These presentations are viewed as effective in part because 'witnessing' draws upon a spiritual tradition with deep meaning for the AA elder audiences and it is appropriate to witness in faith-based and other group settings.

Provides/Arranges Transportation

Noting that lack of affordable transportation represented a barrier for the communities served, 13 programs began providing transportation. Community Health Advisors (CHAs) in the Deep South Network provided information about rideshares with others in their community and provide information about private transportation services. Additionally, the CHAs traveled to rural areas to reach out to residents of the most remote and isolated communities. The Seattle Indian Health Board recognized that the Native American and Alaska Native population that it serves are extremely mobile and may need to travel great distances for service. The Breast and Cervical Cancer Program's medical assistant, who tracks all patients' mammography adherence makes sure that patients have a follow-up exam or subsequent screen scheduled. The medical assistant attempts to have the patient's medical appointment on the same day of the month that the mammography machine is available to reduce transportation barriers to adherence. The Indian Health Service, as another example, designed its Community Health Representative Program in response to the lack of health care services in remote Alaskan villages. Instead of bringing community members to a service, it established a service near them.

Increasing Understanding and Motivation to Seek Services

Many of the strategies described by sites as cultural tailoring reflected a focus on increasing awareness and understanding of cancer, cancer detection, and cancer care for persons from communities of color. A second focus was on motivating individuals to advocate for themselves to obtain all those health care services that they needed. Programs focused on primary prevention or screening education most often adopted these strategies.

Linguistic and cultural translation was often mentioned in the context of understanding and motivation. Clinica Tepeyac, located next to the local church, used staff from the community and conducted all business in Spanish. Moreover, its Reach and Teach project had *promotoras de salud* (community health workers), bilingual women trained in cancer prevention and care. They performed out-reach to women in the community by distributing health information and providing one-on-one and group education programs. Similarly, AAPCHO's CARE program recruited community out-reach workers who came from the same cultural backgrounds and also spoke the languages of the populations served by participating community health centers. The six intervention sites also used the ethnic media to educate their communities.

In another example, the Baltimore Cancer Coalition used a different set of strategies to make program material culturally appropriate. Staff from one of the program's community sites, the Hispanic Apostolate, held focus groups with congregation members and others to develop culturally appropriate educational materials for breast cancer awareness. They learned that the educational materials provided in Spanish from the NCI were uninteresting and unfamiliar to these Latino elders. They reframed the materials as 'fotonovelas' (soap opera stories in comic book format) and added plot lines that responded to real concerns for prospective readers. For example, an older woman in one fotonovela struggles to get her husband's permission for her to go for the screening and eventually convinces him that caring for her health using the best available resources was crucial to the well being of the whole family.

Another strategy that programs used to increase individuals' understanding and motivation involved presenting information in ways participants might find personally relevant. Some programs made an effort to provide culture-specific examples or scenarios in discussions of health risk and treatment. Some others were careful to emphasize health promotion rather than disease prevention. Promoting and improving health made for a much more acceptable topic of discussion than the gloomy topics of disease and illness. Moreover, health promotion presented a much more immediate and compelling goal than prevention of diseases that participants may not yet or may never have. All of the sites targeted to American Indian/Alaska Native, Asian/NHOPI, and Latino groups emphasized the importance of adopting this kind of positive message. For example, the six AAPCHO CARE sites realized that women in the community were often unwilling to come to events specifically focused on breast cancer screening. Participating health centers reported that in order to share information about breast cancer screening in a culturally tolerable fashion, they needed to hold health promotion and wellness events that had recreational and educational components and were inviting for both women and men.

Overcoming Systemic Barriers to Accessing Care

Other cultural tailoring strategies were more closely tied to screening adherence and detection or treatment management programs where staff emphasized assisting elders in overcoming systemic barriers to use of the health care system or in solving other life problems that interfere with cancer prevention, screening, and treatment participation. These programs highlighted the importance of addressing the disconnect between the medical establishment and the needs of elders of color by focusing issues such as translation, solving scheduling problems, and reducing financial barriers.

Several programs employed clinical translation services or sought to provide service in the population's native language in an effort to insure that participants received appropriate care. In the Avon Breast Cancer project, Latina patients requiring diagnostic work-ups and treatment were aided by a Spanish-speaking Breast Health Care Coordinator from the Chelsea Health Care Center in getting referrals and making appointments for care at the Massachusetts General Hospital. Since practitioners at the hospital were rarely bilingual, the program held a dedicated weekly breast clinic with a full-time Spanish interpreter available to help surgical residents communicate with their patients.

Just as important as practitioner/patient communication during a clinical encounter, according to many programs, were record keeping and notification challenges. Many sites found that practitioners needed reminders to conduct some interventions, patients were not scheduled for appropriate follow-up care, or patients never received reminders about appointments. Several sites, such as Harlem's BECH Patient Navigator program, the JTCCP in the Health Choice Network of Miami, and the Avon Breast Cancer project at MGH used innovative information technology to improve the program's capacity to manage care. In JTCCP, practitioners and community health workers were armed with hand-held computers that allowed them to record findings from health risk appraisals and make appointments and referrals as they met with prospective patients. The patient navigators at BECH worked directly with programmers to develop a patient tracking system that reflects the information needs and specific procedures of concern as they facilitate cancer detection and treatment planning processes.

Individuals in the target populations often lacked insurance or struggled with expenses related to co-payments, deductibles, or lack of coverage for select services. Closely related to lack of insurance or an inability to pay for services were the systemic problems created by poverty and unemployment. Several programs responded by assisting participants to solve public and private insurance problems, obtain other public benefits, and address immediate needs for food and shelter. The Baltimore Cancer Coalition's prostate cancer project and Clinica Tepeyac, for example, both provided services to needy members of their communities at low or no cost. A major element of the North General Hospital Patient Navigator program is up-front attention to financial obstacles that might prevent access to services. Upon a patient's arrival at the cancer center, a 'first encounter' staff person conducts a preliminary financial interview and arranges for the hospital's financial office to complete financial assessment and insurance applications. Similarly, the staff of the Boston Public Health Commission's Boston REACH 2010 Program found that most clients needed help with housing and economic security. In addition to being cancer experts, case managers have become housing experts, adept at helping people get onto public-assistance housing waiting lists and into shelters or other interim living conditions.

Engagement Strategies

A growing literature demonstrates that identification, recruitment, enrollment and continued engagement of participants for health promotion or care improvement initiatives can be particularly challenging for organizations targeting traditionally underserved populations. As case studies pursued different overall intervention goals and cultural tailoring strategies, they also developed alternative engagement strategies. Despite their differences in contexts and goals, the case study sites used one of four types of approaches for engaging R/E elders: out-reach, in-reach, combined out-reach and in-reach, and training.

Out-reach Health promotion, screening education, and some screening adherence and detection management sites used an out-reach approach to engagement. They sought to identify and recruit target community members who were not regular users of health service providers that offered consistent cancer prevention and control services. Out-reach approaches were more common in programs with more tenuous ties to specific health care providers. Out-reach, nonetheless, represented a difficult undertaking. Sometimes out-reach workers were unable to attract community members from the target populations to attend educational activities and events. For example, Chicago REACH 2010 held events in AA churches in the hope of attracting low-income AA women to its programs. Despite this culturally savvy approach, this method did not provide the anticipated access to target groups. Although the mainline Protestant churches that agreed to work with the program were in low-income inner city neighborhoods, their members often commuted from higher income suburbs, while most target population members participated in smaller, evangelical congregations that were less willing to participate.

In-reach   Programs that used an in-reach model focused participant identification, recruitment and enrollment efforts only on individuals already receiving care from the sponsoring healthcare provider. For example, one component of the American Cancer Society Heartland Division's Patient Navigator program sought to reduce the time frame between patient referral from a community health center in response to a suspicious screening finding and initiation of treatment or other case resolution by the public tertiary hospital. Referrals from the affiliated health centers, however, were irregular so program staff felt that they were failing to reach many in the target population. Similarly, without an out-reach component, the Boston REACH 2010 hospital based Case Management Component had trouble recruiting participants for case management and was operating well below capacity at the time of our visit. While the program hoped to recruit 600 women of African descent for its case management program, only 78 had been recruited after a year of operations. This program lacked a specific procedure to ensure that all persons non-adherent on screening or with suspicious screening findings were referred for case management.

Combining out-reach and in-reach   Programs that combined out-reach with in-reach activities seemed most successful in overcoming the difficulties faced by programs using only one of these engagement strategies. Combination programs managed not only to recruit participants from the community, but also to bring them into the health system for screening and, in some cases, diagnosis and treatment. They were consistently linked to one or more sponsoring healthcare providers. For example, the Baltimore City Cancer Plan's Prostate Cancer project conducted risk assessments and screening education in multiple community and healthcare contexts and thus met ambitious enrollment targets. The program coordinated and tracked referrals for diagnostic and treatment services using both community-based and hospital based navigators. The program consciously constructed its budget to accommodate expenses for screening, detection services subsequent to positive screens, and treatment for under-insured participants with cancer diagnoses. In this way, the program avoided the problem faced by other sites of educating people about risk but being unable to assist them further. Similarly, the programs at BECH and North General Hospital in Harlem complemented the in-reach engagement strategy of their Patient Navigator initiatives with broad dissemination of cancer screening materials and messages in an effort to promote earlier engagement in cancer prevention and detection.

Training   Instead of focusing on out-reach or in-reach activities, some programs concentrated on training organizations or individuals to perform interventions in their communities. Five of our case study programs emphasized training as their main strategy for engaging members of target communities, with four of these programs based in advocacy agencies and one based in an academic health center.

The AAPCHO CARE program focused on building infrastructure and organizational capacity in its six partner community health centers. The program trained staff at the centers to enhance their existing efforts related to funding, coalition building, assessment of community needs, and participant engagement. The National Center for Farmworkers' Health developed and disseminated a program, Cultivando La Salud for training promotoras de salud. The program employed a training-of-trainers model, providing technical assistance and materials to migrant and community health centers. In participating centers, an Out-reach Director/Lay Health Worker Supervisor is trained as a trainer, who then recruits women farm workers to conduct educational sessions and provide individual assistance with screening adherence. The case study programs focused on training all highlighted their rigorous and demanding curricula and demonstrated the ability to export their training to other multiple sites.

Community Health Workers

Among the programs we studied, community health workers (CHWs) predominated as a key strategy for cultural tailoring of interventions and, often, as the primary personnel responsible for program operation. Nineteen of the 25 programs we studied utilized community health workers. The CHW model has great potential to make the healthcare system more accessible to members of traditionally underserved R/E populations. However, programs have encountered a number of obstacles.

Community health worker roles A number of national organizations are seeking to define the roles of CHWs. The National Rural Health Association has indicated, for example, that a CHW is a public health professional who promotes full and equal access to necessary health and social services by applying his or her unique understanding of the experiences, language and culture of the communities he or she services. This group identifies CHWs as essential for the provision of 'quality health promotion and disease prevention information' as well as to provide the critical link to existing health care services and facilities. The CHW is a member and resident of a community who reaches out, educates, assists and connects individuals and families to the health delivery system.

In our case studies, respondents noted that CHWs bring unique knowledge and understanding of the culture and the health issues, needs and challenges of the communities they serve. Respondents valued these workers because they can create a natural link between community members and the health delivery system. The roles and responsibilities of the CHWs, however, varied enormously. For example, within the case study sites, CHW roles included outreach worker, educator, advocate, translator/interpreter, community organizer, counselor and cultural mediator. Among the various responsibilities, CHWs may assess individuals' needs, coordinate or manage care, educate individuals and families about health promotion, disease prevention, cancer screening, access to care and eligibility for benefits.

CHW training and certification   Training and certification of CHWs constitutes another important issue in developing and sustaining R/E cancer disparity reduction programs. The variety of roles and responsibilities of CHWs complicates the training and certification process of CHWs. Not surprisingly, we found notable variation in the training these workers received. For example of the 19 programs employing CHWs, 16 had a training program, and 12 had an established standardized curriculum. The amount of time spent in training and/or supervised practice for CHWs ranged from 16-80 hours of training, with an average of approximately 60 hours. The costs of training for many programs appeared significant because of their intensity and reliance on multiple professional presenters and trainers.

Most of these training programs focused more on imparting information about health, cancer, and screening, than on inculcating competencies in motivating people to use services, change behavior, or access benefits. The programs seemed to be creating yet another kind of 'cancer expert,' whose own pre-existing skill (or lack thereof) in motivating her peers potentially determined program success. For example, funding changes reduced the Oklahoma City Witness project budget and it was necessary to eliminate the Outreach Coordinator position held by a CHW. While the program continued to train volunteers to be health advisors and Witness Role Models, staff reported that program effectiveness suffered. The volunteers had been trained to lead group sessions, but were not prepared to attract community members to sessions or to perform the critical function of helping people schedule and follow-through on screening. Similarly, even though Chicago REACH 2010 provided formal training for volunteers, this training did not seem to prepare CHWs for their roles as outreach workers and advocates. Site leaders found wide variation among volunteers in commitment to project goals, skills in leading out-reach programs, and level of advocacy activities. This variability in CHW skills and attitudes directly influenced the extent of participation among church members in the health seminars and other activities that the program sponsored. Clinica Tepeyac's Reach and Teach program's experience also bears on this problem. Although the promotoras de salud trained by the program were charged with out-reach, program staff confided that these CHWs seemed to do little more than advise women in the community to access services at the clinic.

In many of the programs that trained CHWs, medical professionals or academics provided training. The trainings tended to build upon the existing competencies in the healthcare system by providing information about disease process and treatments. Only two of the programs we studied made efforts to teach CHWs about engaging community members and motivating them to adopt new behaviors. Both the AAPCHO CARE Program, in its effort to strengthen the organizational capacity of its six participating community centers, and the National Center for Farmworkers Health, in its endeavors to train site staff as trainers, utilized a behavioral change theoretical perspective as part of their curricula. These programs taught workers to assess individuals with respect to their readiness to change and to target their motivational messages and questioning to this stage of change. Upon examination of the CHWs' role and task definitions in the study programs, it seems that curricula that emphasize community organizing, motivation tactics, and accessing public or private benefits would be appropriate additions.

Recruitment and retention of CHWs The discrepancy between need and supply of CHWs constitutes a significant challenge for the model. Many of the programs identified problems with recruitment and retention of CHWs. Since considerable resources were devoted to training, frequent turnover among CHWs had the potential to hurt program effectiveness and was economically costly for programs, which faced the recurrent problem of training and orienting new CHWs. Resource constraints were the primary culprits in this chronic recruitment and retention problem. In many cases, limited funding made programs dependent upon the unpaid labor of volunteers. This model has clear advantages: structuring and delivering services through volunteers involves low cost to the healthcare system and, to the extent that volunteers belong to programs' target populations, provides a convenient method for culturally tailoring services. It is unclear, however, that this volunteer-reliant approach is a sustainable or responsible model for addressing R/E disparities in cancer, especially when socioeconomic inequality, poverty and unemployment, constitute primary barriers to appropriate health service use. It seems unreasonable and unfair to design programs around the expectation that people who are struggling with basic life needs would or should volunteer their time and effort to address issues that may be low on their lists of priorities.

Hiring CHWs did not always solve the recruitment and retention problem for the case study programs. For the most part, programs that hired CHWs did not have the resources to offer them good jobs – jobs with enough hours, competitive pay, and opportunities for advancement and promotion. The tight budgets and grant-funded nature of many of the programs blocked their abilities to design attractive CHW jobs. For example, while the National Center for Farmworkers Health's Cultivando la Salud hired promotoras de salud, these positions paid $8/hour and were only budgeted to last six months, hardly making them attractive long-term job opportunities. In the Alaska Indian Health Services' Community Health program, CHWs were offered CHWs a career ladder with the opportunity for advancement and higher pay than any program in our sample. Nonetheless, many of the CHWs left the program having acquired marketable skills. The stress of being the only primary health care provider and resource in remote areas was cited as another major reason for moving on.

Integrating the CHW role into the health care system An important element in the success of the CHW role is its incorporation into the health care system. Unless the CHW are fully integrated into a health system it is difficult for them to act as effective conduits between the community and that system. For example, several sites noted that traditional health care professionals did not comprehend or value the role of the CHW. As a result, practitioners could fail to communicate or cooperate with the CHW. Recognizing this potential barrier, several programs made substantial commitments to integrating CHWs into the healthcare system. This was often expressed by having program leadership directly involved in selection, training, and supervision of the CHWs or using leading healthcare professionals as advocates for the CHWs in establishing relationships with collaborating organizations. For example in the BECH Patient Navigator program, clinical staff were required to refer all cases to the patient navigators if the Memorial Sloan-Kettering Cancer Center radiologist found suspicion of cancer upon review of a mammogram, a nurse practitioner indicated the need for additional tests based on clinical examination or Pap smear findings, or a surgeon or other physician had scheduled further clinical tests. As a result of the hands-on and detail-oriented approach of the program's founder, Dr. Harold Freeman, the patient navigators have been incorporated into the clinical protocols of the cancer center. At both North General Hospital and MGH/Chelsea clinical and administrative leaders receive regular feedback on the outcomes of the navigation program and work personally with navigators and others to maximize its impacts.

Conclusions

The programs addressing cancer disparities that we examined in our national screening sample and case studies had not been the subjects of comprehensive evaluations of health-related and health care utilization outcomes. Their experiences still point to a number of important lessons for policy and practice. Though many of these same lessons have been noted in other qualitative reports, they must be viewed with some caution. Neither prior research nor the emerging programs we examined provide data that systematically links the design features and implementation experiences of cancer control initiatives targeted to elders and others in traditionally underserved R/E communities to clear evidence for better outcomes, such as lower rates of disease, costs of care, survivorship, or mortality.

It should be noted, however, that the lack of clear impact assessments did not reflect the intentions of program leaders. To the contrary, they often bemoaned lack of support for process and outcome evaluation. Conducting and synthesizing the results of such evaluations are not easy tasks because these programs sought to influence diverse outcomes with multiple determinants. Nonetheless, current approaches to propelling innovation in healthcare miss opportunities to build the needed body of knowledge. Program leaders reminded us that there does not exist a private market to stimulate new attention to engaging elders of color in systems with appropriate attention to delivery of evidence-based health promotion, disease detection, and disease treatment resources. Meanwhile, the public and philanthropic payers for services to these populations and communities have often seemed more interested in high-technology health science initiatives or quick dissemination of educational materials than the difficult work of learning all that we can from careful assessment and replication of existing innovative models. Screening sample and case study programs repeatedly shared difficulties in gaining financial support for implementation and outcomes studies or research on replicating their concepts and strategies in other contexts. Short-term funding, rapidly changing public sector priorities, philanthropic sponsors' apparent obsessions with doing something new and newsworthy, and lack of support for addressing the challenges of building informed community engagement in health program enhancement were repeatedly cited by our study participants as barriers.

As we developed the national screening sample and selected case studies, at least three themes emerged that deserve additional discussion. First, our exploration of emerging models confirmed some of the most striking findings from the literature reviews: initiatives addressing cancer disparities have focused most on breast and cervical cancer screening education for AA women. To date, less attention has been devoted to teaching other R/E groups about detection of these cancers. We also found many instances of fewer instances of initiatives targeted to older women that focused on breast and cervical cancer screening adherence and treatment management; health promotion relevant to other cancers; or management screening, detection, and treatment for other cancers. These findings clearly point to the need for new program initiatives.

A second, though clearly related, theme was also indicated in examining our screening and case study samples. It has been asserted that policy makers, scientists, and funders of emerging programs have achieved little consensus about the causes of cancer disparities and appropriate solutions (DHHS/AHRQ, 2003). Yet in our study, one model – screening education programs that use an out-reach approach to engagement – appeared to dominate among emerging programs. Although teaching traditionally underserved groups about cancer detection has undeniable value, this most prevalent approach embodies a view of the causes of cancer disparities that is neither consistent with the available literature nor with the experiences of program leaders. The available literature describes a cancer prevention, detection, and treatment system that is technologically sophisticated yet socially, culturally under-developed (Freeman, Muth and Kerner, 1995; Freeman and Reuben, 2001). Consistently, the programs we studied had come to view the health care systems as disconnected from elders of color. They gave legion examples of health systems that fail to provide cancer education in ways that engage elders of color in attitudinal and behavioral changes. They observed that target communities faced looming barriers to health system entry and complex financial and care process challenges that make it nearly impossible for elders to maintain long-term relationships with providers or adhere to recommendations. They reported problems with communication and collaboration among providers. To many programs, it seemed that a patient needed to have limitless time, patience and empowerment to overcome system problems. Surprisingly frequent examples of cultural and personally disrespectful treatment by provider representatives and health professionals only deepened target community patients' disaffection from the health system by placing further demands on patients. In this context, projects that exclusively replicate out-reach and screening education strategies are not likely to create lasting impacts on cancer prevention, care and outcome disparities.

We did find examples of programs that seemed to respond to more of the factors that are being linked to R/E cancer disparities among elders. Screening adherence and detection management and treatment management programs typically combined out-reach and in-reach engagement approaches to gain participation both from persons with little ongoing healthcare system contact and from system users at risk for poor quality and continuity of care. These programs sought not only to provide participants with information and motivation to adhere to professional recommendations, but also sought to help them overcome access barriers and system failings by providing concrete assistance in navigating complex multi-step care processes and holding providers accountable for following through on evidence-based care protocols. Such models were designed to forge supportive linkages between traditionally underserved patients and healthcare systems.

Despite differences in program goals and engagement strategies, the third major observation from this review of emerging programs was that almost all adopted a variant of the community health worker model. The use of CHWs was often recommended and endorsed by participants in communal planning initiatives. Their presence was often crucial in bringing community members together to share program activities. CHWs, whether as paid or volunteer staff, were seen as a primary tool in cultural tailoring of cancer prevention, detection and treatment initiatives to reduce R/E disparities. Whether their roles involved helping patients understand treatment options, schedule follow-up visits, address transportation problems, or plan solutions to coverage or financial challenges, the use of CHWs offered a relatively affordable way to enhance the resources of healthcare providers to meet the heightened needs faced by many elders in R/E minority communities. But most of all, CHWs functioned as cultural translators and brokers. They offered a human link between programs and targeted communities and created new lines of communication between community members and health systems.

References

Blankertz, L. (1998). The value and practicality of deliberate sample for heterogeneity: a critical multiplist perspective. *American Journal of Evaluation*, 19(3): 307-324.

Department of Health and Human Services; Agency for Healthcare Research and Quality. (2003). National Healthcare Disparities Report. http://www.qualitytools.ahrq.gov/ disparitiesreport/download report.aspx. Chapter 5: 1-64.

Freeman, H., Muth, B. and Kerner, J. (1995). Expanding access to cancer screening and clinical follow-up among the medically underserved. *Cancer Practices*, 3(1): 19-30.

Freeman, H. and Reuben, S. (2001). *Voices of a Broken System: Real People, Real Problems*. Bethesda, MD: President's Cancer Panel, National Cancer Program, National Cancer Institute, U.S. National Institutes of Health.

Glasgow, R., Lichtenstein, E. and Marcus, A. (2003). Why don't we see more translation of health promotion research to practice? Rethinking the efficacy-to-effectiveness transition. *American Journal of Public Health*, 93(8): 1261-1267.

Appendix 8.1

Summary Characteristics of the Case Study Sites

Access Community Health Network, Chicago, IL
- Project: Chicago Racial Ethnic Approaches to Community Health 2010 (REACH 2010);
- Setting: Community health center network;
- Goal: Screening education;
- Population target: African American, Hispanic, Immigrant;
- Condition target: Breast and cervical

American Cancer Society Heartland Division, Kansas City, MO
- Project: Hospital/Community health center network; Advocacy network
- Setting: Patient Navigator Program
- Goal: Treatment management
- Population target: All R/E Groups, Elderly, Medicaid, Low income, Immigrant
- Condition target: Multiple

Asian and Pacific Islander American Health Forum, San Francisco, CA
- Project: Advocacy network
- Setting: Asian American and Pacific Islander National Cancer Survivors Network (APICSN), Asian American and Pacific Islander Tobacco Education Network (APITEN)
- Goal: Health risk management
- Population target: Asian, Alaskan/Pacific Islander
- Condition target: Multiple

Association of Asian Pacific Community Health Organizations, Oakland, CA
- Project: Advocacy network
- Setting: The Community Approach to Responding Early (CARE)
- Goal: Screening education
- Population target: Asian, Immigrant
- Condition target: Breast and cervical

Baltimore Cancer Coalition, Baltimore, MD
- Setting: Hospital/Community health center network Advocacy network, Baltimore City Cancer Plan (BCC)
- Goal: Health risk management, screening education, screening adherence, treatment management,
- Population target: All R/E Groups, elderly, low income, immigrant
- Condition target: Multiple

Boston Public Health Commission
- Setting: Boston, MA, Government/Hospital/Community health center network, Racial Ethnic Approaches to Community Health 2010 (REACH) Case Management Component
- Goal: Screening education, screening adherence, treatment management
- Population target: African American, elderly, immigrant
- Cancer target: Breast and cervical

Clinica Tepeyac Denver, CO
- Setting: Community health center network, Reach and Teach Project
- Goal: Screening education, screening adherence
- Population target: Hispanic
- Cancer target: Multiple

Community Health Services Division of the Oklahoma Department of Public Health Oklahoma City, OK
- Setting: Government/Human service agency, Oklahoma City Witness Project
- Goal: Screening education
- Population target: African American, Caucasian, elderly, immigrant
- Cancer target: Breast and cervical

Dana Farber Cancer Institute (DFCI), Boston, MA
- Setting: Hospital/AHC Community health center network, Cancer Prevention Through Small Business Project (CPTSBP)
- Goal: Health risk management
- Population target: All R/E Groups
- Cancer target: Multiple

Deep South Network for Cancer Control, Birmingham, AL
- Setting: Hospital/AHC, Academic institution, Deep South Network Community Health Advisors Program
- Goal: Screening education
- Target population: African American, rural, low income
- Cancer target: Breast and cervical

Elder Voices, Inc., Albuquerque, NM
- Setting: Advocacy/network, Public Benefits Counseling Program (PBC)
- Goal: N/A
- Target population: Native American
- Cancer target: Multiple

Grace Hill Centers, St. Louis, MO
- Setting: Community health center/network, Assistance and Self-Help to End Smoking Project (ASHES), Mammography and Pap Project (MAP)

- Goal: Health risk management, screening education, screening adherence
- Population target: African American, low income
- Cancer target: Breast and cervical

Health Choice Network (HCN), Miami, FL
- Setting: Community health center network, Healthy Body, Healthy Soul, Jessie Trice Cancer Prevention Project (JTCPP)
- Goal: Health risk management, screening adherence, treatment management,
- Population target: All R/E groups, low income, immigrant
- Cancer target: Lung cancer

Indian Health Service, Alaska
- Setting: Government/HIS, Community Health Representative Program (CHR)
- Goal: Health risk management, screening adherence
- Population target: Alaskan/Pacific Islander
- Cancer target: Multiple

Lahey Clinic, Burlington, MA
- Setting: Community health center network, Wellness for Seniors Collaborative Program
- Goal: Health risk management
- Population target: Caucasian, elderly
- Cancer target: Multiple

Massachusetts General Hospital/Chelsea Health Care Center, Boston/Chelsea, MA
- Setting: Hospital/AHC, community health center network, Avon Breast Cancer Project
- Goal: Screening adherence, treatment management
- Population target: African American, Hispanic, low income, immigrant
- Cancer target: breast and cervical

National Center for Farm-workers Health, Buda, TX
- Setting: Advocacy/network, Cultivando La Salud
- Goal: Screening education, screening adherence
- Population target: Hispanic, rural, immigrant
- Cancer target: Breast and cervical

North General Hospital/Breast Examination Center of Harlem, Harlem, NY
- Setting: Hospital/AHC, community health center network, patient navigator programs
- Goal: Screening adherence, treatment management
- Population target: African American, Hispanic, Medicaid, low income
- Cancer target: Breast and cervical

Planned Parenthood, Bridgeport, Ct
- Setting: Human service agency, Witness Project of Connecticut
- Goal: Screening education
- Population target: African American, elderly
- Cancer target: Breast and cervical

Seattle Indian Health Board Seattle, WA
- Setting: Community health center network, Breast and Cervical Cancer Health Program and the Nutrition Program
- Goal: Health risk management, screening education, screening adherence
- Population target: Alaskan/Pacific Islander, Native American, low income
- Cancer target: Breast and cervical

Senior Services of Seattle/King County, Seattle, WA
- Setting: Human service agency, Senior Wellness Program (SWP),
- Goal: Health risk management, all R/E Groups
- Population target: Elderly, Medicaid, low income, immigrant
- Cancer target: Multiple

Texas Cancer Council, Houston, Dallas and Tyler, TX
- Setting: Government/African American Breast Cancer Outreach Program
- Goal: Screening education, screening adherence
- Population target: African American
- Cancer target: Breast and cervical

University of Arizona at Tucson/Mariposa Community Health Center Nogales, AZ
- Setting: Hospital/AHC, community health center network, Juntos Contra el Cancer Prevention Program
- Goal: Screening education, screening adherence
- Population target: Hispanic, rural, immigrant
- Cancer target: Breast and cervical

University of Colorado, Denver, CO
- Setting: Academic institution, Native American Women's Wellness Through Awareness (NAWWA)
- Goal: Screening education, screening adherence
- Population target: Native American
- Cancer target: Breast and cervical

University of Kentucky Center for Rural Health, Hazard, KY
- Setting: Hospital/AHC, community health center network, Kentucky Homeplace and Southeast Kentucky Community Access Program (SKYCAP)
- Goal: Health risk management, screening adherence, treatment management
- Population target: Caucasian, rural, low income
- Cancer target: Multiple

Chapter 9

Opportunities for Reducing Cancer Disparities: New Directions for Medicare

The preceding reviews of published literature and survey of emerging programs provide a perspective on current understandings of racial/ethnic (R/E) disparities in cancer care and outcomes for Medicare beneficiaries. Our work also offers insights about the challenges and opportunities facing the US health care in its efforts to eliminate cancer disparities and other health inequalities. In this chapter, a synthesis of our findings serves as the basis for recommending new research areas and opportunities to apply current knowledge to cancer prevention, detection, and treatment for traditionally underserved elders.

Our findings point to continuing opportunities to better understand the epidemiology and biology of carcinogenesis and the technologies of cancer detection and treatment. For some cancers, current research has yet to identify individually modifiable risk factors or how macro-individual policy or program initiatives might reduce population risks. In other cases, consensus has not been achieved on efficacious and affordable detection and treatment regimens. To some extent, efforts to reduce or eliminate R/E cancer disparities through public health population-level initiatives and payer-initiated improvements in health care for individual elders will require continuing progress in these technical areas. But R/E health disparities do not pose primarily technical bio-medical challenges. Our findings support the conclusion that among elders in the United States, existing prevention, detection, and treatment technologies are not provided equally across the lines of R/E and correlated socio-economic factors. Although population group variations in prevalence were noted for several cancer sites, our evidence reviews indicated that a considerable share of the R/E gradient in cancer outcomes is created and sustained by how health care practitioners, provider organizations and systems behave.

Viewing cancer disparities as a challenge to health care organization and delivery suggests that at least two kinds of innovations are needed: (1) strategies that promote more consistent application of consensus cancer control technologies to elders in underserved communities of color; and (2) new approaches to service delivery that can respond to both the heightened needs among underserved R/E elders and their historic and current of disconnection from the health system.

The evidence reviews, signal the need for re-thinking cancer control at the individual level using the framework of chronic disease management. Cancer is traditionally conceptualized as an acute condition, but the evidence reviewed here indicates that at the individual level, cancer control has more in common with extremely common conditions such as diabetes and hypertension. Chronic conditions, according to consensus recommendations, require engagement and monitoring of patients in multiple clinical activities and self-care efforts over time. For cancer, as for other conditions, increased incidence and prevalence within the US reflects both improved detection and improved survivorship. But long-term continuity of individual care is becoming a feature of cancer control for other reasons. Cancer etiology and relapse are at least partially linked to individually modifiable behaviors. Cancers with consensus screening programs can be detected and pre-cancerous conditions can be addressed through ongoing comprehensive tracking. Potentially co-morbid conditions can be identified and managed. For these reasons, individual level cancer control needs to empower both practitioners and patients to work together to minimize risks and maximize appropriate adherence to broadly inclusive health promotion and disease prevention recommendations over time. Like a chronic condition subject to acute exacerbations and varying needs for healthcare intervention, cancer detection and treatment occurs in complex interactions among different types and levels of health care organizations. Our reviews and interviews indicate just how complex cancer detection, primary treatment, and adjuvant therapies have become: they involve the patient with multiple providers, seen repeatedly and in varied locations, and intense demands on physical, social-emotional, and economic resources. A chronic disease model for cancer control recognizes the need for careful attention to helping individual patients make it through this demanding process through maintenance of formal relationships and nurturing of informal coordination links.

Summary of Findings and Conclusions

The preceding chapters were developed using a conceptualization of cancer control as a sequence that includes: identification and management of risk factors: screening and detection, diagnosis, primary treatment and adjuvant treatments, and relapse monitoring. Our reviews produced varied accounts of the causes and consequences of R/E disparities across cancer sites. Much less research was identified on addressing R/E disparities in cancer care than existed for risks and screening, but replicable frameworks for reducing disparities were noted throughout the cancer control sequence.

Identify and Manage Cancer Risks

Our review of reports on cancer risk factors and R/E differences in modifiable risks found evidence linking one or more of the behavioral risks to each of the cancers. For example, there is consensus from epidemiological studies that tobacco use increases risks for prostate, lung, stomach, head and neck, and pancreatic cancers, while obesity is linked to prostate, colorectal, and pancreatic cancers. For other cancers, these primary behavioral factors have not been consistently associated with cancer onset in epidemiological studies. In several cases, these behaviors have been linked to post-treatment overall or disease-free survival. At the same time, other behaviors (hormone use) and environmental factors that increase risks have also been identified for breast, cervical, and other cancer sites. Pre-cancerous conditions that are treatable were noted as risks for cervical, colorectal, prostate and other cancer sites. R/E, social class, education remain as socio-economic risk factors after controlling for known behavioral and environmental factors. Nonetheless analyses of the 1999/2000 and other sources found that many of the potentially individually modifiable risk factors are more prevalent among elders of color: African Americans, Latinos, and American Indian/Alaska Natives reported higher rates than whites or Asian Americans for multiple behavioral risks. There are also broad differences in risk behaviors among groups within these pan-ethnic populations. Although epidemiologists conclude that behavioral risk factors account for some of the group differences in cancer prevalence and interact with R/E group or associated factors, the research remains inconsistent on these questions. Further, cancer for several sites was particularly more prevalent for African American men than other groups and these differences are not well explained by the currently identified modifiable behavioral risk patterns. With few exceptions, research on cancer risks has not adopted a lifespan developmental approach, and thus issues related to the relative influence of current and cumulative behavioral risks and ages of onset or modification of specific behavioral risk factors on cancer prevalence have not been examined consistently.

Cancer Prevention Strategies and Racial/Ethnic Elders

There appear to be no intervention studies that demonstrate a link between behavior change and cancer incidence in elders, but studies of smoking cessation and reduction in lung cancer in younger populations are relatively conclusive. Prevention of breast, cervical, and colorectal cancer reoccurrence through risk factor modification (weight loss, exercise etc) for general populations is receiving increasing support as appropriate and cost-effective for older adults. In part, these limited positive findings also reflect the impacts of these same behavior changes on potentially co-morbid health conditions. But rates of participation in behavioral risk management, cancer prevention, or other chronic condition self-management activities differ by R/E groups, with whites in more affluent urban and suburban communities demonstrating markedly higher rates of participation. Owning a Medicare supplemental insurance policy, having a usual source of care in a community primary care setting, higher education, and higher income and assets seem to be the strongest predictors of adherence to behavioral risk management and preventive services guidelines. There is also consistent evidence for the impacts of primary care provider organization resources and systems to promote adherence. Unfortunately, elders of color are less likely to receive care from providers with these resources. These findings indicate the need for more initiatives aimed at engaging elders of color in consistent primary care and accelerating the adoption by primary care providers who serve older R/E minorities of chronic disease management models of cancer prevention, risk modification, and early detection.

There are very few studies of physical activity, nutrition/weight management, and multi-component interventions with elders of color. There appear to be no published reports on health risk appraisal/multi-component behavior change programs, smoking cessation and alcohol use reduction interventions for elders of color groups. Nonetheless, there are many examples of linguistically and culturally adapted materials and programs, as well as guidance for healthcare, social service, community and religious organizations on their implementation. These materials often reflect the view that intervention approaches that are working in general populations need only minimal adjustments to be effective with elders of color. Many reports now emphasize the need for practitioner competence in cross-cultural encounters. But recent findings in cultural adaptation of cancer materials (Kreuter, Steger-May, Bobra, et al., 2003) and marketing materials more generally (Briley, Morris, and Simonson, 2000) suggest that viewing culture in terms of specific beliefs, context-independent values, or behavioral dispositions does not produce materials or provider behaviors with significantly improved efficacy among elders of color. There is little evidence that broad scale dissemination of these materials gets them in the hands of target audiences or leads to behavior change. Tailoring health promotion and disease prevention initiatives to elders of color requires more inclusive attention to how culture, socio-economic status, prior healthcare experiences, and institutional barriers to receipt of healthcare interact with other individual, care system, and community features.

There is also clear need for new research on how to engage and maintain participation of elders of color in effective and efficacious physical activity, nutrition/weight management, smoking cessation, and multi-component interventions. Available studies from both elders of color and other populations underscore the challenges associated with engaging persons in behavioral risk management and suggest the use of motivational interviewing and other techniques that individualize messages about prevention based on stages of change and related frameworks. Primary care practitioners often miss opportunities to encourage or support elder patients in deciding to use formal behavior modification resources or maintain lifestyle changes. Programs that draw on personnel more closely connected to target populations and those that respond to the symbol systems and preferred social patterns in target communities appear more effective.

Racial/Ethnic Disparities in Cancer Incidence and Outcomes

Our literature review of R/E differences in cancer incidence and outcomes showed significant differences across cancer sites in the patterning of R/E differences. African Americans (AAs) and other traditionally underserved groups are at greater risk for getting cancer, having poorer treatment and, having worse survival outcomes. In general, differences between AAs and whites in incidence are smaller than differences in outcomes. For breast cancer, AA women had lower incidence and higher mortality, while this pattern of lower incidence but higher mortality was seen for AI/AN and Hispanics for several cancer sites. For the five better-studied and most deadly cancers – breast, cervical, prostate, colorectal, and lung – there was evidence that R/E differences in stage at the time of diagnosis accounted for a significant share of mortality or survival disparities. For cervical cancer, outcomes were worse for AA and Hispanic women than for whites at each stage of diagnosis.

Consensus recommendations for use of screening methods were found for breast, cervical, colorectal, and oral cancers and consensus recommendations on timing of screening were found for breast and cervical cancers. Prostate cancer screening remains controversial but there is evidence for targeted screening for some high-risk groups, particularly AA men with family histories of prostate cancer. There is broad support for a new focus on informed decision-making and closer targeting for PSA testing. For the other cancer screenings, population programs for elders are recommended because of the potential to identify cancers in earlier, more treatable stages. But screening also facilitates detection and treatment of pre-cancerous lesions, particularly in colorectal and cervical cancers. Treatment of these pre-cancerous lesions is generally curative, but needs to be followed by careful monitoring for recurrence. This suggests that these cancers are nearly entirely preventable and that continued higher rates among older people of color represent a failure of primary care. Rates of adherence to colorectal screening protocols are lower than desirable for all Medicare beneficiaries, but notably lower for persons of color. Similarly, prostate cancer screening rates are lower than recommended for AA men. There is broad consensus that increasing adherence to screening guidelines for these cancers by R/E minority elders could reduce stage-at-diagnosis differences between groups and thus contribute to reducing disparities in cancer outcomes. For cancers without accepted screening mechanisms, however, it appears that addressing the stage-at-diagnosis differences requires ensuring medical care use and attention on the part of both patients and practitioners to health risk management or testing in response to prior exposures or epidemiological risks.

For breast, cervical, colorectal, and prostate cancer, there are reports of culturally tailored interventions to increase screening that typically involve use of community health workers to conduct educational programs using culturally and linguistically adapted materials. In some multiple component programs, education is linked to operational enhancements that address access barriers. Our meta-analysis of these studies shows that culturally tailored programs yield modest, significant effects but they are heterogeneous in their findings. Projects that combined CHWs, communal planning and delivery of services, and other operational enhancements to reduce barriers to access appeared more effective. There were insufficient culturally tailored prostate and colorectal screening to support meta-analysis, but qualitative reviews indicated that there was at least some evidence that techniques similar to those used to increase breast and cervical screening by women of color could be adapted to other screening tests. There have been few prior discussions of whether or not programs targeting all cancers with consensus screening recommendations and insurance coverage.

For each of the cancers examined, final diagnosis, staging and treatment requires a multi-step process involving multiple tests, procedures, and professional consultations. For breast, cervical, colorectal, lung, and prostate cancers, there is evidence that women of color and AA men are less likely to receive a complete screening follow-up and diagnostic process. Specific evidence of less use and less timely use of diagnostic procedures with AA women and other Medicare beneficiaries of color were noted for all of these sites, except lung cancer. No less important than complete diagnosis is timely completion of all recommended primary and secondary treatments. These findings underscore the potential to improve cancer survivorship by ensuring that patient and practitioners complete the process. Yet for all of the cancers studied there is consensus that in many treatment contexts elders of color, but especially African Americans receive less appropriate primary and secondary treatment, less use of appropriate adjuvant therapies, and lower participation in clinical trials where new, promising therapeutic approaches are being tried. In sharp contrast to the breast and cervical cancer screening participation initiatives for women of color, these reviews did not locate experimental studies of initiatives to ensure higher adherence to diagnostic, treatment and aftercare guidelines in care for elders in underserved R/E groups.

Emerging Interventions to Reduce Racial/Ethnic Disparities in Cancer

Findings from 26 case studies of interventions intended to reduce R/E cancer disparities, identified through screening interviews with 115 emerging models, showed broad consensus among site leaders with respect to the causes of cancer disparities and some of the components of potentially effective approaches. These programs were selected in part because they had not yet been the subjects of comprehensive evaluations. Nonetheless, our case studies found that like many prior initiatives to reduce R/E health disparities, none of these programs had been designed in ways to ensure eventual availability of cost-effectiveness data. Their implementation experiences still offered some important lessons. Most of the case study sites viewed R/E disparities in cancer care as the joint product of systems of care and underserved groups experiences with these systems. They attributed disparities to a bi-directional process creating a disconnection between the target populations' cultural perspectives on cancer and health services and current health care practices. Many sites reported the R/E elders were unlikely because of past experiences of discrimination to challenge (primarily white, high-status, young) practitioners. Yet these elders were less likely to adhere to medical recommendations when providers appeared disrespectful of their worldviews and life experience. Poverty, unemployment and associated problems further compounded barriers to appropriate care for elders of color. Following through on cancer detection and treatment or dealing with time-consuming medical recommendations may be particularly demanding for elders of color facing intergenerational family responsibilities and practical barriers to using care. Among these practical barriers were transportation and other limits to the accessibility of services, lack of supplemental insurance and other financial barriers to care, and difficulties negotiating bureaucratic barriers to insurance coverage or care completion.

Although the lions' share of emerging programs focused on breast and cervical cancer education, the models we examined also explored comprehensive health promotion/disease prevention, screening adherence and follow-up facilitation, and treatment and aftercare facilitation goals. The adoption of goals beyond screening education reflected perceptions that changes in health care practitioner, organization, and system behavior were needed to address disparities in addition to changes in elder R/E minority attitudes towards screening. While programs focused exclusively on screening education tended to use out-reach methods to recruit participants, programs that adopted broader goals also tended to combine out-reach with in-reach and training strategies for engaging participants. Case study programs also adopted a variety of strategies for 'cultural tailoring' their interventions. Most programs cited two related strategies: community members as program staff and communal approaches to planning and implementation. Community health workers (CHWs) – as paid or volunteer staff – were central to the interventions adopted by most of the emergent programs. These programs viewed CHWs as able to form cultural and linguistic links between health care systems and individuals in target communities. Their use was often recommended as an essential strategy for engaging elders of color in appropriate cancer prevention, detection, and care through communal planning processes that engaged members of target communities in detailing barriers to use of services and adherence to other health promotion recommendations. For many sites, communal implementation of cancer-related activities was an additional way to share project resources with the community.

Yet our case studies also suggested that CHWs are an underutilized resource. We found that most programs trained CHWs to perform a very narrow scope of service – focusing on screening education without attention to ensuring individual follow-through – specific perhaps to one disease or one population. CHWs clearly could potentially do more. In one or more case study sites, CHWs assisted with each of the goals of health risk management, screening education, screening adherence, and treatment facilitation. The supply of CHWs was most often cited as the major factor limiting their broader participation in reducing R/E cancer disparities. Traditional funding streams for health care are not designed to compensate either for this kind of worker, nor for the services they deliver.

Opportunities for Reducing Cancer Disparities Among Elders

Two recent reports provide specific recommendations for addressing R/E disparities in cancer. The Trans-Health and Human Services Cancer Health Disparities Progress Review Group (PRG) developed 14 recommendations for alleviating the unequal burden of cancer, including (Department of Health and Human Services, 2004). The PRG recommendations are shown in Table 9.1. Over a 3-year period, these proposals would launch initiatives to discover, develop, and deliver 'evidenced-based' programs to reduce cancer disparities by race/ethnicity and other socio-economic factors. Specific programmatic changes for Medicare or other health financing and quality assurance programs were not articulated. The

Intercultural Cancer Council, a national group of government, academic, and healthcare experts on cancer control disparities endorsed the PRG recommendations in their preliminary report *From Awareness to Action: Eliminating the Unequal Burden of Cancer* (ICC, 2004). ICC makes specific health-care financing recommendations as well, calling for: 1) passage and implementation of a 2002 legislative proposal for demonstrations of patient navigator/community health worker models (H.R. 5187); 2) increased Federal funding for the CDC breast and cervical cancer screening programs and similar initiatives; 3) funding for tobacco control programming tailored to communities of color; 4) restored alignment between Medicare and private insurance coverage for cancer care in specialty settings and participation in clinical trials, eliminated through the 2003 Medicare reforms; 5) fund and implement a demonstration program for Medicare reimbursement of orally-administered chemotherapy drugs, and 6) achieve universal health insurance coverage by 2010.

Both sets of recommendations clearly address some of the most pressing systemic barriers to appropriate cancer control services for R/E minority elders and others in traditionally excluded socio-economic groups. Implementing the PRG and ICC plans would produce a major re-orientation of Federal research and service expenditures towards addressing cancer disparities, focus new attention and resources on communities facing the greatest cancer disparities, and direct new resources to the goal of creating a healthcare work force that is both diverse and culturally competent. Despite the clear evidence for disparities in cancer control, finding the resources and political will to implement these agenda is uncertain.

Many policy makers and thought leaders may view these proposals as overly broad or overly costly given current US federal deficits and other budget priorities. Advocates for market-oriented reforms to healthcare will be troubled by a sense that these recommendations speak to a greater governmental role in health care financing and delivery, even as we pursue efforts to transform Medicare and other public programs into fixed-dollar benefits administered privately. Still others may see a lack of attention to addressing the root causes of cancer inequalities. It is also unclear whether or not these proposals have been framed in ways that will garner public or professional commitment to their implementation. Beyond these political questions, however, our evidence review and survey of emerging programs indicates that implementing the health care service components of these recommendations will require knowledge gap-filling investments in demonstration and evaluation efforts focused on how to improve the accessibility and appropriateness of cancer control services for elders in traditionally underserved R/E groups.

Table 9.1   Recommendations from the Trans-Health and Human Services Cancer Health Disparities Progress Review Group*

1) Conduct a program and budget review of all relevant HHS programs to shift and realign support where possible to evidence-based programs that are effective in addressing health disparities.
2) Assemble a Federal Leadership Council on Health Disparities led by the HHS Secretary.
3) Implement in all HHS agencies recommendations from the Institute of Medicine Report entitled: *Unequal Treatment: Confronting Racial and Ethnic Disparities in Healthcare.*
4) Evaluate specific grant and contract processes to determine what additional steps are needed to enhance peer review panels for cancer health disparities.
5) Establish new approaches to data collection and sharing to aid in the study of cancer and race, ethnicity, and socio-economic status.
6) Increase the proportion of HHS agency support targeted to disease prevention, health promotion, and translational research on cancer health disparities.
7) Establish partnerships for sustainable community-based networks for participatory research in areas of high cancer disparities.
8) Develop and implement a new trans-HHS initiative to qualify high disparity geographic areas for special program designation.
9) Develop, implement, and carefully evaluate education and training programs designed to create a diverse and culturally competent cancer care workforce.
10) Implement evidence-based tobacco control strategies including those that create financial disincentives for tobacco consumption and those that provide social reinforcement for not smoking.
11) Ensure that populations at highest risk have access to age – and gender – appropriate screening and follow-up services for breast, cervical, and colorectal cancer. Expand to include these services for additional cancers.
12) Support culturally, linguistically, and literacy specific approaches for eliminating cancer health disparities.
13) Ensure that every cancer patient has access to state-of-the-science care.
14) Collaborate with private and voluntary health sectors to ensure that all Americans receive the full range of services, and care from cancer prevention to diagnosis to treatment.

Source: Department of Health and Human Services. (2004). *Making Cancer Health Disparities History: Report of the Trans-HHS Cancer Health Disparities Progress Review Group*. http://www.chdprg.omhrc.gov/pdf/chdprg.pdf.

As noted in the PRG and ICC reports, these gaps in the evidence base have been known for some time. For example, in proposing passage of the HR 5187, the patient navigator legislation, ICC is endorsing 5-year NCI and AHRQ intervention and evaluation programs closely linked to premiere cancer care centers and academic institutions. While of undeniable value, concepts emerging from this discovery and development strategy would still require additional demonstration in the context of Medicaid or Medicare to explore the mechanisms of delivery, reimbursement, and quality assurance across diverse settings. The need for exploration of new cancer disparity reduction strategies within the context of current healthcare financing systems was reflected in the December 2000 BIPA legislation (Section 122), 'Cancer Prevention and Treatment Demonstrations for Ethnic and Racial Minorities' that requires the Centers for Medicare and Medicaid Services (CMS) to conduct demonstrations that explore how Medicare might reduce racial and ethnic (R/E) minority group disparities in cancer prevention, treatment, and outcomes. According to Section 122, the goals of the demonstrations are to:

• Improve the quality of items and services provided to target individuals in order to facilitate reduced disparities in early detection and treatment of cancer;
• Improve clinical outcomes, satisfaction, quality of life, and appropriate use of Medicare-covered services and referral patterns among those target individuals with cancer;
• Eliminate disparities in the rate of preventive cancer screening measures, such as pap smears and prostate cancer screenings, among target individuals; and
• Promote collaboration with community-based organizations to ensure cultural competency of health care professionals and linguistic access for persons with limited English proficiency.

The legislation further called for an evaluation of the cost-effectiveness, quality of care, beneficiary satisfaction, and provider satisfaction in the demonstrations. CMS has interpreted this legislation as directing demonstration efforts to Medicare fee-for-service (FFS) settings. Both because the reviews reported here were developed to guide development of this demonstration and because the reviews found clear evidence for the disparities targeted by these objectives, the recommendations we present are intended to respond to these goals. Our recommendations also fill in some of the 'how' for implementing the PRG and ICC recommendations. As was the case for major components of the evidence reviews, the recommendations have been refined since initial presentation to the Expert Panel. Draft proposals were presented to 25 potential participating organizations (community health centers, managed care plans, comprehensive cancer centers, Indian Health Service providers, and public hospital systems) and their reactions with taken into account. We also try to reflect continuous change in scientific literatures and policy contexts.

The policy context has changed with the release of the PRG and ICC cancer control disparities recommendations and the passage of the Medicare Prescription Drug, Modernization and Improvement Act of 2003 with its renewed focus on promoting managed care plans. As a result, our proposals call for addressing R/E cancer disparities both in the fee-for-service (FFS) settings where most elders receive healthcare and in Medicare and Medicaid managed care environments. Although our reviews found no studies specifically focused on cancer care disparities for Medicare beneficiaries in managed care, there is ample evidence for R/E disparities in cancer care for younger populations (Yood and Johnson, 1999; Lafata, Cole, Johnson et al., 2001; Legoretta, Liu, and Parker, 2000). It has been argued that Medicare already reimburses MCOs for offering an integrated and coordinated package of covered services in the context of incentives to provide comprehensive preventative and disease management services to all members and thus should not receive demonstration funding to better achieve related goals. On the other hand, many of the not-for-profit plans, particularly those that retain staff models, have strong traditions of demonstrating new approaches to patient management. As 'managed' care organizations, such plans should be in a good position to organize and implement interventions – and many may already have years of experience in offering components of the intervention. Further, several of the areas with high rates of Medicare MCO penetration also have concentrations of elders of color (e.g. south Florida and California), some Medicaid/Medicare dual-eligible plans have been particularly successful in targeting elders of color (e.g. Texas STAR), and many MCOs have sufficient stability of member and provider participation and concentrations of beneficiaries from the targeted racial and ethnic groups. Finally, including managed care plans in the proposed demonstrations would not require separate reimbursement strategies since, as described below, we propose a partial capitation reimbursement for the recommended out-patient Medicare services that could readily be added to current payment approaches.

In addition to broadening the demonstration efforts to include Medicare managed care programs, our evidence reviews and proposals from other groups have highlighted at least three other features that should be incorporated in CMS demonstrations and subsequent program enhancements that were not features in prior discussions. First, communal participation in planning and governance of demonstrations targeting R/E minority elders – sometimes called community participatory approaches – should be incorporated. Communal participation appears to be required not only to win trust and legitimacy from targeted communities but also to design interventions that respond to the lived experiences of elders in these communities. Organizations participating in the demonstration should explicitly detail how elders from the communities they serve will be empowered to shape specific protocols and ongoing monitoring and re-adjustment of program activities. A real willingness to share the control over demonstration resources with persons in targeted communities is the central component of this participatory approach. Second, priority in selection of demonstration sites should be given to communities where cancer care and outcome disparities are most pronounced and to organizations with demonstrated broad commitments to reducing health disparities. In many cases, this prioritization will mean that community health centers, public 'safety net' hospitals, and related providers in medically under-served and economically under-developed communities would be specifically encouraged to participate. In the long run, if these interventions prove successful, it may be more useful to envision the Medicare enhancement being demonstrated not as general expansions of the healthcare insurance entitlement but as specialty programs limited to providers and communities with elevated needs and ongoing strategies for to cancer control disparities reduction. Third, the demonstration should follow the lead of the HRSA Health Disparities Collaboratives and many privately supported healthcare improvement initiatives by including a strong technical assistance program into the demonstration. This component could foster new learning, capacity building, and comparability among the demonstration sites. Technical assistance program will provide opportunities for site personnel to learn from each other and to cooperatively shape the demonstration. The demonstration plan should incorporate sufficient lead-time for site development so that these program-wide consultation processes have sufficient time to influence site operations.

Since we identified evidence for disparities at each phase in the cancer control process, the proposed demonstration services also highlight identification and management of cancer risks, screening adherence and follow-up, and treatment and aftercare facilitation. Because elders of color experience particular difficulties as they move between levels of the health system, there are some overlaps in the activities proposed under each of the new benefits. The three new Medicare services are summarized in Table 9.2 and discussed below, followed by crosscutting considerations related to implementation, quality assurance, and evaluation.

Health Risk Management

Our reviews found considerable support from epidemiological studies for the importance of individually modifiable behavioral risks in cancer etiology and severity but almost no experimental evidence that altering behaviors influence cancer rates or outcomes. Findings from the equal treatment studies, however, indicate that R/E group differences in the management of chronic health problems other than cancer, such as cardiovascular diseases, diabetes, and depression, in part determine R/E disparities in cancer outcomes. Since effective self-management of these conditions includes addressing a range of behavioral and lifestyle risks, it seems likely that increasing the engagement of R/E elders in management of behavioral risks and other modifiable determinants of health can alleviate some R/E disparities in cancer and health.

Health risk management (HRM) encompasses approaches that increase elders' participation in primary care linked to comprehensive health promotion and disease prevention programs. Having a usual source of care in a community-based primary care setting has been linked to engagement in activities that can reduce the risk of cancer. Consistent primary care and associated health promotion activities can also influence the development and course of other chronic conditions. This in turn can reduce morbidity and mortality for cancer patients and potentially reduces need for other health services. Effective HRM will promote smoking cessation, physical activity, and nutrition/weight management. It would also include multi-component health promotion interventions such as chronic disease self-management.

Table 9.2   Three Medicare demonstration services for reducing racial/ethnic disparities in cancer: service descriptions and recommended requirements

Type of Service	Health Risk Management (HRM)	Screening Adherence and Detection Facilitation (SADF)	Treatment and Aftercare Facilitation (TAF)
Primary Role	Performs Health Risk Assessment (HRA), conducts motivational interviewing, tailors lifestyle counseling, assists with benefit coordination, refers to primary care and screening, and refers to social and prevention services	Maintains individual record of adherence to all Medicare-reimbursed screens, sends personalized reminder letters, arranges for service on schedule, follows-up on missed visits, facilitates referral to other providers for cancer care, and tracks patient till definitive resolution	Maintains individual record of progress and facilitates access to standard of care services from suspicion of cancer through definitive diagnosis, primary and secondary treatments, adjuvant care and reoccurrence monitoring. Assists with benefits coordination, health and +social service referrals
Organizational Affiliation	Community health center, group practices, outpatient clinics	Cancer screening provider, comprehensive cancer center, community health center	Hospital, safety net health system, cancer center
Operational Supports	Patient registry, MIS to track service referrals, actions and follow-up, computerized HRA, adapted health education materials	MIS to track use and completed referral, personalized letters, links to financial offices, interpreter services, adapted health education materials	MIS to track use and completed referrals, decision supports to track standard of care completion, interpreter services, adapted health education/discharge summary materials
Training/ Certification	40-60 hours in class plus extra training in motivational/tailoring techniques and use of computerized HRA and registries	40-60 hours in class plus extra training in screening issues and MIS use; extra clinical training re screens and benefits	40-60 hours in class plus extra training in screening issues and MIS use; extra clinical training re cancer treatment and benefits

Type of Service	Health Risk Management (HRM)	Screening Adherence and Detection Facilitation (SADF)	Treatment and Aftercare Facilitation (TAF)
Intensity	4-9 hours per year per eligible person	2-3 hours per year per eligible person	10-15 hours per eligible person for primary and secondary treatment, 2-3 hours per year for relapse monitoring
Immediate Outcome Measures	% of HRAs with tailored action plans; % with usual source of care; % of cases engaged in behavior change; % adherent to overall lifestyle recommendations.	% of cases adherent on all screens; % of cases brought to resolution; % of cases with standard-of-care detection and prevention services, faster case resolution; and improved patient satisfaction health-related quality of life.	% of cases completing standard-of-care diagnosis and treatment; time to completed treatment; % of cases tracked annually, and improved patient satisfaction and health-related quality of life.

Based on experiences in several of the emerging programs and our meta-analysis of culturally tailored screening education programs, it seems likely that the use of CHWs could be an effective component of these demonstrations. In this context, CHWs could not only perform outreach roles, seeking to engage elders in primary care programs, they could also serve important roles in program implementation, such as helping participants remain motivated and documenting adherence to preventive care guidelines. Available studies from both elders of color and other populations underscore the challenges associated with engaging elder persons in behavioral risk factor management and suggest the use of motivational interviewing and techniques that individualize messages about prevention based on stages of change and related frameworks. CHWs could be trained to apply these techniques. Further, for elders of color, health promotion interventions seem more effective when they highlight health improvement and when they can be individualized to preferences on activities, group participation, timing, and effort. CHWs could play primary roles in this process of cultural and individual tailoring.

Provider organizations would be paid for HRM using a partial capitation payment approach with periodic interim payments adjusted for actual costs within established limits. The payment would be structured to offer incentives to providers to engage patients who had not been receiving regular primary care visits and completion of all appropriate preventive services covered currently by

Medicare, to engage patients with identified individually modifiable health risks in behavior change (e.g. smoking cessation), and to engage patients with heightened cancer or other disease risks from modifiable behaviors or other exposures in targeted cancer detection services (e.g. lung scans for former tobacco users). Provider organizations would receive payment for HRM programs in addition to any current payments for primary care or preventive health services. Providers would be expected to develop computer-assisted systems for maintaining a patient health risk management registry linked to a management information system that supports care management. To be reimbursed, providers would enroll individuals in a health risk management program. Enrollees would complete a health risk appraisal and work with a primary care practitioner and CHW to develop an individualized action plan to receive appropriate Medicare preventive services (such as, breast, cervical, colorectal, and prostate cancer screening, vaccinations, glaucoma screening, diabetes-related counseling) address individually modifiable health risks (such as, lack of supplemental insurance, high risk health behaviors, lack of adherence to regimens for hypertension or diabetes), and identify past behavioral or environmental exposures that increase their risks for disease. Participants would also receive written and telephone contacts to increase participation in scheduled services, reinforce self-efficacy in behavior change, and address emergent health or social challenges. Written materials and other communications would be linguistically and culturally tailored.

Participating organizations would offer or support referrals to community programs to support behavior changes. Based on findings in case study sites offering comprehensive health promotion/chronic disease self-management programs, individuals might require 3-5 hours of individual attention annually from CHWs, although providers would face additional costs for information system enhancements, supervision of CHWs, and mounting group programs to support behavior change. For individuals whose conditions require more focused or sustained attention to behavior change or who have difficulties meeting the objectives in their action plans, HRM providers would offer more intensive tailored assistance with specific behavioral changes or chronic condition self-management. Given the difficulties faced by many in achieving and maintaining health promoting behaviors and the heightened prevalence of one or more behavioral risk factors among R/E minority elders, it seems likely that a majority of enrolled participants will make some use of the intensive HRM services, requiring an additional 1-4 hours of individualized or group services.

Although the justifications for HRM – as for prevention and chronic condition management in general – are strong, this proposed Medicare enhancement represents a higher risk strategy than do the screening or treatment proposals presented below. First, Medicare demonstrations typically adopt a short time horizon, 2-3 years, while the positive benefits of behavior change may take longer to emerge. For example, in the case of smoking cessation, despite its obvious long-term benefits, 3-5 years are considered the minimum before a smoker's disease risks begin to equal those of non-smokers. Second, healthcare practitioners and provider organizations have much more experience in exhorting patients to make behavior changes than in assisting individuals in maintaining motivation or newly adopted behavior patterns over time. Providers functioning in the current Medicare environment and those serving less affluent patients have had relatively little experience with proactively tracking adherence over an extended period or addressing barriers to adherence. They have not taken responsibility for helping patients adhere to challenging behavior modification and disease self-management protocols. Thus, while apparently of modest scope with individual annual costs comparable to one or two home health visits, the HRM intervention will demand a major shift in practice patterns.

Screening Adherence and Detection Facilitation

Our reviews of available research establish the need among elders from traditionally underserved R/E groups for services that ensure screening adherence and facilitation of cancer detection (SADF). As did prior reviews, we found that cancer prevalence and outcome disparities are largely shaped by group differences in detection and cure of pre-cancerous lesions and group differences in the stage-at-diagnosis. For cancers without accepted screening mechanisms (lung, stomach) addressing R/E stage-at-diagnosis differences requires ensuring medical care use and attention on the part of both patients and practitioners to health risk management. But cervical and colorectal cancers can be prevented by identification and treatment of pre-cancerous lesions, while breast, cervical, colorectal, and aggressive prostate cancers can be identified through periodic screening at earlier stages with higher potential for efficacious treatment. Overall screening rates need improvement, but this is particularly true for colorectal cancer. Because risks for all cancers increase with age, screening may be particularly important for Medicare populations. Yet elders in traditionally underserved R/E groups participate less in screening and are less adherent to the recommended schedules for screening, although patterns of adherence differ by screening test and population. We found that although breast and cervical screening education programs had significant positive impacts, emerging programs that sought to ensure screening adherence that specifically linked patients to provider organizations and addressed practical barriers to utilization were considered more effective. Screening adherence programs aimed at R/E minorities for colorectal and prostate cancer have received much less attention. Further, we found no published reports or emerging programs that sought to engage elders in adhering to all recommended screening.

Our reviews suggested that even the best screening adherence programming might not be adequate to reduce R/E disparities in stage-at-diagnosis. We found that some of the differences in cancer treatment and survival appear to occur because of failure to complete follow-up of suspicious lesions and associated diagnostic work-ups. Published reports and interviews with emerging programs leaders repeatedly noted that a sizable proportion of elder patients from under-served groups were lost to follow-up after a suspicious screening, while in other cases, a failure to fully stage disease and asses other aspects of health status prevented appropriate treatment planning. Interventions that increase the likelihood that patients and practitioners follow up on suspicious screening findings, perform complete diagnostic work-ups, and follow standards of care for diagnosis and treatment, appear largely missing in the literature for R/E elder populations. To meet this objective, practitioners and provider organizations need to learn ways to share with patients the responsibility for screening adherence and complex follow-up processes. This will be challenging for providers holding traditional understanding of the distribution of health-relevant responsibility between patients and providers. By contrast, this proposal endorses, for elders of color, a mix of roles that places more responsibility on provider organizations for record keeping, communicating effectively across lines of difference, and maintaining a health promoting relationship.

We propose that SADF be offered by provider organizations that can deliver or arrange for the full range of cancer screenings appropriate for elders, typically hospitals, comprehensive cancer centers, and specialty outpatient departments. As in the HRM service, SADF would be reimbursed on a partial capitation basis with a negotiated annual rate per enrolled beneficiary. This payment would be in addition to any existing reimbursement for screening, detection, and diagnostic services. While well-financed academic health centers, large practices, and managed care plans may have systems in place for many of these functions, they may not be working well for elders of color. For other institutions, the largely clerical aspects of screening adherence record keeping are daunting given other demands. Both kinds of institutions have expressed interest in this activity. Programs would recruit enrollees through community events and other outreach efforts, while also developing systems of referral from primary care providers and public health initiatives. Programs would need to develop information exchange agreements with these providers and specialty practitioners. For each enrolled person, an individual record of screening participation would be developed, shared with the patient, and also maintained by site. Patients would receive reminders for all scheduled screenings and telephone assistance in scheduling and attending appointments. Patients with missed appointments would be rescheduled. The SADF provider would adopt a specific protocol for follow-up services in response to suspicious screening findings for cancer site and these decisions would be reflected in a clinical information system. Individual SADF enrollees with suspicious findings would receive assistance in scheduling and maintaining all needed appointments for follow-up services until a definitive diagnosis or other resolution is obtained. Helping enrollees complete follow-up diagnostic services may involve not only providing assistance with transportation or other practical barriers to adherence, but also addressing psychosocial barriers to adherence. CHWs would also continue tracking of documentation of completion of follow-up tasks and transfer of case responsibility for treatment. Based on experiences in the patient navigator programs we studied in New York, Kansas City, and Boston, it seems likely that the SADF function would require an average of 2-3 hours of CHW time annually, far less for those who are adherent to screening protocols and have no suspicious findings, but much more for those who face psychosocial barriers to screening adherence or who need assistance working through a response to positive screening findings.

Treatment and Aftercare Facilitation

No less important than complete diagnosis is timely completion of all recommended primary and secondary treatments. Practitioners and patients can enhance cancer survivorship by ensuring adherence to state-of-the-science protocols during primary treatments and completion of aftercare services. Current healthcare systems provide neither incentives nor requirements for treatment and aftercare facilitation, and the providers uses by urban or rural communities of color may be unprepared to ensure continuity and quality of services. Bickell and Young (2001), for example, in case studies of 6 New York hospitals found that the hospitals had no systematic way of tracking patients as the progressed, or dropped out of cancer treatment. With the goals of efficient cancer care and improved cancer survivorship, a treatment and aftercare facilitation (TAF) intervention would combine using a community health worker, serving as a patient navigator, with improved clinical information systems, enhanced practitioner decision support, and linguistically/culturally appropriate patient educational materials. Although demonstrations and evaluations of cancer treatment management services, such as navigators, were not identified in the US literature, there is a body of literature that shows positive effects of coordinating treatment.

The TAF benefit would be available to patients with cancer diagnoses and treatment plans. Because acute care providers of primary oncology treatments are reimbursed on the basis of diagnostically related groups (DRG) in the Medicare FFS program, it would be difficult to link reimbursement for TAF to the administrative component of the DRG rate. Rather, the service would be reimbursed as a supplemental payment to the physician or department providing outpatient adjuvant therapy serving a cancer patient whose medical or psychosocial status suggested the need for care coordination. Again, a partial capitation payment would be negotiated and subject to review based on costs within established limits. Provider organizations or physicians offices would enroll patients in the TAF program. The CHW assigned to the TAF program would work with patients throughout the treatment process to facilitate their understanding of treatment and aftercare choices and the implications of adherence or non-adherence to recommendations. The CHW would develop with the patient and practitioner of record a treatment plan that reflects provider organization adopted primary, secondary, and adjuvant interventions for each cancer diagnosis. With input from the provider and patient, this plan would be continuously updated during the treatment process. CHWs would work with patients post-discharge to ensure completion of recommended chemotherapy or radiotherapy, and to schedule and ensure adherence to protocol-specific follow-up visits for relapse monitoring and addressing any treatment complications over time. The partial capitation payment would reflect an estimate for 10-15 hours of CHW time for each case during the initial treatment and aftercare period and a lower level of 2-3 hours annually to ensure compliance with relapse monitoring.

TAF programs would have four primary functions: 1) maintain individual record of progress and facilitate access to standard of care services from suspicion of cancer through definitive diagnosis, primary and secondary treatments, adjuvant care and reoccurrence monitoring; 2) Address barriers to treatment, including the use of interpreters wherever appropriate and access to same language providers where possible, benefits coordination, and arranging for such things as transportation and childcare when needed; 3) Assist patients and families with treatment adherence in a culturally appropriate manner; 4) Assist patient to make informed choices about their treatment through use of adapted educational materials and culturally tailored learning methodologies.

Crosscutting Concerns in Demonstration Design

Demonstration Scope and Recruitment: BIPA 2000, Section 122 called for spending $25 million dollars from the Medicare trust fund for design and implementation of demonstrations at no less than nine sites (based on four R/E minority populations, urban and rural settings, and programming in Guam) to address R/E disparities in cancer control. The possibility exists for additional funding if the demonstration proves successful. While substantial, this investment pales in comparison to the ICC call for spending $500 million on a demonstration to improve access to oral chemotherapy administration. Given the success of emerging programs in finding sources of financing for chemotherapy for persons without adequate insurance protection and ongoing concerns with exploitative pricing of these medications, it may be more useful to focus resources on solving the organizational and delivery challenges in cancer prevention and screening for traditionally underserved groups than on drug financing objectives at this time.

The model adopted in the HRSA Health Disparities Collaboratives that allows for small introductory projects in many sites could be accommodated in the Section 122 demonstrations, but it seems that this model makes it difficult to adequately assess the impacts of programs or issues related to their full incorporation by large and complex health systems. At this point, the potential of these new benefits has been established and policy development requires a greater understanding of the cost and health outcome implications of their implementation in diverse settings. On the other hand, the average direct costs for each of these interventions at several hundred dollars per enrollee per year and the relatively small and concentrated populations to be targeted in some cases suggests that it would be possible to mount up to 20 individual sites, serving 100-500 patients/year, or a total demonstration population of around 25,000 beneficiaries over the course of a 3-year demonstration. Although CMS may face such severe constraints on evaluation resources that they need to internally direct some of the Section 122 funding for evaluation and develop a smaller demonstration, multiple sites, site samples of this size and a longer demonstration time horizon are all probably needed to adequately assess the implications of new prevention, treatment, and aftercare management strategies on cancer care outcomes and costs.

Given the well-documented difficulties in recruiting women and R/E minorities in health services demonstrations and research and in cancer trials in particular, it seems possible that these site sample expectations are ambitious. These sample targets, however, could obtained by building on the experiences of emerging programs and incorporating recommendations from efforts in other areas

(Curry and Jackson, 2003; NIH, 1994). Foremost among these learnings is the need to build trust in healthcare providers within target communities and addressing practical barriers to service use. Some trust-building strategies that might be incorporated into demonstration designs include using CHWs and other intermediaries who act as cultural and linguistic translators; involving the community in the planning of the demonstration and establishing a community advisory board; providing language and literacy appropriate education/information about the services; using carefully phrased, literacy and cultural appropriate language in invitation letters or consent forms; matching the gender and race/ethnicity of the recruiter to that of the potential participant. Strategies to overcome practical barriers to service use include: monetary incentives to cover transportation and cost of the service being offered as well as participation time and effort, providing transportation, providing literacy, language and cultural appropriate recruitment materials, and offering assistance in acquiring health insurance coverage and social services such as housing and childcare. Achieving the desired samples may also require adopting strategies to overcome practitioner and provider organization barriers to program participation by offer multicultural sensitivity training to providers, providing translation services, involving other staff in identification of clients in need of services, monetary incentives for additional time required to identify eligible clients

Community Health Workers

Requirements for operational enhancements, such as new clinical information systems, decision supports for practitioners, linguistically and culturally tailored patient reminder letters and educational materials, have been as administrative costs in prior CMS demonstrations. But reimbursing for CHW delivery of services to Medicare beneficiaries is an untried and unique proposal. Several factors need to be considered in this context.

In the past, when CHWs have provided services like those proposed here, they have worked as volunteers or been paid through project grants. We found no prior instances of direct Medicare reimbursement of paraprofessionals. Given the need to integrate CHWs into cancer prevention, detection, and treatment teams, such direct reimbursement seems unwarranted. Demonstration sites would need to develop clear job specifications. CHWs in this context appear most comparable to home health aides, and would be compensated by provider organizations reimbursed for delivery of a package of services rather than for the time spent by individual workers. The proposed demonstrations do not create a new class of Medicare-reimbursed professionals, but rather call on provider organizations to explore employing community members as part of their services to typically underserved communities. This approach places the onus on demonstration programs, to establish standards for the competencies and training processes for CHWs. Among the states, Texas stands alone as having an established CHW/promotoras de salud certification process. Demonstrations in other states would need to rely on standards established by their Medicaid programs, the Indian Health Service, the community health centers, or national organizations advocating further professionalizing of the CHW role. In this context, programs would need to carefully configure training to match job demands. Unlike the approaches advocated by many of the emerging programs, this might entail a greater focus on motivational interviewing and other behavior modification strategies and less attention to the biology of cancer.

Assessment of Program Impacts

Current data are inadequate to assess the cost implications of unequal treatment for cancer for older adults in the United States. Disparities in cancer are clearly expressed by lower utilization of Medicare-covered primary care and preventive services. Disparities in cancer care mean that elders of color are often first diagnosed at less treatable stages, face poorer outcomes, and more invasive treatments, these patterns may be associated with lower total costs because of lower overall survival. Similar points could be made with other acute and chronic health conditions. The tragic human costs of health and healthcare disparities are clear, yet inadequate attention to primary and preventive services and tertiary care access barriers may generate greater short-term expenditures. With all factors considered, financing systems probably still save costs by continuing patterns of unequal care. From this perspective, the major new costs associated with the proposed interventions are likely to be associated with induced utilization and costs for primary care, preventive services, cancer treatment and aftercare, and co-morbid condition care. With these expected program outcomes, demonstrations to reduce R/E cancer control disparities need to be examined within a cost-effectiveness framework that values each life equally (after appropriate adjustment for quality of life) and assesses new interventions in relation to the potential costs for treating underserved groups comparably to whites with similar illness patterns.

The principle hypothesis to be explored is that provision of demonstration interventions around health risk management, Medicare preventive services and cancer detection, and cancer treatment can facilitate increased receipt of standard of care interventions and improved quality and acceptability of care for Medicare beneficiaries in the targeted, currently underserved racial and ethnic minority groups. Evidence in support of this hypothesis would be derived from treatment and co-ethnic control group member differences at baseline and follow-up on measures of:

- Patient adherence to screening recommendations for breast, cervical, colorectal, and prostate cancer;
- Patient adherence to prevention goals as indicated by smoking status, BMI, and physical activity;
- Patient completion of cancer detection/prevention services subsequent to a positive screening finding
- Cancer stage at diagnosis;
- Patient completion of state-of-science protocols for cancer treatments and aftercare;

- Overall utilization and costs for Medicare-reimbursed services;
- Health related quality of life; and
- Satisfaction with care.

Incremental Solutions to R/E Cancer Control Disparities

We believe that adopting a chronic disease management approach to cancer control may be helpful for all elders (Ko and Chaundry, 2002). Nonetheless, the incremental changes in Medicare services we propose based on a disease management perspective may generate diverse reactions. This approach is likely to be viewed as unnecessary by elders with strong financial and social resources or by those familiar with well-financed, premiere or academically linked health systems with adequate resources for care management. But adopting a chronic disease management perspective in cancer control seems central to reducing or eliminating R/E care and outcome differences because more elders in traditionally underserved groups have increased cancer risks and potential co-morbid conditions as well as increased likelihood of prior and ongoing experiences of mistrust, disrespect or disconnection from health care. The health care system role in reducing and eliminating R/E cancer disparities as envisioned by these recommendations is not confined, however, to adopting a chronic disease conceptualization. Our evidence review highlighted the need for new kinds of human linkages between communities of color and health systems, including personnel with strong ties to targeted communities and new communal approaches to program planning and implementation. These approaches share some of health care institutions' resources and prestige with traditionally under-served communities and create new bonds of individual and institutional trust.

Our proposals to develop health risk management, screening adherence, and treatment facilitation assistance to elders of color, reflect an understanding of the long-term, dynamic, and multifaceted qualities required for chronic disease management. The proposals for new interface roles filled by community health workers and operational enhancements for provider organizations reflect an understanding of the crucial role of culturally mediated and relationship-intensive approaches required to sustain effective management of chronic conditions. Provider organizations that serve more concentrated populations of elders from traditionally excluded R/E communities and safety net providers would be particularly encouraged to take on these responsibilities. If Medicare and other payers concerned can implement these ideas successfully with fair service provision to elders of color, they can serve as a blueprint for broader efforts to achieve just and affordable healthcare.

Given lofty goals such as changing how health care providers conceive of cancer control for individual Medicare beneficiaries and participatory, inclusive reframing of their relationships with target communities, the specific Medicare benefit and quality assurance initiatives proposed here are relatively modest. Neither the state of current knowledge nor the contentious context of Medicare policies at this time seemed to support broader proposals. The absence of adequate data on the financial consequences of cancer control disparities for the Medicare program is one of the most pressing knowledge gaps. Without data to assess the contributions to overall Medicare costs of complex interactions of prevalence, stage at diagnosis, treatment, and survival patterns by race/ethnicity, it is difficult to gauge how cancer disparity reduction will be compared with other Medicare priorities. Demonstrations of these modest Medicare enhancements must be sufficiently large and adopt sufficiently comparable strategies to support evaluation of their cost implications as well as to increase current knowledge about implementation. With the passage of the 2003 Medicare reform legislation that includes new prescription drug coverage and an ambitious program to entice elders away from traditional fee-for-service Medicare to a new breed of private plans, health care for elders in this country will be in such a state of flux in coming years that it will be difficult to focus policy and program attention on even these modest enhancements. For us, it seems reasonable to frame R/E cancer disparities as an expression of historical and current patterns of socio-economic injustice that require major economic and political restructuring to address comprehensively. And moving the US healthcare towards a single payer universal coverage policy would address many of the challenges to equitable care that we have reviewed. Nonetheless, our evidence review indicates that incremental changes have the potential to address rapidly some of the sources for cancer prevention, detection, and treatment disparities among older people. We are concerned that feasible improvements in quality and quantity of life elders in underserved R/E groups will be lost in the debates over longer-term solutions. In the end, the recommended strategies though incremental seem to represent needed initial steps that could also add to the knowledge base for designing larger efforts.

References

Bach, P., Schrag, O., Brawley, A. et al. (2002). Survival of blacks and whites after a cancer diagnosis. *Journal of the American Medical Association*, 287: 2106-2013.

Ben-Menachem, T. and Morlock, R.J. (2001). Sociodemographic differences in the receipt of colorectal cancer surveillance care following treatment with curative intent. *Medical Care*, 39(4): 361-372.

Bickell, N.A. and Young, G.J. (2001).Coordination of care for early-stage breast cancer patients. *Journal of Internal Medicine*, 16(11): 737-742.

Briley, D., Morris, M. and Simonson, I. (2000). Reasons as carriers of culture: Dynamic vs. dispositional model of cultural influence on decision making. *Journal of Consumer Research*, 27 (2): 157-178.

Curry, L. and Jackson, J. (2003). The science of including older ethnic and racial group participants in health-related research. *Gerontologist*, 43(1): 15-17.

Ko, C. and Chaudry, S. (2002). The need for a multidisciplinary approach to cancer care *The Journal of Surgical Research*, 105(1): 53-57.

Kreuter, M., Steger-May, K., Bobra, S. et al. (2003). Sociocultural characteristics and responses to cancer education materials among African American women. *Cancer Control*, 10(5 Suppl.): 69-80.

Legorreta, A., Liu, X. and Parker, R. (2000). Examining the use of breast-conserving treatment for women with breast cancer in a managed care environment. *American Journal of Clinical Oncology*, 23(5): 438-441.

National Institutes of Health. (1994). Guidelines on inclusion of women and minorities as subjects research in clinical research. *Federal Register*, (59) No. 14508.

Pearson, D., Jackson, L., Winkler, B. et al. (1999). Use of an automated pharmacy system and patient registries to recruit HMO enrollees for an influenza campaign. *Effective Clinical Practice*, 2(1): 17-22.

Ross, S., Grant, A., Counsell, C. et al. (1999). Barriers to participation in randomized controlled trials: a systematic review. *Journal of Clinical Epidemiology*, 52(12): 1143-1156.

Yood, M. and Johnson, C. (1999). Race and differences in breast cancer survival in a managed care population. *Journal of the National Cancer Institute*, 91(17): 1487-1491.

Zhu, K., Hunter, S., Bernard, L. et al. (2000). Recruiting elderly African-American women in cancer prevention and control studies: A multifaceted approach and its effectiveness. *Journal of the National Medical Association*, 92(4), 169-175.

Index